PEDIATRIC
PEARLS

PEDIATRIC PEARLS

THE HANDBOOK OF PRACTICAL PEDIATRICS

FOURTH EDITION

Beryl J. Rosenstein, MD
Professor of Pediatrics
The Johns Hopkins University School of Medicine;
Director, Cystic Fibrosis Center
The Johns Hopkins Hospital
Baltimore, Maryland

Patricia D. Fosarelli, MD
Assistant Professor of Pediatrics
The Johns Hopkins University School of Medicine;
Professor of Spirituality and Practical Theology
The Ecumenical Institute of Theology
Baltimore, Maryland

M. Douglas Baker, MD
Professor of Pediatrics
Yale University School of Medicine;
Chief, Pediatric Emergency Medicine
Yale-New Haven Children's Hospital
New Haven, Connecticut

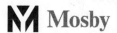 Mosby

An Imprint of Elsevier Science

St. Louis   London   Philadelphia   Sydney   Toronto

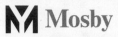

Mosby

An Imprint of Elsevier Science

The Curtis Center
Independence Square West
Philadelphia, Pennsylvania 19106

Pediatric Pearls: The Handbook of Practical Pediatrics   0-323-01498-4
Copyright © 2002, Mosby, Inc. All rights reserved.

Notice

Pediatrics is an ever-changing field. Standard safety precautions must be
followed, but as new research and clinical experience broaden our
knowledge, changes in treatment and drug therapy may become necessary
or appropriate. Readers are advised to check the most current product
information provided by the manufacturer of each drug to be administered
to verify the recommended dose, the method and duration of administration,
and contraindications. It is the responsibility of the licensed prescriber,
relying on experience and knowledge of the patient, to determine dosages
and the best treatment for each individual patient. Neither the publisher nor
the editor assumes any liability for any injury and/or damage to persons or
property arising from this publication.

Previous editions copyrighted 1997, 1993, 1989

Library of Congress Cataloging-in-Publication Data

Rosenstein, Beryl J.
  Pediatric pearls : the handbook of practical pediatrics / Beryl J. Rosenstein,
Patricia D. Fosarelli, M. Douglas Baker.—4th ed.
    p. ; cm.
  Includes bibliographical references and index.
  ISBN 0-323-01498-4 (alk. paper)
  1. Pediatrics—Handbooks, manuals, etc. I. Fosarelli, Patricia D. II. Baker,
M. Douglas. III. Title.
  [DNLM: 1. Pediatrics—Handbooks. WS 39 R815p 2002]
  RJ48 .R67 2002
  618.92—dc21   2002024410

Acquisitions Editor: Dolores Meloni
Publishing Services Manager: Pat Joiner
Senior Designer: Mark A. Oberkrom

CL/QWF
Printed in the United States of America

Last digit is the print number: 9 8 7 6 5 4 3 2 1

CONTRIBUTORS

Carl R. Baum, MD
Assistant Professor of Pediatrics
Yale University School of Medicine;
Director, Medical Toxicology
Yale-New Haven Children's Hospital
New Haven, Connecticut

Paul D. Sponseller, MD
Professor and Head
Pediatric Orthopaedics
The Johns Hopkins Hospital
Baltimore, Maryland

PREFACE

It is hard to believe that we have just completed the fourth edition of *Pediatric Pearls*. When we wrote the first edition, we envisioned it to be a handbook of practical diagnostic and therapeutic points for the practitioner who cared for children and adolescents. Now, 15 years later, the book is much longer because it is much more encompassing than our original vision.

As with earlier editions, we have rewritten and updated existing chapters based on our clinical experience, current literature, and discussion with colleagues. These chapters have been reviewed by pediatricians who are experts in their respective fields. Bibliographies have been updated, certain sections (e.g., the section on HIV infection) have been greatly expanded as our knowledge has evolved, and other sections have been shortened or deleted. In the third edition, we added two chapters (Common Behavioral Problems and School Health Issues) to address the "new morbidity" issues that pediatric health care professionals now face. Because of the very favorable feedback on these chapters, in this fourth edition we have added a chapter addressing the physical, psychological, and spiritual needs of chronically ill, catastrophically injured, and dying children and their families.

Also, with this edition, we welcome Doug Baker as a co-editor. Doug is a former colleague at the Johns Hopkins Hospital, who now serves as Chief of Pediatric Emergency Medicine at the Yale–New Haven Children's Hospital.

We are grateful to all who made the first three editions of *Pediatric Pearls* so successful. We hope this edition will be even more useful to students, house officers, and practitioners responsible for the care of young patients, as well as to all the young people who are the recipients of their knowledge, skill, and caring.

Beryl J. Rosenstein
Patricia D. Fosarelli
M. Douglas Baker

ACKNOWLEDGMENTS

We are indebted to all of the Chief Residents of the Harriet Lane Home, Outpatient Department, who nurtured this project during its embryonic stages, and to Catherine DeAngelis, MD, and the late Frank A. Oski, MD, for their early encouragement and support. We are grateful to a number of our colleagues who reviewed sections of this edition of the handbook: Nancy Barnett, Bernard Cohen, Emily Germain-Lee, Sharon McGrath, Alicia Neu, Ambadas Pathak, Michael Repka, Linda Resar, Janet Serwint, David Tunkel, and Eileen Vining. Francine Cheese and Linda Packham provided excellent secretarial support. Their ability to decipher and decode our corrections was a source of constant relief and amazement. We thank Edward D. Miller, MD, CEO, Johns Hopkins Medicine, and George Dover, MD, Chairman of the Department of Pediatrics at Johns Hopkins, for allowing us to use the Johns Hopkins Children's Center logo on the cover. Last, but certainly not least, we thank Dolores Meloni, Andrea Bucci, Pat Joiner, Mark Oberkrom, and Adria Harris at Elsevier Science, and Jody McBride at Clarinda Publication Services for their editorial, organizational, and moral support in bringing this project to completion.

Beryl J. Rosenstein
Patricia D. Fosarelli
M. Douglas Baker

CONTENTS

ABBREVIATIONS

ABD	abdominal
ABG	arterial blood gas
ABO	blood groups
ACE	angiotensin-converting enzyme
ACTH	adrenocorticotropic hormone
ADD	attention deficit disorder
ADHD	attention deficit hyperactivity disorder
AFB	acid-fast bacilli
AGN	acute glomerulonephritis
AgNO$_3$	silver nitrate
ALT	alanine transferase (SGOT)
ALTE	apparent life-threatening event
AN	anorexia nervosa
ANA	antinuclear antibody
ANC	absolute neutrophil count
AOM	acute otitis media
AP	anteroposterior
ASA	acetylsalicylic acid
ASAP	as soon as possible
ASO	antistreptolysin-O
AST	aspartate transferase
A-V	atrioventricular
AV	arteriovenous
AZT	zidovudine
BAL	dimercaprol
BC	blood culture
bid	twice a day
BM	bowel movement
BN	bulimia nervosa
BP	blood pressure
BPD	bronchopulmonary dysplasia
bpm	beats per minute
BRATS	banana, rice, applesauce, toast, saltines
BUN	blood urea nitrogen
C	centigrade
C3	serum complement
Ca	calcium
Ca:Cr	calcium:creatinine
Calcium EDTA	calcium disodium edetate
CBC	complete blood count
cc	cubic centimeter
CCB	calcium channel blocker
CDC	Centers for Disease Control and Prevention
CF	cystic fibrosis
CFU	colony-forming unit
CHD	congenital heart disease
CHF	congestive heart failure
CIE	counterimmunoelectrophoresis
cm	centimeter
CMV	cytomegalovirus
CNS	central nervous system
CO	carbon monoxide
CO$_2$	carbon dioxide

Col	colonies
CPAP	continuous positive airway pressure
CPK	creatine phosphokinase
CPR	cardiopulmonary resuscitation
Cr	creatinine
CRP	C-reactive protein
C&S	culture and sensitivity
CSF	cerebrospinal fluid
C-spine	cervical spine
CT	computed tomography
CV	cardiovascular
CVA	costovertebral angle
c/w	compared with
CXR	chest x-ray
d	day
D/C	discontinue
DDAVP	desmopressin
DDH	developmental dysplasia of the hip
ddI	dideoxyinosine
DEA	Drug Enforcement Agency
DIC	disseminated intravascular coagulation
diff	differential
DKA	diabetic ketoacidosis
dL	deciliter
DMSA	2,3-dimercaptosuccinic acid
DMT	dimethyltryptamine
DNA	deoxyribonucleic acid
DNR	do not resuscitate
DPI	dry powder inhaler
DTaP	diphtheria-tetanus-acellular pertussis
DTP	diphtheria-tetanus-pertussis
DTR	deep tendon reflex
D_5W	5% dextrose in water
$D_{25}W$	25% dextrose in water
Dx	diagnosis
EBV	Epstein-Barr virus
ECG	electrocardiogram
ECHO	echocardiogram
ED	emergency department
EDTA	ethylenediaminetetraacetic acid
EEG	electroencephalogram
ELISA	enzyme-linked immunosorbent assay
EM	erythema multiforme
ENT	ear, nose, and throat
EOS	eosinophils
EP	erythrocyte protoporphyrin
ESR	erythrocyte sedimentation rate
ET	endotracheal
ETT	endotracheal tube
F	Fahrenheit
FB	foreign body
FDA	Food and Drug Administration
Fe	iron
FEP	free erythrocyte protoporphyrin
FEV_1	forced expiratory volume in 1 second
FHx	family history
FSH	follicle-stimulating hormone

FTA-ABS	fluorescent treponemal antibody absorption (test)
FTT	failure to thrive
F/U	follow-up
Fx	fracture
g	gram
G−	gram negative
GABHS	group A β-hemolytic streptococcus
GC	gonococcal
G-CSF	granulocyte colony-stimulating factor
GE	gastroenteritis
GER	gastroesophageal reflux
GGT	gamma-glutamyltransferase
GI	gastrointestinal
GnRH	gonadotropin-releasing hormone
G-6-PD	glucose-6-phosphate dehydrogenase
gt	drop
gtt	drops
GU	genitourinary
GYN	gynecology
h	hour
Hb A$_{1c}$	glycosylated forms of hemoglobin that can be separated from the main Hgb fractions Hb A$_1$ and Hb A$_2$
HbCV	*Haemophilus influenzae* b conjugate vaccine
HBIG	hepatitis B immune globulin
HBsAg	hepatitis B surface antigen
HBV	hepatitis B virus
HC	head circumference
hCG	human chorionic gonadotropin
HCO$_3$	bicarbonate
Hct	hematocrit
HDCV	human diploid cell vaccine
HDL	high-density lipoprotein
HEENT	head, eyes, ears, nose, and throat
Hg	mercury
Hgb	hemoglobin
HIB	*Haemophilus influenzae* type B
HIV	human immunodeficiency virus
H/O	history of
H$_2$O$_2$	hydrogen peroxide
H&P	history and physical
HPF	high-power field
HPV	human papilloma virus
hr	hour
HR	heart rate
hs	at bedtime
HSP	Henoch-Schönlein purpura
HSV	herpes simplex virus
HUS	hemolytic-uremic syndrome
Hx	history
IBD	inflammmatory bowel disease
ICH	intracranial hemorrhage
ICP	intracranial pressure
I&D	incision and drainage
IDDM	insulin-dependent diabetes mellitus
IFA	immunofluorescent antibody
IgA	immunoglobulin A
IgG	immunoglobulin G

IgM	immunoglobulin M
IM	intramuscular
INH	isoniazid
IO	intraosseus
I&O	intake and output
IPV	inactivated polio vaccine (Salk)
ITP	immune thrombocytopenic purpura
IU	international unit
IUD	intrauterine device
IV	intravenous
IVIG	intravenous immune globulin
IVP	intravenous pyelogram
JRA	juvenile rheumatoid arthritis
K	potassium
Kcal	kilocalories
KCl	potassium chloride
KD	Kawasaki disease
KOH	potassium hydroxide
KPO_4	potassium phosphate
KS	ketosteroid
kV	kilovolt
LATS	long-acting thyroid-stimulating hormone
LDH	lactic (acid) dehydrogenase
LDL	low-density lipoprotein
LET	lidocaine, epinephrine, tetracaine
LFTs	liver function tests
LH	luteinizing hormone
LP	lumbar puncture
LSD	lysergic acid diethylamide
LTB	laryngotracheobronchitis
max	maximum
MCHC	mean corpuscular hemoglobin concentration
MCV	mean corpuscular volume
MDA	methylenedioxyamphetamine
MDI	metered dose inhaler
mEq	milliequivalent
μg	microgram
mg	milligram
Mg	magnesium
min	minute
mm	millimeter
MMR	measles-mumps-rubella
mo	month
Monos	mononuclear cells
MRI	magnetic resonance imaging
Na	sodium
NAC	N-acetyl-L-cysteine
$NaHCO_3$	sodium bicarbonate
Neg	negative
NF	neurofibromatosis
NG	nasogastric
NH_3	ammonia
NH_4	ammonium
NIDDM	non–insulin-dependent diabetes mellitus
NP	nasopharyngeal
NPO	nothing by mouth
NSAID	nonsteroidal antiinflammatory drug

NTM	nontuberculous mycobacteria
O_2	oxygen
OCD	obsessive-compulsive disorder
OGES	oral glucose-electrolyte solution
25-OH-D	25-hydroxyvitamin D
OM	otitis media
OME	otitis media with effusion
OPV	oral polio vaccine (Sabin)
OR	operating room
OTC	over-the-counter (drug)
oz	ounce
P	phosphorus
PA	posteroanterior
Pb	lead
PCA	patient-controlled analgesia
Pco_2	partial pressure of carbon dioxide
PCP	phencyclidine
PCR	polymerase chain reaction
PE	physical examination
PEFR	peak expiratory flow rate
PET	positron emission topography
PID	pelvic inflammatory disease (salpingitis)
PMI	point of maximal impulse
PMNs	polymorphonuclear cells
PO	by mouth
Po_2	partial pressure of oxygen
PO_4	phosphate
PPD	purified protein derivative
PPD-B	purified protein derivative–Battey
prn	as needed
PTSD	post-traumatic stress disorder
pt	patient
PT	prothrombin time
PTT	partial thromboplastin time
PUD	peptic ulcer disease
PVC	premature ventricular contraction
q	every
qd	once a day
qid	four times a day
qod	every other day
qxh	every "x" hours
RA	rheumatoid arthritis
RAIU	radioactive iodine uptake
RAST	radioallergosorbent test
RBC	red blood cell
RDW	red cell distribution width
RE	racemic epinephrine
REM	rapid eye movement
RF	rheumatic fever
rhG-CSF	recombinant human granulocyte-colony stimulating factor
RIA	radioimmunoassay
RIG	rabies immune globulin
RLQ	right lower quadrant
RMSF	Rocky Mountain spotted fever
R/O	rule out
RPR	rapid plasma reagin
RR	respiratory rate

RSV	respiratory syncytial virus
RTA	renal tubular acidosis
RUQ	right upper quadrant
RVA	rabies vaccine adsorbed
Rx	prescription, drugs, medication
SaO_2	oxygen percent saturation (arterial)
SBE	subacute bacterial endocarditis
SBI	serious bacterial infection
SCD	sickle cell disease
SCFE	slipped capital femoral epiphysis
SIADH	syndrome of inappropriate antidiuretic hormone
SIDS	sudden infant death syndrome
Sig	directions
SJS	Stevens-Johnson syndrome
SLE	systemic lupus erythematosus
SMA	sequential multiple analyzer
SOB	shortness of breath
SOM	serous otitis media
S/P	status post
spec. gr.	specific gravity
SQ	subcutaneous
SS	sickle cell
S&S	signs/symptoms
SSD	sickle-cell disease
STD	sexually transmitted disease
STS	serologic test for syphillis
Sx	symptoms
T	temperature
T_3	triiodothyronine
T_4	free thyroxine
T&A	tonsillectomy and adenoidectomy
TAC	tetracine, adrenaline, and cocaine
TAR	thrombocytopenia, absent radii
TB	tuberculosis
TC	throat culture
3TC	lamivudine
TCA	tricyclic antidepressant
TEF	tracheoesophageal fistula
THC	tetrahydrocannabinol
TIBC	total iron-binding capacity
tid	three times a day
TM	tympanic membrane
TMP/SMZ	trimethoprim-sulfamethoxazole
TORCH	toxoplasmosis, other (viruses), rubella, cytomegalovirus, herpes simplex virus
TPN	total parenteral nutrition
TRH	thyroid-releasing hormone
Trich	*Trichomonas*
TSH	thyroid-stimulating hormone
tsp	teaspoon
Tx	treatment
U	unit
U/A	urinalysis
URI	upper respiratory infection
US	ultrasound
UTI	urinary tract infection
VCUG	voiding cystourethrogram

VDRL	Venereal Disease Research Laboratory
VGE	viral gastroenteritis
VP	ventriculoperitoneal
vs	versus
VZIG	varicella-zoster immune globulin
WBC	white blood cell
WHO	World Health Organization
w/u	work-up
yr	year
ZnPP	zinc protoporphyrin
1°	primary
2°	secondary
$\approx$	approximately
$\geq$	equal to or greater than
$\leq$	equal to or less than

PEDIATRIC PEARLS

THE HANDBOOK OF
PRACTICAL PEDIATRICS

GENERAL APPROACH TO THE PATIENT

MEDICAL ASSESSMENT

A. HISTORY

1. A careful, pertinent, and thorough history is an essential first step in understanding the problems of any patient. In addition to the chief complaint and current illness of the patient, explore the medical history, past and current medications (including nonprescription medications), immunizations, hospitalizations, previous surgeries, transfusions, previous major illnesses and accidents, recent exposures, family history, social situation, and sources of medical care. Record this information so that it is both available and useful in the future. Be sure to talk to the person most knowledgeable about the medical history of the patient.

2. Be alert for the "hidden diagnosis"; the complaint of the patient or family member may have little or nothing to do with the actual problem. Try to determine what really is troubling the patient or family member; open-ended questions may be especially helpful.

   Example: Chief complaint: stomach pains. Actual diagnosis: school phobia or sexual abuse.

3. Also include the following in the history:
   a. Address and telephone number (or nearest telephone) of the patient
   b. Name of a parent or guardian
   c. Names and addresses of other physicians from whom and locations at which the patient receives medical care
   d. Insurance information

B. PHYSICAL EXAMINATION

1. Obtain weight, length, and vital signs (temperature, HR, RR; BP in children and adolescents); determine head circumference, if appropriate (e.g., in infants or toddlers).

2. The PE should include pertinent positive and negative findings. Do not limit the PE to the organ system that is the basis for the chief complaint. Carefully observe the child to ascertain the degree of discomfort (if any) experienced during the PE, which is especially important when the diagnosis is uncertain or when the chronicity or reported severity of the symptoms does not match the physical appearance of the child. Be sure to record a description of the child's appearance. Terms such as "well-developed, well-nourished white female" might not completely describe the child's "true" appearance. For example, you might ask, was she happy or sad? Did she look her age or older? Younger? Was she cooperative with you? With her parent?

Did she seem to understand your directives during the PE? Was she clean or soiled? Remember, your description might be of great use to the *next* person who examines the child; therefore your records should be as complete as possible.

3. Depending on the degree of emotional or physical discomfort, performing a PE on a child is sometimes difficult. Therefore it is important to explain what you will be doing as you proceed or in response to questions. In the long run, a hurried attitude hurts the examiner, the patient, and the parent. Sometimes children need to be distracted during the PE so that they do not "help" (e.g., during the assessment of the patellar tendon reflex) or "hinder" (e.g., during the examination of the lungs or heart when silence is needed). Patience and a gentle explanation of what is needed usually secure better conditions for true assessments, especially with children older than toddlers. Sometimes the PE needs to be performed while the child is sitting on a parent's lap or while the parent is holding the child's hand; so be it. If the child starts to cry or feels uncomfortable with what is happening, that part of the PE should not be forced at that time *unless it is truly an emergency.*

4. The feelings and concerns of the child should always be heard and respected. There might be major reasons (of which you are unaware) the child does not want a certain procedure to be performed. For example, a child who screams and cries when the examiner attempts to visualize the genitalia might be reliving an abusive situation. Therefore be sensitive to what is communicated both verbally and nonverbally. Do not be afraid to back off or to get assistance when needed. The older child and adolescent should be asked if he or she prefers the parent to be in or out of the room during the PE. Respect the wishes of the patient. If the parent is not in the room, a chaperone should be present when the genitalia are being examined, regardless of whether the patient is male or female.

C. LABORATORY TESTS

1. Order only those tests that will affect patient management. Costly laboratory testing is not indicated every time a diagnosis is uncertain. It is imperative to follow up on the results. Failure to do so is not good medical practice and may leave the examiner open to legal action if a test result dictates a certain action that is not taken because the examiner is unaware of the result.

2. The suggested laboratory tests for each discussed entity are presented in this book. When you promise to notify the parent (or patient) of the test results, make sure that you do so in a timely fashion; document the communication.

MEDICAL ASSESSMENT BY TELEPHONE

A. GENERAL PRINCIPLES

1. Identify yourself.
2. Request identification of the child, the caller, and the caller's relationship to the child.
3. Ascertain the age and approximate weight of the child.
4. Listen to the parent's story.
5. When asking questions, wait for the answer to one question before going on to the next one.
6. Remain courteous and calm (even if the parent is neither).
7. Avoid using ambiguous or medical terms that might confuse the parent.
8. Identify the child's problem to your satisfaction before rendering advice; plainly state what you believe the problem to be.
9. If the child does not need to be seen, explain why not and give the parent specific therapies to try; give advice on what to do if these measures fail.
10. Instruct the parent about the symptoms that are part of the natural course of the illness and those that warn of a worsening condition. Indicate which symptoms warrant medical attention.
11. Ask the parent to repeat all the instructions you have given, and ask whether there are any questions.
12. Encourage the parent to call back if he or she has questions or if the condition of the child worsens.
13. Follow up on any child who has symptoms that concern you (do not depend on the parent to call back). If the family has no telephone, obtain the telephone number of a relative or friend. Briefly document the content of all calls; it is imperative to document calls when a medication (prescription or OTC) is ordered or when the parent is urged to bring the child into the office to receive medical attention.

B. SPECIAL PRINCIPLES FOR THE MOST COMMON COMPLAINTS*

1. Respiratory complaints
a. Does the child have a cold? Is it getting better or worse? In what way?
b. Does the child have a fever? How high is the temperature?
c. What medications (how much, for how long, and how often) have been used for the fever and the cold?
d. Does the child have a cough? Is the child also vomiting?
e. Does the child have a runny nose? What color is the nasal discharge?
f. Does the child seem to breathe more noisily than usual?
g. When the child breathes, can you see the ribs?
h. Is any area of the body blue?

*Modified from DeAngelis C: *Pediatric primary care,* ed 3, Boston, 1984, Little, Brown.

1

GENERAL APPROACH TO THE PATIENT

   i.   Do the nostrils move with each breath?

   j.   Can the parent count the child's breaths? (If a watch or clock with a second hand is not available, the parent can count out loud while you time the breaths.)

   k.   Is there a hoarse cry or barky cough?

   l.   Is there a rash?

   m.   Is the child vomiting or having diarrhea?

   n.   How is the child acting, eating, and sleeping?

   o.   What is the child doing now?

2.   Fever

   a.   Did the parent take the child's temperature, or did the child just feel warm to the touch?

   b.   What was the temperature? Which method was used to take the temperature: rectal, oral, axillary, or aural?

   c.   Has the child been given medicine to reduce the temperature? Which one, how much, and how often? When was the last dose?

   d.   Does the medicine seem to bring down the temperature?

   e.   What else has the parent tried to make the child better?

   f.   What other signs of illness are there (e.g., respiratory problems, rash)?

   g.   How is the child acting, eating, and sleeping?

   h.   Has the child received an immunization? What type? When?

   i.   Does the child seem to be in pain? How so?

   j.   Does anyone who has been in contact with the child have similar complaints?

3.   Dermatologic problems

   a.   How long has the child had the rash, and where did it first appear?

   b.   Where is the rash now? Is it on the palms and soles?

   c.   What color is the rash, and how large are the individual spots?

   d.   Can the parent feel and see the rash?

   e.   Does the rash disappear with pressure?

   f.   Does any part of the rash have blisters or crusts?

   g.   Does the rash itch, burn, or hurt?

   h.   Has the child had a similar rash in the past?

   i.   Has the child been around anyone else with a similar rash?

   j.   What other signs of illness does the child have?

   k.   How is the child acting, eating, and sleeping?

   l.   Does the child have a high temperature?

   m.   Has the child recently taken or is the child currently taking any medications? Which ones?

   n.   Has the child been exposed to any new allergens? Which ones?

4.   Trauma

   a.   What type of injury did the child sustain (e.g., fall, laceration, burn, or bite)?

      (1)   How and when did it occur?

      (2)   Which body part sustained injury?

- b. If the child struck his or her head:
  - (1) Did the child lose consciousness, vomit, or have a seizure afterward?
  - (2) How is the child acting now?
  - (3) If another body part was injured, is the child using it normally now?
  - (4) What has the parent done for the injury?
- c. If the child sustained a laceration:
  - (1) Is the laceration still bleeding?
  - (2) How large is the laceration?
  - (3) Is the blood bright red and spurting?
  - (4) What has the parent done to stop the bleeding?
  - (5) What is the child doing now?
  - (6) When did the child last have a tetanus shot?
- d. If the child was burned:
  - (1) What part of the body was burned?
  - (2) How large an area is involved?
  - (3) Is there an area of redness, or are there blisters? Have the blisters broken?
  - (4) Does the child complain of pain at the burn site?
  - (5) What has the parent done for the burn?
  - (6) How is the child acting?
  - (7) When did the child last have a tetanus shot?
- e. If the child was bitten:
  - (1) What bit the child?
  - (2) If the bite was from a dog, is the dog known to the family?
  - (3) Has the dog been behaving abnormally?
  - (4) Has the dog had its shots?
  - (5) Was the dog provoked?
  - (6) If the bite was from a wild animal, what type of animal was it?
  - (7) Has the animal been captured?
  - (8) When did the child last have a tetanus shot?
  - (9) What has the parent done for the bite?
  - (10) What area of the body was bitten, and how does the area look?
  - (11) How is the child acting?
5. GI complaints
- a. Is the child experiencing diarrhea, vomiting, or both?
- b. For how long?
- c. If vomiting, is the child merely coughing up phlegm, spitting up after feeding, or actually vomiting?
- d. When does the vomiting occur in relation to meals?
- e. Can the child eat certain foods without vomiting? Which ones?
- f. Can the child drink anything without vomiting?
- g. Could the child have accidentally ingested a household product or medication?

h. Does the vomiting occur forcefully or effortlessly?
i. Does the child seem hungry or in pain?
j. How many bowel movements has the child had today? Yesterday?
k. How many times has the child vomited today? Yesterday?
l. Is the vomitus red or green?
m. Is the stool red or green? What does the stool look like? Does it have any formed elements in it?
n. Is the child taking any medication?
o. What has the parent done for the illness, including dietary and medicinal regimens?
p. Is the child getting better or worse?
q. Is the child's mouth wet?
r. Has the child been urinating the usual number of times and in the usual amounts?
s. What other signs of illness are present (e.g., rash, respiratory symptoms)?
t. Has the child had a fever? How high was the temperature? Which method was used to take the temperature: rectal, oral, axillary, or aural?
u. How well is the child sleeping?
v. How is the child's appetite for foods and liquids?
w. What liquids and foods has the parent given to the child today? How well were they tolerated?
x. How is the child's activity?
y. Does anyone who has been in contact with the child have similar complaints?
z. What is the child doing now?

THERAPEUTICS
A. MEDICATIONS

1. Consider the following: whether the drug is really indicated, what therapeutic effects to expect, side effects (may differ according to the age of the child), half-life, dosage, cost (use the generic form when possible), interactions with other drugs (e.g., erythromycin and theophylline), and the risk of poisoning. Be especially aware of unnecessary antibiotic use (leading to resistant strains of bacteria).
2. Consider the most appropriate form of administration (e.g., tablet, capsule, liquid, or suppository).
3. Consider the frequency and periodicity of administration (qid generally means 8 AM, noon, 4 PM, and 8 PM; q6h is 8 AM, 2 PM, 8 PM, and 2 AM). Simplify regimens as much as possible; make them convenient with school, day-care, sleep, and other activities.
4. Arrange to follow blood levels when necessary (e.g., with anticonvulsants).
5. Consider the ability of the parent and child to adhere to the regimen. It decreases as the number of medications or modalities increases and when specified times for administration are inconvenient.

6. Teach the parent or child about the indications, effects, and side effects of the medication; how to administer and accurately measure it; and how to prevent an inadvertent overdose.
a. Have the parent or child repeat what you have stated.
b. Special instructions should always be written down.
c. Explain to the parent that the medication must be taken for the full course, even if the symptoms disappear in several days.
7. Document that you have explained to the parent or child the action and any common side effects of the drug. In addition, document any adverse drug effects reported by the parent or child and report them, if applicable, to the FDA.

B. PRESCRIPTIONS

1. Be sure that the parent or child is able (i.e., has the money, time, and transportation) to get the prescription filled. Assume nothing!
2. Write legibly. Not only is it inconsiderate to write illegibly, it is also potentially dangerous because prescriptions can be filled incorrectly. If you cannot write clearly, print. Use only standard abbreviations.
3. Include all pertinent information.
a. Name, address, and age of the patient.
b. Name and form of the drug (e.g., tablet, liquid, or capsule) and dosage or concentration (e.g., 500-mg tablet, 500 mg/5 ml, 250 mg/5 ml).
c. Amount to dispense, such as the number of tablets or amount of liquid. Remember, some medications come in standard amounts, such as 150 ml; thus the drug might be more expensive if the pharmacist must "break" the bottle to comply with your prescription (e.g., the medication comes in a standard size of 150 ml and you prescribe 130 ml). The policies of pharmacists vary in this regard; know what the pharmacists in your area do in such situations.
d. Directions (sig) such as amount, frequency, route, and duration (e.g., 5 ml q4h PO × 7 days). Do not use teaspoon measurements; prescribe a syringe for accurate dosing.
e. When a refill is necessary, indicate how many, spelling out the number, if any (e.g., a controlled substance); if no refill is desired, write "zero" after "refill."
f. Do not forget your signature and DEA number when prescribing a controlled substance.
4. Include all prescription data (name of drug, form, dosing regimen, and amount dispensed) in the patient's medical record.

C. COUNSELING PATIENT AND FAMILY ABOUT AN ILLNESS OR CONDITION

1. Counseling is *essential* for physician and patient rapport. Counseling improves communication and understanding of the illness, improves compliance with follow-up and medication, alleviates fears and misconceptions, and prevents mismanagement at home. The patient

1

GENERAL APPROACH TO THE PATIENT

and family will also know what to expect and when to return if certain signs or symptoms develop. Nurses can teach temperature measurement and fever management and review the physician's instructions with the parent or patient.

2. In general it is better to contact the family for telephone follow-up than to expect a parent to call you. Arrange a time when and a telephone number where a parent can be reached. Keep track of patients in need of telephone contact so that they do not fall through the cracks.

D. DOCUMENTATION

1. Be sure to document adequately and legibly the results of the history and PE, laboratory tests ordered, test results, clinical impression(s), therapeutic modalities suggested, and medications prescribed or OTC medications recommended. Also document when a return visit or follow up by telephone is necessary.
2. Although thorough documentation is a great deal of work, it will assist the *next* person who sees the patient and can be a saving grace if litigation is threatened.
3. Be aware of confidentiality in any electronic documentation you may send or receive, by fax or e-mail; this is especially important if you are communicating with a parent or patient by e-mail.

E. BIBLIOGRAPHY

Schmitt B: *Pediatric telephone advice,* Boston, 1980, Little, Brown.

CARDIOPULMONARY RESUSCITATION

Most pediatric cardiopulmonary arrests begin with respiratory insufficiency. Cardiac standstill is usually a secondary event. As a result, recovery rates for children who are apneic but not yet pulseless are much better than those for children who are both apneic and pulseless. To achieve success, intervention must be properly organized, quickly initiated, and appropriately focused (ABCs).

2

A. ORGANIZATION

It is essential to maintain an organized approach during resuscitation. Resuscitation responsibilities should be established well in advance of any need. Team members must be skilled at their jobs and must know the limitations of their responsibilities and skills. The leader must clearly communicate to the entire team his or her thought processes and orders. Once a decision is made, there is no room for ambiguity. Although resuscitations can be effectively conducted by a smaller group of health care professionals, whenever possible, it is best to have available the following personnel.

1. One person to direct and monitor (oversees entire procedure)
2. One person to maintain a patent airway and ensure proper oxygenation and ventilation
3. One person for cardiac massage
4. One or two people to establish venous access and draw blood
5. One person to prepare medications
6. One person to record medications, procedures, and pertinent occurrences
7. One person to get equipment, supplies, and other personnel if needed

To facilitate efficiency, the resuscitation "crowd" must be kept under control. Those not immediately involved with the resuscitation should remain out of the way and quiet. The team leader should use his or her discretion to limit the number of participants. Regardless of the cause of the underlying disease (e.g., trauma, sepsis), it is advisable to approach resuscitation by first performing a primary survey, followed by a secondary survey, and then definitive care.

B. ALPHABET OF RESUSCITATION (ABCDE): THE PRIMARY SURVEY

The primary survey is the "automatic" component of resuscitation during which life-threatening disorders are corrected. Every child in need of resuscitation should receive every component of the primary survey. The primary survey is also referred to as the ABCs.

1. **A**irway: Airway obstruction is commonly the precipitating event in a pediatric cardiopulmonary arrest. Restoration of adequate oxygenation

and ventilation is essential if resuscitation is to be successful. Clear the oropharynx of secretions and vomitus (use large-bore suctioning); this procedure should not be done blindly. Open the airway using the chin-lift or jaw-thrust technique. In general, and especially in the injured child, maintain the cervical spine in an in-line (neutral) position; *do not* hyperextend the neck. An oral or nasal airway may be inserted to prevent the tongue from obstructing the airway. The tip of the oral airway should just approximate the angle of the mandible. Pliable nasal airways are more comfortable for the patient. The preferred nasal airway should measure in length from the nostril to the tragus of the ear. The caliber of the artificial airway should be that which fits comfortably within the nostril.

2. Breathing: With the exception of total airway obstruction (which occurs with aspiration of a foreign body and in some anatomic abnormalities), any child's lungs can be effectively ventilated by way of the bag valve mask (BVM) technique. This technique should be used for those children who require only a short period of positive-pressure oxygenation and ventilation. For those who require extended assistance, BVM should be used until the placement of an ETT is feasible. ETT size (internal diameter [ID]) is best approximated using a simple mathematical age-based formula (Table 2-1). Uncuffed ETTs should be used in children under 8 years of age. The ETT should be inserted beyond the teeth to a depth (centimeters) of about three times its internal diameter (millimeters). Watch the chest for good expansion; note any improvement in perfusion and pulses. The trachea should be intubated if the BVM technique is insufficient or if adequate and spontaneous respirations cannot be maintained. Muscle relaxants may be needed to facilitate intubation and are discussed later in this chapter.

   After intubation, assess the lungs bilaterally for equal breath sounds, and assess the adequacy of ventilation and perfusion. If available, capnometry and pulse oximetry should be used to help make this assessment.

3. Circulation (Table 2-2): Once a patent airway has been established and gas exchange restored, attention should be directed toward the circulatory system. Conventional resuscitation techniques still call for mechanical chest compressions as the preferred way to augment tissue perfusion. Chest compressions should be initiated for patients with absent pulses, infants with measured HRs less than 60 beats per minute, and children with detectable but ineffective pulses (poor tissue perfusion). To best facilitate this, follow these guidelines:

a. Make sure a firm board is under the chest for effective closed-chest cardiac massage.

b. Give one breath per 5 compressions (the ratio remains the same, regardless of age and size), and approximately 100 compressions per

TABLE 2-1

GUIDELINES FOR ENDOTRACHEAL TUBE (ETT) SIZE IN CHILDREN

	ETT Internal Diameter (ID)
Newborns	3.0-3.5 mm (ID)
Infants and children	$ID(mm) = \dfrac{Age(yr) + 16}{4}$

Uncuffed tubes should be used for children under 8 years of age (ID <6 mm).

TABLE 2-2

GUIDELINES FOR CHEST COMPRESSIONS IN CHILDREN

	Newborn	Child	Adult
Compression (rate/min)	120	100	80
Depth of compression (in)	0.5-1	1-1.5	1.5-2
Ventilation (rate/min)	20	16	12

minute. The AHA further recommends that for children over 8 years of age who have "unprotected airways," 2 breaths per 15 compressions should be delivered.

c.   The time of compression should equal the time of compression release for best cardiac output.

d.   Whenever possible, synchronize compressions with respirations (ventilate as compression is released).

e.   Compressions should be applied evenly over the midsternum; the proper hand placement for compressions is one fingerbreadth below the area where the transnipple line intersects the sternum.

f.   Check the efficacy of CPR. Palpate peripheral pulses (femoral, brachial, and carotid) while pumping. Assess perfusion (capillary refill should be <2 seconds), ventilation, and pupil reactivity.

4.   **D**rugs: As many as 20 different medications have been recommended as useful adjuncts for pediatric resuscitation. Although most of these are not commonly required, it is essential to know the indications, effects, and dosages of a few first-line resuscitation drugs. These drugs are also summarized in *The Harriet Lane Handbook.* Their use is described in more detail subsequently. You do not need to wait for an ECG or arterial blood gas results before giving drugs. Establish good vascular access as soon as possible. Peripheral access remains the first-line approach. In the sickest patients, however, such access might be difficult to achieve. If a percutaneous venous line cannot be established quickly (within 2 minutes), consider alternate routes (e.g., intraosseous [by way of the proximal tibia], central line using the Seldinger technique, central line by cutdown).

It is important to remember that four useful resuscitation drugs (**l**idocaine, **a**tropine, **n**aloxone, **e**pinephrine) may be given by way of an ETT. Endotracheal doses of lidocaine, atropine, and naloxone are the same

2

CARDIOPULMONARY RESUSCITATION

as IV-IO doses. The ET dose of epinephrine, however, is 10 times the IV-IO dose.

a. Most Commonly Used Resuscitation Drugs

   (1) **Adenosine** has become the agent most commonly used to chemically convert SVT in children. It is an extremely short-acting agent (half-life of 10 seconds) that slows sinus rate and AV nodal conduction velocities, and commonly causes transient asystole. Although vagal maneuvers can first be attempted to reverse SVT, adenosine remains the *drug* of choice for that purpose. Adenosine should be administered as a 0.1-mg/kg (maximum 6 mg) rapid intravascular bolus that may be doubled for the second dose (maximum 12 mg).

   (2) **Amiodarone** is newly recommended for a wide range of atrial and ventricular arrhythmias in children. As is lidocaine, amiodarone should be considered for reversal of ventricular tachycardia, especially when cardioversion with electricity has failed. Amiodarone is also recommended as a remedy for ectopic atrial tachycardia and junctional ectopic tachycardia. For refractory pulseless ventricular tachycardia or ventricular fibrillation, a 5-mg/kg dose should be administered as a rapid intravascular infusion. For perfusing supraventricular and ventricular rhythms, a loading dose (5 mg/kg) may be administered over 20 to 60 minutes and repeated to a maximum dosage of 15 mg/kg/day.

   (3) **Atropine sulfate** is recommended as an effective agent for reversal of symptomatic bradycardia (including patients with evidence of AV block) that is unresponsive to initial treatment with supplemental oxygen, proper ventilation, and administration of epinephrine. Atropine is not recommended for this purpose in newborns (epinephrine is preferred). Atropine is one of four resuscitation drugs that may be administered by way of an ETT. Intravascular and endotracheal doses are the same (0.02 mg/kg). The minimum single dose is 0.1 mg. The maximum single doses are 0.5 mg for a child and 1.0 mg for an adolescent. The maximum total doses are 1.0 mg for a child and 2.0 mg for an adolescent.

   (4) **Epinephrine** is, exclusive of oxygen, the single most commonly used drug during resuscitation. Epinephrine is a combination alpha- and beta-adrenergic agonist that reliably stimulates cardiac contractions, increases HR, increases cardiac contractility, and causes vasoconstriction. It is a useful adjunct for treatment of asystole, pulseless arrest, symptomatic bradycardia, hypotension, and hypoperfusion. Some controversy exists regarding the preferred dosing of epinephrine for patients with pulseless arrest. Absent complete uniformity of opinion, current standards call for the following approach. After initiation of basic life support (including oxygenation, ventilation, and chest compressions), an

initial bolus of epinephrine should be administered either intravascularly in a dose of 0.01 mg/kg (0.1 ml/kg of 1:10,000 solution) or by way of an ETT in a dose of 0.1 mg/kg (0.1 ml/kg of 1:1000 solution). Subsequent intravascular boluses of epinephrine can be given of either the same or higher (0.1 to 0.2 mg/kg) doses. All ETT doses should be 0.1 mg/kg (0.1 ml/kg of 1:1000 solution). For patients with symptomatic bradycardia, all intravascular doses should be 0.01 mg/kg (0.1 ml/kg of 1:10,000 solution) and all ETT doses should be 0.1 mg/kg (0.1 ml/kg of 1:1000 solution). Epinephrine can also be administered by continuous infusion (0.1 to 1.0 μg/kg/min). Epinephrine can cause tachyarrhythmias, and high-dose infusions can produce significant vasoconstriction that can compromise tissue perfusion. Epinephrine should not be mixed with sodium bicarbonate and is contraindicated in the treatment of ventricular tachycardia secondary to cocaine.

(5) **Lidocaine** is also an alternative treatment for wide-complex tachycardia, ventricular fibrillation, or pulseless ventricular tachycardia. As can atropine, naloxone, and epinephrine, lidocaine can be given by way of an ETT and intravascularly. Both the intravascular and ETT bolus dose is 1.0 mg/kg (IV-IO as a rapid push). After return of spontaneous circulation, lidocaine can be given as a continuous infusion (20 to 50 μg/kg/min) for recurrent ventricular tachycardia, ventricular fibrillation, or ventricular ectopy, especially if associated with myocarditis or structural heart disease.

(6) **Oxygen** is the most important and most commonly required resuscitation drug. It should be administered to all children during resuscitation. Oxygen should always be given in the highest available concentration and in humidified form if possible.

b. Other Resuscitation Drugs

(1) **Bretylium** has been removed from the list of commonly considered drugs for pediatric advanced life support. Nevertheless, it can be used in certain circumstances. Bretylium has been used as a supplemental agent (after lidocaine and other standard interventions) for chemical conversion of ventricular arrhythmias. For ventricular fibrillation, a rapid intravascular infusion of 5 mg/kg is recommended. For ventricular tachycardia, 5 to 10 mg/kg is the recommended dose. Bretylium can cause hypotension, especially in patients who have hypovolemia.

(2) **Calcium** (10% calcium chloride or calcium gluconate) is useful for reversal of hypocalcemia and hyperkalemia and potentially useful for managing hypermagnesemia or calcium channel blocker overdose. Calcium can increase myocardial contractility but can also cause significant bradycardia, especially if infused rapidly. The recommended dose of calcium chloride is 10 to

20 mg/kg or 0.1 to 0.2 ml/kg IV, infused *slowly* (preferably through a central line) to avoid bradycardia. The recommended dose of calcium gluconate is 60 to 100 mg/kg or 0.6 to 1.0 ml/kg of a 10% solution. Remember to clear the IV line of sodium bicarbonate (because $NaHCO_3$ + Ca = chalk). Calcium is not recommended for routine treatment of asystole or electromechanical dissociation.

(3) **Dextrose** is indicated for documented hypoglycemia and is best administered as a 5 ml/kg bolus of 10% dextrose. A bolus of 25% dextrose (2 ml/kg) can be used but may result in rebound hypoglycemia if not followed by glucose infusion.

(4) **Dobutamine** is an inotropic agent, usually used to treat cardiogenic shock, particularly in patients with high vascular resistance and adequate intravascular volume. Dobutamine is administered as a continuous infusion (2 to 20 mcg/kg/min), usually initiated at 5 to 10 mcg/kg/min and then titrated to effect. Dobutamine can produce or exacerbate hypotension or tachyarrhythmias and should not be mixed with sodium bicarbonate.

(5) **Dopamine** has many effects that are dose dependent (see the following points). Before using dopamine, expand intravascular volume in shock states secondary to hypovolemia. Dopamine has minimal toxicity when used at reasonable doses. However, it can produce tachyarrhythmias, high blood pressure, and local vasoconstriction (during extravasation). During high infusion rates (>20 mcg/kg/min), peripheral, renal, and splanchnic vasoconstriction can result. As with dobutamine, dopamine should not be mixed with sodium bicarbonate.

    (a) Dosage ranges

        (i) Low dosage: 1 to 7 mcg/kg/min; increases renal blood flow.

        (ii) Moderate dosage: 7 to 20 mcg/kg/min; promotes vasoconstriction; increases cardiac output and blood pressure.

        (iii) High dosage: 20 to 30 mcg/kg/min; causes systemic vasoconstriction; decreases renal blood flow.

(6) **Etomidate** is an ultra–short-acting nonbarbiturate, nonbenzodiazepine sedative–hypnotic agent with no analgesic properties. It produces rapid sedation without causing cardiovascular or respiratory depression and is the sedative of choice for patients with multiple trauma or hypotension. Etomidate will also decrease intracranial pressure (ICP), cerebral blood flow, and cerebral basal metabolic rate. Etomidate can also cause myoclonic activity and can exacerbate focal seizure disorders. For rapid sedation, a dosage of 0.2 to 0.4 mg/kg

infused over 30 to 60 seconds will act quickly and last for 10 to 15 minutes. Etomidate is relatively contraindicated in children with known adrenal insufficiency or known focal seizure disorders.

(7) **Isoproterenol** infusion has been removed from the list of commonly considered drugs for pediatric advanced life support. Nevertheless, it is still considered useful for selected patients with status asthmaticus unresponsive to other measures, and for those with bradycardia unresponsive to other measures (especially for patients with bradycardia accompanied by heart block). Isoproterenol has several potent cardiovascular effects: increased HR, increased myocardial contractility (resulting in increased myocardial oxygen demand), and increased arterial and venous vasodilation. Isoproterenol is contraindicated in patients with ischemic heart disease (including aortic stenosis) and in patients with hypovolemia. Isoproterenol is administered as a constant infusion, beginning with 0.1 mcg/kg/min. Dosage may be further increased by 0.1 mcg/kg/min every 15 minutes until improvement or toxicity occurs; the usual maximum dosage is 1.5 mcg/kg/min. Because of its potent effects, isoproterenol should be used with caution. Establish two IV lines when initiating isoproterenol infusions in patients with asthma, because the abrupt cessation of this drug (such as that which occurs with IV malfunction) may result in a quick return of severe bronchospasm. Isoproterenol also increases myocardial oxygen consumption, which may be dangerous if Pao_2 is less than 60 mm Hg. Patients receiving isoproterenol should have continuous cardiac monitoring to detect possible arrhythmias or ST-segment changes.

(8) **Magnesium sulfate** is useful for management of torsades de pointes ventricular tachycardia, suspected hypomagnesemia, or status asthmaticus unresponsive to beta-adrenergic agonists. For treatment of either torsades de pointes or asthma, a bolus dose of 25 to 50 mg/kg (maximum 2 g) is given over 10 to 20 minutes. Rapid boluses can possibly cause hypotension or bradycardia. In patients with renal failure, magnesium should be used with caution.

(9) **Naloxone (Narcan)** is a narcotic antagonist and is particularly useful for reversal of narcotic-induced respiratory depression. The recommended dose is 0.1 mg/kg, which can be readministered every 2 to 3 minutes. Many physicians use a standard 1- to 2-mg dose for all ages. Naloxone may be given by way of the ETT at the same dose.

(10) **Prostaglandin E_1** is used to maintain patency of the ductus arteriosus in newborns with cyanotic congenital heart disease and ductal-dependent pulmonary or systemic blood flow. It is given as

2

CARDIOPULMONARY RESUSCITATION

a continuous infusion, initiated at 0.05 to 0.1 mcg/kg/min and titrated to effect. PGE_1 can cause vasodilation, hypotension, apnea, hyperpyrexia, jitteriness, seizures, hypoglycemia, and hypocalcemia.

(11) **Sodium bicarbonate** is useful for reversal of metabolic acidosis in patients with adequate ventilation. In patients with inadequate ventilation, administration of sodium bicarbonate will result in increased levels of serum carbon dioxide. During resuscitation, small doses (1 mEq/kg) should be used. When given to newborns, half-strength solutions (0.5 mEq/ml) should be used but only after adequate ventilation is established. The adult dose is 1 to 2 ampules (44 mEq/ampules).

Note: Be sure to clear any IV line of sodium bicarbonate after its administration. Agents such as epinephrine, dobutamine, and dopamine are less effective in alkaline solutions; when mixed together, calcium and bicarbonate will form concretions.

5. Exposure (of the patient) and Environment, ECG, and Electricity:

a. Exposure of the patient in a patient-friendly environment is an essential step in the resuscitation process. Clothing should be removed to maximize the perspective of the resuscitation team. The environment for the exposed child, however, should be warm and comfortable. The smaller the child, the greater the ratio of body surface area to body mass and thus the greater the insensible losses of body heat and water. Cover or otherwise warm the child whenever possible.

b. Similarly, it is essential to assess the cardiac status of the child throughout the resuscitation and postresuscitation period. Continuous cardiac monitoring and periodic ECG interpretation are critical.

c. When ventricular fibrillation or pulseless ventricular tachycardia is detected, electrical defibrillation is required. Synchronized cardioversion is the treatment of choice for tachyarrhythmias (SVT, VT, atrial fibrillation, or atrial flutter) that cause cardiovascular compromise.

(1) **Proper paddle position and skin interface** greatly affect success. Place one paddle to the right of the upper sternum and below the clavicle; place the other paddle to the left of the left nipple in the anterior axillary line. On small children and infants, place the paddles on the chest and back directly over the heart. The dose of electricity varies according to weight.

(2) **Defibrillation doses** are 2 J/kg for children who weigh less than 50 kg, and 200 J for those who weigh 50 kg or more. Initially, up to three shocks may be given in rapid succession (2, 2 to 4, and 4 J/kg), followed by CPR, epinephrine, and additional electricity (4 J/kg). If ineffective, the sequence of CPR, drug, and electricity can be repeated, substituting amiodarone or lidocaine for epinephrine.

(3) **Synchronized cardioversion** is provided by delivering smaller doses of electricity. Using the synchronized (sync) mode,

0.5 J/kg are given initially. Second and subsequent energy levels are 1.0 J/kg. If this sequence does not work, reevaluate the rhythm.

C. RAPID-SEQUENCE INTUBATION

Rapid-sequence intubation (RSI) is an organized, controlled approach to intubation that involves the use of chemical agents. Premedications are indicated to facilitate intubation for patients with increased muscle tone or seizures or patients struggling with respiratory failure. Various combinations of agents can be used for this purpose. Most protocols call for a combination of a sedative-hypnotic agent (usually a benzodiazepine or barbiturate) and a neuromuscular blocking agent, with or without cardiovascular adjuncts.

RSI follows a stepwise approach:
1. Preparation of equipment and medications
2. Placement of monitoring devices
3. Preoxygenation
4. Administration of premedications
5. Application of cricoid pressure
6. Administration of sedative agent
7. Administration of paralytic agent
8. Intubation
9. Postintubation observation and monitoring

It is best to establish a protocol for RSI before its use. Only agents known to the user should be used. All resources to provide positive-pressure oxygenation and ventilation must be immediately available in the event that intubation is unsuccessful. The following is a sample RSI protocol:
a. Provide preoxygenation with 100% humidified oxygen by BVM.
b. Administer atropine, 0.02 mg/kg (minimum 0.1 mg), to inhibit bradycardia.
c. Apply cricoid pressure (Sellick maneuver) to prevent gastroesophageal reflux and to facilitate intubation.
d. Administer thiopental (2 to 4 mg/kg) or midazolam (0.1 to 0.2 mg/kg, maximum 4 mg) or ketamine (1.0 to 4.0 mg/kg).
e. Administer succinylcholine (1.0 mg/kg in children, 2.0 mg/kg in infants) or vecuronium (0.1 to 0.2 mg/kg) or rocuronium (0.6 to 1.2 mg/kg). Before administering succinylcholine, some physicians advise giving a small dose of pancuronium (0.01 mg/kg) to prevent fasciculations.
f. Intubate with ETT of appropriate size while maintaining cricoid pressure.
g. Reassess the patient and confirm successful intubation.

Remember, succinylcholine is contraindicated in a number of different situations: in patients with hyperkalemia, crush injuries, trauma or burns more than 48 hours old, glaucoma, or penetrating ocular injuries, and at times in the presence of severe increased ICP. Beware of the potential

2

CARDIOPULMONARY RESUSCITATION

complications of muscle relaxants in the patient with an upper airway obstruction.

D. SECONDARY SURVEY AND DEFINITIVE CARE

Once the initial lifesaving components of resuscitation (primary survey) have been accomplished, a more individualized secondary survey should be conducted. In this portion of resuscitation, a careful and thorough stepwise examination of the child should be performed. Portions of the physical examination conducted during the primary survey should be repeated. During each phase of the examination, useful diagnostic tests should be ordered and appropriate therapeutic care initiated. All diagnostic and therapeutic decisions should be tailored to the specific needs of the patient. This approach differs from that of the primary survey, in which every child is managed uniformly.

The secondary survey should be followed by formulation of plans for definitive care, including identification of the physician(s) and in-patient facility that will receive the patient after resuscitation. At this time the status of the patient should be communicated to the primary physician, if this has not been done already.

E. PRESENCE OF FAMILY MEMBERS

The inclusion of family members in the resuscitation process is a topic of debate. Communication of the status of the patient to parents and other family members should be expected as a bare minimum standard. Involvement of family members beyond that standard varies from center to center. Although it is desirable to have family members comfort a dying child, it is essential that they not interfere with any part of the resuscitation process, including the ability of the managing physicians to candidly discuss the course of events. A number of centers have made available to family members medical "interpreters," who accompany family members when they are in the resuscitation bay.

F. BIBLIOGRAPHY

American Heart Association/American Academy of Pediatrics. In Chameides L, editor: *Pediatric advanced life support,* Dallas, 1997, AHA Publication.

Carpenter TC, Stenmark KR: High-dose epinephrine is not superior to standard-dose epinephrine in pediatric in-hospital cardiopulmonary arrest, *Pediatrics* 99:403, 1997.

Ludwig S, Fleisher GR: Pediatric cardiopulmonary resuscitation: a review and a proposal, *Pediatr Emerg Care* 1:40, 1985.

Nadkarni V et al: Paediatric life support: an advisory statement by the Paediatric Life Support Working Group of the International Liaison Committee on Resuscitation, *Resuscitation* 34:115, 1997.

O'Rourke PP: Outcome of children who are apneic and pulseless in the emergency room, *Crit Care Med* 14:466, 1986.

Schoenfeld PS, Baker MD: Management of cardiopulmonary and trauma resuscitation in the pediatric emergency department, *Pediatrics* 91:726, 1993.

Scribano PV et al: Factors influencing termination of resuscitative efforts in children: a comparison of pediatric emergency medicine and adult emergency medicine physicians, *Pediatr Emerg Care* 13:320, 1997.

Stewart RD, Lacovery DC: Administration of endotracheal medications, *Ann Emerg Med* 14:136, 1985.

Torres NE, White RD: Current concepts in cardiopulmonary resuscitation, *J Cardiothorac Vasc Anesth* 11:391, 1997.

Yamamoto LG et al: Rapid sequence anesthesia induction for emergency intubation, *Pediatr Emerg Care* 6:200, 1990.

Zaritsky A: Pediatric resuscitation pharmacology. Members of the Medications in Pediatric Resuscitation Panel, *Ann Emerg Med* 22:445, 1993.

2

CARDIOPULMONARY RESUSCITATION

ABUSE

3

A. CHILD ABUSE

1. Abuse may be active (physical, sexual, or psychological abuse) or passive (physical, emotional, medical, or educational neglect). Physical injury is the easiest to discern; psychological injury is the hardest.

2. If there is suspicion that a child has been abused, health-care providers are *legally* obligated to report it to the proper authorities (usually Child Protective Services or Social Services). Remember, the abuse is being reported to safeguard the child and other at-risk children from further harm.

3. Always supplement medical input with input from social workers, when available. Social workers have expertise in interviewing skills that permits them to discover information that might otherwise remain hidden.

4. Approach the person accompanying the child nonjudgmentally. Ask open, not leading, questions. Do not demonstrate personal prejudices, anger, or disgust. Be as compassionate as possible.

5. If the child has an injury, determine whether the explanation for the injury fits the injury and the child's physical condition and developmental level. If it does, the injury *could* have happened that way; if it does not, the injury *could not* have happened that way.
   a. Was there a delay in seeking medical attention? Why?
   b. Who was supervising the child at the time of the injury?
   c. Has the child sustained burns, lacerations, head trauma, or fractures in the past? If yes, when and what caused these injuries?

6. Determine the child's health status and the family's living conditions.
   a. Where does the child receive well-child care? Are immunizations up to date?
   b. Determine whether the child has a chronic medical condition.
   c. To what support systems does the family have access?
   d. Are the parents employed? Do they have sufficient money for food, clothing, and shelter?
   e. How many persons live with the child?
   f. How many siblings does the child have? What are their ages? Do they live with the child?

7. Determine the child's psychosocial milieu.
   a. Was the child planned?
   b. Who are the usual caregivers? Is the child in day-care? If yes, which one?
   c. What is the child's best characteristic? Worst characteristic?
   d. What does the child do that merits discipline? How is the child usually disciplined?
   e. Does domestic violence occur? Against whom?

f. Do any family members have difficulty with alcohol or drug abuse? Who?

g. If the child is over 2 years of age, is he or she toilet trained? If yes, does he or she ever have accidents? If yes, how is he or she treated afterward?

Note: Many children are abused in conjunction with toilet training, incontinence, meal battles, and sleep problems.

8. While performing the PE, look for both overt and subtle signs of abuse.

a. Is the child clean or dirty?

b. Fearful or calm?

c. Clingy or aggressive?

d. Verbal or silent?

e. Does the child make eye contact with the parent? With the examiner?

f. Does the child want to be held by the parent, or prefer to go to the examiner?

g. How does the parent react to the child's cries or requests?

Note: Psychologically abused children may be timid or aggressive; both behaviors relate to their poor self-image. Neglected children may actually prefer the examiner to their parents.

9. A *thorough* PE is performed; particular attention should be given to the following:

a. Skin markings: lacerations, burns, ecchymoses, linear contusions (that could have been made with a belt or strap), contusions with definite shapes (made with a coat hanger or belt buckle), circular contusions on trunk or limbs (may indicate finger pressure points), bites, and other markings.

b. Oral trauma: torn frenulum (often a result of forced bottle-feeding or pacifier insertion in infants or toddlers), contused gums, and loose teeth (could result from a blow to the mouth).

c. Nasal trauma.

d. Ear trauma.

e. Eye trauma: hyphema, periorbital hematomas, and hemorrhage. Check fundi for retinal hemorrhages.

f. Chest injuries.

g. Blunt abdominal trauma.

h. Genital trauma (see Section B).

i. Limb trauma: asymmetries, fractures, dislocations, the inability to walk, and other signs of trauma.

j. Head trauma: hematomas, lacerations, and deformities. Document positive and negative findings.

k. Growth parameters (plot on growth curves).

10. Laboratory tests should be dictated by the medical history and findings on PE.

a. U/A is indicated when there is evidence of acute genital, abdominal, or back trauma.

b. Evidence of active bleeding, ecchymoses, or blunt abdominal trauma dictates a CBC with platelets and clotting studies.

c. Deformed or tender limbs; tender ribs; and abdominal, head, or chest trauma dictate x-ray examinations. Trauma surveys (to determine past or occult fractures) are useful mainly in preverbal children and mentally limited patients and should be performed in children under 3 years of age suspected of being physically abused.

11. Photographs (labeled with the date, patient's name, and photographer's name) of suspicious skin markings should be obtained and included in the medical record.

12. The child's disposition should be based on both medical and social concerns.

a. Children with moderate to severe injuries, unstable neurologic or cardiovascular results, or acute psychological disturbances should be admitted to the hospital.

b. When the child is not admitted to the hospital, a decision must be made as to where the child may be discharged. If the suspected abuser lives with the child, the child might be sent to another relative or foster care. If the suspected abuser does not live with the child, the child might be sent home with the parent. Immediate placement is made by the social service agency. Ultimate placement is at the discretion of the judicial system.

c. Siblings and other children exposed to the alleged abuser should also be promptly examined and removed from the home if necessary. In such a case, solicit assistance from social services, police, or both.

B. SEXUAL ABUSE

1. Sexual abuse involves actively or passively engaging a child in masturbation; fondling; voyeurism; pornography; or oral, anal, or genital intercourse. The use of bribes, gifts, or compliments to engage a young child in a sexual act should be regarded as forced sexual abuse.

2. A social worker should always be involved at the onset of the evaluation. Some communities have designated sexual assault and rape centers. If the patient is in no other medical distress and if the rape, genital trauma, or sexual assault is recent (<72 hours), he or she should be transported to one of these centers under police escort for evaluation. If the patient is too unstable for referral, perform a complete evaluation and therapy at the hospital.

3. Careful documentation is mandatory and includes a detailed history of the event written as quotations of the parent or, if appropriate, in the patient's words. Be aware that obtaining an accurate history may be difficult, and disclosure might not be immediate. Children may be afraid to reveal the details or name of the assailant.

a. Who is the alleged assailant?

b. When and where did the episode occur?

c. Did penile or other penetration occur?

d. Did other trauma occur? What was it?

e. Who (name and relationship) is now accompanying the patient?

4. A complete PE is necessary. A careful skin examination is also necessary. A PE by an experienced examiner (perhaps with the child under sedation or anesthesia) may be necessary, especially if active bleeding is present.

a. Place special emphasis on the oral, perineal, and anal areas for signs of old or new trauma, pharyngitis, mouth lesions, urethral or vaginal discharge, patulous anus, anal discharge or lesions, or a tender rectum.

b. Document positive findings with properly labeled photographs or drawings.

c. Record the appearance of the hymenal opening in a prepubertal child. To visualize the hymen, either separate the labia and gently pull posteriorly at a 45-degree angle *or* place traction on the labia by gently grasping the labia and pulling toward the examiner. Do not force an examination in a frightened or uncooperative patient; consider the use of sedation or referral.

5. If very recent (<72 hours) sexual abuse is suspected, obtain the following specimens when possible and place in the appropriate containers (forensic kit if available). Alternatively and preferably, send the patient to a sexual assault center if available. These centers are specially equipped to collect the following specimens, which are sent to a forensic laboratory for processing:

a. Hair, if any, combed from the pubic area.

b. Vaginal fluid: wet mount of material examined immediately for motile sperm.

c. Gonococcus culture (throat or mouth, rectum, cervix and vagina, penile urethra) as appropriate.

d. *Chlamydia* cultures of genital secretions as appropriate; if cultures are unavailable, nucleic acid amplification tests are acceptable but should be verified with a second test.

e. Wet mount and culture of vaginal swab for evidence of *Trichomonas vaginalis, Candida albicans,* or bacterial vaginosis.

f. Swab of vaginal secretions mixed in a test tube with 2 ml of normal saline solution. The sample is sent on ice immediately to the laboratory for an acid phosphatase test for semen. The laboratory may also be able to test sperm for DNA pattern. This test may be available only through a police laboratory via a sexual assault center.

g. Scrape from skin or clothing any areas that may represent dried semen for acid phosphatase testing or DNA typing.

h. Obtain blood and urine tests as follows:

(1) Serologic tests for syphilis, HIV, and hepatitis B. Because traumatized children might selectively remember the "blood test" or "needle," be as gentle as possible.

(2) These tests should be repeated in 2 weeks; tests for syphilis and HIV should also be repeated 6, 12, and 24 weeks after the assault. Again, keep in mind that young patients might remember the "blood test" most vividly.

(3) Toxicology screen if appropriate.

(4) Pregnancy test as appropriate. Pregnancy can be detected as early as 9 days after fertilization.

(5) U/A.

6. If sexual activity occurred at least several days before, perform the following (consult a knowledgeable physician if there are *any* questions):

a. A complete PE plus an external genital examination, with specific regard to the vaginal introitus and rectum. If appropriate, diagram abnormal findings on the patient's record.

b. A gonococcus culture from the vagina, throat, and rectum. Obtain specimens to test for syphilis and chlamydia.

c. Pregnancy test if appropriate.

d. U/A.

e. Baseline HIV and hepatitis B tests.

7. An empirical antimicrobial regimen for chlamydia, gonorrhea, trichomonas, and bacterial vaginosis is recommended. Prophylaxis for HIV exposure is discussed in Chapter 22.

a. Ceftriaxone, 125 mg, IM once *plus.*

b. Metronidazole, 2 g, PO once *plus.*

c. Azithromycin, 1 g, PO once *or* doxycycline, 100 mg, PO bid for 7 days.

8. Arrange appropriate follow-up care for the child and family. A social worker can arrange shelter if needed. Prompt individual or group psychological counseling can be very reassuring to the child and can assist in a more complete healing.

9. Parents, foster parents, or guardians should be counseled to not make a bad situation worse by using such terms as *ruined, violated,* or *dirty* around the child. A child's emotional reaction to sexual abuse is magnified by the imposition of adult values and may lead to anxiety, feelings of guilt and worthlessness, depression, and suicide ideation or attempts by the child. Caretakers can themselves benefit from psychological support and counseling.

C. BIBLIOGRAPHY

Adams J: Sexual abuse and adolescents, *Pediatr Ann* 26:299, 1997.

American Academy of Pediatrics—Committee on Child Abuse and Neglect: Guidelines for the evaluation of sexual abuse of children: subject review, *Pediatrics* 103:186, 1999.

American Academy of Pediatrics—Committee on Child Abuse and Neglect: Shaken baby syndrome: inflicted cerebral trauma, *Pediatrics* 92:872, 1993.

American Academy of Pediatrics Section on Radiology: Diagnostic imaging of child abuse, *Pediatrics* 105:1345, 2000.

Atabaki S: The medical evaluation of the sexually abused child: lessons from a decade of research, *Pediatrics* 104:178, 1999.

Botash A: Examination for sexual abuse in prepubertal children, *Pediatr Ann* 26:312, 1997.

Feldman K: Patterned abusive bruises of the buttocks and the pinnae, *Pediatrics* 90:633, 1992.

Frasier L: The pediatrician's role in child abuse interviewing, *Pediatr Ann* 26:306, 1997.

Hymel K, Jenny C: Child sexual abuse, *Pediatr Rev* 17:236, 1996.

Leder MR, Knight J, Emans J: Sexual abuse: management strategies and legal issues, *Contemp Pediatr* 18:77, 2001.

Leder MR, Knight J, Emans J: Sexual abuse: when to suspect it, how to assess for it, *Contemp Pediatr* 18:59, 2001.

Leventhal J et al: Fractures in young children, *Am J Dis Child* 147:87, 1993.

McClain P et al: Estimates of fatal child abuse and neglect: US 1979-1988, *Pediatrics* 91:338, 1993.

Sirotnak A: Testing sexually abused children for sexually transmitted diseases: who to test, when to test, and why, *Pediatr Ann* 23:370, 1994.

Sirotnak A, Krugman R: Physical abuse of children: an update, *Pediatr Rev* 15:394, 1994.

Stewart G et al: Trauma in infants less than 3 months of age, *Pediatr Emerg Care* 9:199, 1993.

COMMON BEHAVIORAL PROBLEMS

A. AGGRESSIVENESS

1. Children often express frustration through hostility, combativeness, or quarreling. Such behavior usually peaks around age 2 (the "terrible two's") as children kick, stomp, jump up and down, throw themselves on the floor, hold their breath, pull, struggle, throw objects, bite, hit, scream, and cry. Such behavior generally subsides as a child learns how to handle frustration in a more socially acceptable manner.

2. Some children continue these behaviors well beyond the preschool years. Children with the aggressive syndrome exhibit arguing, screaming, temper outbursts, loudness, bullying, threatening comments, cruelty to other people or to animals, fighting, stubbornness, irritability, or mood swings. Approximately 50% of all children with this syndrome show social impairments, psychiatric disorders, or criminal behavior as adults.

3. Hypotheses regarding why certain children are aggressive include a dysfunctional response to frustration (either innate or learned), learned behavior from role models (parents and peers), victimization (i.e., abuse), a biochemical imbalance, and genetic or anatomic "set-ups" such as chromosomal abnormalities or defects in certain areas of the brain.

4. A complete history is mandatory when evaluating a child with aggressive behavior. The aggressiveness must be delineated regarding types of behavior, onset, the settings and situations most likely to elicit aggressiveness, school performance (cognitive limitations), parental response and disciplining style, history of child abuse or substance abuse, persons from whom the child models his or her behavior, and environmental factors fostering the behavior. Children with learning problems or with ADD/ADHD are often aggressive in response to their own frustration and low self-esteem as well as in response to teasing by others.

5. Treatment modalities include parent management training (i.e., the parent learns to handle the child in a more effective manner), cognitive therapy in which the child is taught new coping skills, family therapy, individual counseling, and psychopharmacologic interventions. The earlier the intervention, the more likely it is to be successful. School personnel must also be enlisted in these interventions so that a more uniform approach is presented to the child; this is especially true if significant bullying or aggressive behaviors are occurring at school. Highly aggressive children and adolescents or those who threaten violence to others should be taken seriously. They should be managed by a psychiatrist or a psychologist, especially if drug therapy is used.

B. AUTISM

1. *Autism* is defined as a behavioral syndrome (part of the spectrum of pervasive developmental disorders) in which there is qualitative impairment in reciprocal social interactions, impaired verbal and nonverbal communication and imaginative activity, and a markedly restricted repertoire of activities and interests. To be classified as autistic, an individual must have been symptomatic since infancy or early childhood. The incidence is 5 to 15 per 10,000 children, with boys outnumbering girls 4 to 1.

2. In the area of impaired social interactions, autistic children can be either aloof and unreachable (even to their own family), unaware of others' feelings or social cues (either positive or negative), remote but reachable with a great deal of effort, or, on the opposite end of the scale, superficially social (pseudosocial).

3. In the area of impaired communication, autistic children have impaired comprehension and expression of language. They may use nonsense syllables or bits of words from a number of sources that when strung together make no sense. They may demonstrate echolalia, repeating favored expressions repeatedly or answering a question with the same question. They seem to have an inability to use nonverbal gestures when communicating and have no understanding of the nonverbal cues of others. They might speak in a monotone and fail to understand normal variations in speech, or alternatively, they may speak in a sing-song fashion.

4. In the area of restricted activities and interests, autistic children regularly display repetitive movements from which they are not easily dissuaded, such as rocking, head banging, staring at an object, singing the same song repeatedly, doing the same activity repeatedly, and twisting hair.

5. Autistic children have IQs that range from mental deficiency to superior intelligence. Although the mean IQ is low, at least 33% have IQs higher than 70, and 5% are "autistic savants" with unusual rote memory or visual skills.

6. Autistic children tend to have flat affects and respond little to either praise or punishment. However, some autistic children have very labile affects, even without a discernible external cause.

7. Autistic children might have either a very short or an abnormally long attention span. In the latter, an autistic child might stare at the same object for hours without evidence of boredom.

8. Many autistic children have sensorimotor abnormalities such as clumsiness, drooling, a heightened or absent response to loud noises, a fascination with certain visual stimuli, and insensitivity to pain.

9. Seizures are common.

10. The differential diagnosis includes autism and mental deficiency in low-functioning children, language disorder in younger high-functioning

children, and schizophrenia in high-functioning adolescents and young adults.

11. The history should be complete and should elicit the presence of the features and behaviors previously described.

12. The PE should be complete and focus on signs of any disease that might otherwise explain the child's symptoms. The examiner should attempt to engage the child in play or conversation to determine his or her responses firsthand.

13. An awake and sleep EEG is indicated; neuroimaging studies are not indicated because the presence of structural abnormalities does not alter the child's therapy.

14. Seizures should be treated with anticonvulsants; ADD/ADHD should be treated appropriately. No drug has demonstrated effectiveness in improving the symptoms of autism. Many autistic children have been overmedicated in an effort to control their behaviors, but such a practice often leads only to a somnolent child, not a treated one. Be sure to ask about any herbal or complementary modalities that parents may be using in an effort to treat autism.

15. The best treatment currently available is long-term special education. However, the ultimate prognosis is not predictable even when such education is offered continuously and is begun at an early age.

C. COLIC

1. *Colic* describes persistent crying in early infancy (i.e., the first 3 months of life). Although all infants cry, many cry for prolonged periods each day, adding another stressor to the parents' lives. Whether an anxious, stressed parent leads to a stressed infant or vice versa, the result is the same: an infant who is experiencing some level of distress and a parent whose self-esteem suffers because of an inability to console the infant.

2. By definition, infants with colic cry inconsolably more than 3 hours per day at least 3 days per week and for at least 3 weeks. This behavior peaks between ages 6 and 8 weeks and wanes by approximately 3 months. Using this definition, approximately 10% of all infants are colicky. Colic is unrelated to gender, feeding method, or birth weight but is more common in firstborns.

3. Colicky infants typically have bouts of intense crying in which their legs are drawn up to their abdomen; these bouts of crying are often associated with skin color changes and the passage of flatus. Such infants may be poor sleepers and hypersensitive to external stimuli.

4. The evaluation of a colicky infant should include prenatal, perinatal, medical, family, social, and developmental histories. The timing, duration, and type of symptoms that occur during a crying episode should be noted. The feeding history, in terms of overfeeding, underfeeding, or maladaptive feeding, is especially important. Ask questions regarding formula preparation, timing of feedings, behavior

COMMON BEHAVIORAL PROBLEMS

4

and interest during feedings, position during feedings, frequency of burping, amount taken and the time in which it is taken, and parental reaction to feeding.

5. The PE is usually normal, but a careful search for subtleties that might indicate other reasons for excessive crying (e.g., occult fractures or occult organ trauma) is indicated. Observing a feeding may produce valuable information unavailable from the history.

6. The differential diagnosis includes immaturity of the nervous system or the GI tract, food allergy, GER, difficult temperament, and parental anxiety.

7. Laboratory tests generally are not helpful.

8. Treatment of colic consists of supporting both the parent and infant. Counseling should be provided regarding coping strategies and techniques for calming or feeding the infant and for ameliorating environmental conditions that might exacerbate crying. Dietary manipulations, if used at all, should be held to a minimum; each formula change should be evaluated for 10 to 14 days before deciding on its role in colic. No drug for colic has been proven effective *and* safe.

D. CONVERSION REACTIONS

1. A conversion reaction is a mechanism by which an unconscious idea or wish is expressed in bodily terms and is experienced as a physical symptom that has specific but unconscious and symbolic meaning to the patient. Any bodily process can serve as the focus of the conversion symptom; the somatic symptoms of relatives or close friends can also serve this purpose. Although conversion symptoms have no organic basis, their perpetuation may result in biochemical or physiologic changes.

2. A complete history and PE are essential. A clue to the diagnosis of a conversion reaction is the observation that a patient's symptoms do not fit the classic physical, biochemical, or physiologic manifestations of the condition in question. In addition, the patient's reaction to the symptom(s) may be completely inappropriate.

3. Adolescents with conversion reactions are often egocentric, emotionally labile, dramatic, attention seeking, pseudomature, or sexually provocative. Such adolescents are often overprotected by their parents.

4. Individuals with conversion reactions experience both primary gain (the extent to which the symptom decreases the unpleasant emotion and symbolically communicates the forbidden but unconscious wish) and secondary gain (removal from a conflict or uncomfortable situation).

5. The precipitation of a conversion reaction may result from an acute or long-standing stress such as unresolved grief or anger.

6. The differential diagnosis includes hypochondriasis, malingering, psychosis, and psychophysiologic disorders. With hypochondriasis, the patient is filled with concern when the diagnosis of an organic disease

is entertained; a patient with a conversion reaction is indifferent. With malingering, patients *consciously* try to avoid unpleasant situations by attempting to feign illness and are aloof or hostile to physicians. In contrast, individuals with conversion symptoms are interested in seeing a medical provider. With psychosis, bizarre symptoms are reported (e.g., "my brain is shrinking"); plausible symptoms are reported by an individual with a conversion reaction.

7. With psychophysiologic disorders, the patient has an identifiable unpleasant affect that activates the autonomic neuroendocrine system and results in such signs as tachycardia, sweating, or hyperperistalsis. The patient experiences these signs as palpitations, sweating, or diarrhea. Thus the trigger is emotional and the expression of it is clearly organic. Sometimes it is difficult to distinguish between psycho-physiologic disorders and conversion reactions.

8. The treatment of conversion reactions may be carried out by the primary medical provider alone (if he or she has the expertise, time, and interest to do so) or together with a mental health professional. It is essential that the primary medical provider conduct the initial evaluation (history, PE, warranted laboratory tests) and discuss the results with the parent and patient. It is vitally important to state at the onset of the discussion that many physical problems have both physical and emotional causes and that each person's body has a certain physical way of reacting to stress. Such a concurrent physical-psychological approach better prepares all concerned for any eventual outcome. There are no magical drugs for the treatment of conversion reactions, and in an adolescent, drugs might do more harm than good. The best success follows repeated sessions in which the patient can talk about his or her feelings.

9. Treatment of psychophysiologic symptoms includes relaxation therapy, biofeedback, cognitive therapy (e.g., learning coping skills for times of stress), environmental manipulation (e.g., altering the environment, if possible, to reduce the individual's stress), and individual or family therapy.

E. DEPRESSION

1. The diagnosis of a major depressive illness requires five or more of the following symptoms: depressed mood, loss of interest or pleasure, significant weight loss or gain, failure to make expected weight gains for age, insomnia or hypersomnia, psychomotor agitation or retardation, fatigue or loss of energy, feelings of worthlessness or excessive inappropriate guilt, decreased concentration, and recurrent thoughts of death or suicide (especially with plans).

2. Almost 2% of preschool-age children and 5% of adolescents are clinically depressed; some investigators estimate that almost 10% of all children suffer some form of depression by age 12.

3. Most at risk for depression are children and adolescents who have one or more of the following factors:
   a. Depressed parents
   b. Divorced parents
   c. Hospitalized siblings
   d. ADD/ADHD
   e. Incarceration
   f. Mild mental retardation
   g. Lower socioeconomic status
   h. Chronic illness
   i. Pregnancy or children of their own

4. Although the classic presentation of depression is a sad, weepy child with psychomotor retardation, a depressed child may be hyperactive and aggressive. Many runaways run because they are depressed about their home situation, peer relationships, or school performance.

5. Children with depression generally look sad, have a negative self-image, lack a sense of fun in their lives, experience pathologic guilt, have few friends or social contacts, are poor students (either an acute onset or a long-standing problem), are chronically fatigued, and have sleep and appetite disturbances, psychomotor retardation, or morbid thoughts.

6. Depressed children have a sense of loss of an object, a person, or their own self-esteem; the last is especially true of children who fail at school or in peer relationships.

7. A meticulous history and PE are indicated for children and adolescents with depression. The history should highlight precipitating episodes, duration and progression of symptoms, family history of depression, school performance, peer relationships, and recent traumatic events in the family, neighborhood, school, or peer group. The parents should be asked about other unusual symptoms (e.g., new-onset clumsiness) that might point to an organic process. It is important to talk with the child about the depression and whether he or she has suicidal or homicidal thoughts. The PE should be thorough to rule out an organic process (e.g., a brain tumor) as the cause of the depressive symptoms.

8. Laboratory tests should be kept to a minimum; however, drug testing and a pregnancy test should be considered.

9. Serious depression, especially together with suicidal or homicidal ideation, requires inpatient hospitalization to protect both the child and others. Outpatient therapy is preferable for children and adolescents with mild to moderate depression. If the primary medical provider lacks the training, time, or expertise, he or she *must* consult with or refer the depressed child or adolescent to a mental health professional.

10. Psychotherapy has produced good results in treating child and adolescent depression. Also useful are tricyclic antidepressants, monoamine oxidase inhibitors, and lithium carbonate. Drug therapy should be carefully monitored because all of these drugs have potent

side effects. Before the initial drug administration, CBC, BUN, electrolytes, thyroid function tests, LFTs, creatinine, and an ECG should be obtained. Because the tricyclics (notably imipramine) have potent cardiac effects, parents and patients should be warned, and resting pulse rates should be monitored periodically. Plasma drug levels, BP, and ECGs (to look for prolongation of the QRS complex or PR interval) should be monitored.

F. EATING DISORDERS

1. General
a. Even young children are conscious of their body image; children as young as 8 to 10 years of age have reported dieting. The perception that children who are obese have fewer friends prompts most children to avoid obesity at all costs.
b. Chronic dieting is particularly common in girls whose body habitus does not match the ideal figure touted by the media. Methods to keep weight down include bulimia (self-induced vomiting) or the use of diet pills, diuretics, ipecac, or laxatives.
c. Children and adolescents who are chronic dieters often come from families in which weight and body appearance are of paramount importance. Because there is a genetic component to body habitus, children of parents who are (rightly or wrongly) concerned about their own weight see the parents' attitudes as models for their own.
d. Risk factors for eating disorders include female gender; menstrual irregularities (interplay of hormones and physical activity); compulsive athletic activity; chronic stress, especially that imposed by perfectionism; and compulsive stereotypic behaviors related to eating (e.g., chewing each bite 100 times).
2. Bulimia nervosa (BN)
a. BN is a syndrome in which there is binge eating (i.e., rapid ingestion of a large amount of food in a short period of time) at least two times a week and in association with the following:
   (1) Self-induced vomiting, severe food restriction, cathartic or laxative abuse, strenuous exercise, and weight fluctuations
   (2) Fear of loss of control regarding eating and purging behaviors
   (3) A heightened concern with body shape and weight accompanied by dissatisfaction, depression, and self-deprecation
   (4) No known physical abnormality to account for these findings
b. Binge eaters are often unaware of being hungry before eating but cannot stop once they start. It is an addiction. In contrast to those with anorexia nervosa, binge eaters are aware of their feelings.
3. Anorexia nervosa (AN)
a. AN is a syndrome that includes the following:
   (1) A marked fear of fatness, a disturbed perception of body size (even if underweight), and an obsessive desire to lose increasing amounts of weight

4

COMMON BEHAVIORAL PROBLEMS

      (2)   Self-starvation with marked weight loss (greater than 15% of body weight) or a failure to gain weight

      (3)   Amenorrhea (no bleeding for three or more menstrual cycles) and other physiologic signs associated with starvation

      (4)   Hyperactivity and sleep disturbances

      (5)   Bizarre attitudes regarding food and a denial of illness

      (6)   No known physical cause to account for these findings

b.   With AN, hunger may be diminished or increased. Patients with AN often are immature, fearful of growing up, perfectionistic, and lack control in their lives so that all of their efforts are placed on controlling their weight. Such patients are stunted physically, socially, and emotionally.

c.   AN and BN are more prevalent in affluent societies in which food is plentiful. Both conditions are more common in female patients (BN—F:M = 5:1; AN—F:M = 9:1), especially in those who have been sexually abused. At least 10% of individuals with AN engage in bulimic behavior, but those with BN do not usually have symptoms of AN. AN begins earlier (between ages 12 and 16) than BN (between ages 15 and 20).

d.   The initial presentation of AN is usually marked weight loss or amenorrhea. Pubertal progression may be arrested. In BN, any symptom might be the presenting one, and sometimes patients seek help on their own accord because they are frightened by their own lack of control.

e.   Findings vary by disease.

      (1)   With AN, cachexia is obvious. There may be hypothermia, bradycardia, and hypotension, all of which are signs of physiologic accommodation to starvation. Loss of scalp hair and the presence of lanugo and skin mottling are common. Bones may "stick out," and the thyroid might appear prominent because of the loss of subcutaneous tissue. Abrasions of the palate, buccal mucosa, and the dorsum of the hands indicate self-induced vomiting. Repeated vomiting may also lead to parotid or submandibular gland swelling. Pretibial and ankle edema, mitral valve prolapse, and cardiac arrhythmias may be present. Patients may be hyperactive, restless, and irritable or, alternatively, hypoactive, sluggish, and slow in thinking.

      (2)   With BN, the patient might be underweight, overweight, or of normal weight. Depending on the severity of illness, physical signs can be minimal or marked. If vomiting is a common occurrence, oral abrasions and salivary gland enlargement are present. Dehydration (with concurrent hypotension and tachycardia) may be present.

      (3)   With AN, laboratory findings include a low WBC, platelet count, and Hct (bone marrow suppression); hypokalemia; low serum Mg and P (late finding); and ECG abnormalities (sinus bradycardia, inverted T waves, A-V block, arrhythmias, low voltage).

Electrolytes are otherwise normal unless dehydration, vomiting, and laxative/diuretic abuse are present. X-ray studies may reveal osteoporosis, gastric distension, and a narrow cardiac silhouette. Cerebral atrophy might be evident on a CT scan.

(4) With BN there is often evidence of either hypochloremic alkalosis as a result of repeated vomiting or metabolic acidosis as a result of laxative abuse. Hypokalemia, hypomagnesemia, and hypocalcemia are common. The ECG shows evidence of hypokalemia (arrhythmias, U waves, depressed T waves). X-ray studies show gastric distension and evidence of paralytic ileus.

f. The differential diagnosis includes IBD, achalasia, thyroid disease, adrenal disease, and malignancy (CNS or otherwise).

g. Treatment

(1) With AN the patient is terrified of eating, and therefore a sympathetic but firm approach is useful. Expect setbacks; they will occur. Candidates for outpatient management include those whose disease has been in place for no more than 3 or 4 months; those who do not binge, purge, or use laxatives or diuretics; those whose families are relatively well functioning; and those who want help and seem eager to cooperate in their treatment. Indications for hospitalization are severe weight loss, outright starvation, drug use, CHF, metabolic derangements, abnormal ECG, or severe depression. All patients with AN must learn that their disease is controlling them and not the other way around. The disease is also in control of their family, social, and scholastic lives. Regular weigh-ins are mandatory; a weight gain of 0.2 kg/d is desired. Consultation and shared management of the patient with a mental health professional and a nutritionist are necessary.

(2) With BN, immediate hospitalization is needed if there are metabolic or cardiac derangements. The patient should be managed together with a mental health professional and a nutritionist.

4. Overeating

a. A proper diet and activity level are important both to prevent eating disorders and to treat individuals who are overweight or overfat. The term *overweight* refers to individuals whose weight exceeds 120% of that expected for height; this condition may be a function of both body frame and adiposity. Determining whether an individual is overfat is best accomplished by using the triceps skinfold measurement.

b. In the absence of serious physical disease, no child or adult loses weight unless he or she wants to. Therefore the first goal of therapy is to enlist the patient's (and family's) support and cooperation. The medical provider should remind parents that the obese child may be the object of teasing, embarrassment, and self-shame and that all family members need to maximally support the child while he or she is attempting to lose weight.

4

COMMON BEHAVIORAL PROBLEMS

    c.   The goal for an actively growing child may be weight maintenance rather than weight loss, especially if the child has only mild to moderate obesity. For each 20% increment in excess of ideal weight, 1 to 2 years of weight maintenance are required to achieve the ideal weight. The loss of 1 pound each month is a reasonable goal when weight loss is required in young children.

    d.   A food intake diary can be used to identify both problem foods to be eliminated or reduced and problem times during which eating in the absence of hunger is likely. Reduced fat intake and reduced total calorie intake are important. However, highly restrictive diets should be instituted only when there is a serious medical reason and in consultation with a dietician.

    e.   Increased activity is important but cannot be the only technique because excess caloric intake is at least as important a factor as insufficient exercise. Children and adolescents should be encouraged to exercise regularly and to spend less time in sedentary activities such as watching television or videos or using a computer.

    f.   Behavior modification is also important, especially when it focuses on the positive rather than on the negative. For example, the focus can be on the amount of weight that the child has lost, the child's adherence to the diet, or the child's increased physical activity rather than on the amount of weight regained or still left to lose, the child's failure to adhere to the diet, the child's reluctance to become more active, the predictions of the morbidities that the child will experience if he or she fails to lose weight, or the insinuation that the child lacks friends because of his or her weight. In some cases, the eating habits of the entire family should be changed for the health of everyone concerned.

G. FEARS/PHOBIAS/PANIC ATTACKS

1.   Young children have many fears, which vary by age.

a.   Infants are usually afraid of loud sounds, bright lights, sudden movements, strangers, animals, heights, and separation. All such stimuli represent a threat to the infant, who cannot make sense of them.

b.   In addition to many of the feared items from infancy, toddlers fear new situations, the dark, and water. Because toddlers do not yet understand size relationships, they cannot understand that they cannot be flushed down the toilet or go down a drain. Fear of the dark occurs because children of this age are beginning to develop an imagination, and who knows what lurks in the darkness?

c.   Children between 3 and 5 years of age commonly have night fears and nightmares (a combination of the darkness and imagination), a fear of death, a fear of separation, and phobias (see Point 3).

d.   Children between 6 and 12 years of age develop sophisticated fears about their local and universal world, such as school fears, a fear of new social situations, and a fear of harm to self and to loved ones.

e.   Some fears are universal (e.g., fear of falling).

2. Fears are usually transient and diminish over time. However, the following techniques are helpful:

a. Infants: Avoiding sudden changes in sound or lighting; permitting infants to *gradually* become accustomed to sounds, lights, or persons that will be a part of their lives; urging strangers not to overwhelm infants with kisses and hugs nor to pick them up against their will (to combat stranger anxiety); encouraging infants to be with adults other than the parents for brief periods of time (to combat separation anxiety); *gradually* introducing infants to a potentially scary situation (e.g., a dog) by demonstrating bravery with it (to decrease fear of new objects).

b. Toddlers: Using a night-light or transitional object to help soothe fear of the dark; encouraging water play to minimize fear of water; permitting toddlers to become accustomed to periods of separation from parents; encouraging toddlers to pretend they are the feared animal, person, or object.

c. Preschool-age children: Using a night-light and gentle bedtime routines to minimize night fears; avoiding stimulating activities or shows before bedtime; talking honestly about death when it comes up in conversation; preparing children for a separation from a parent by talking about it beforehand and even enlisting their help in planning the return.

d. School-age children: Communicating with children about their fears and wishes; empathizing with fear about school or peers; appropriately praising them for the good things they can do; minimizing parental pressure to excel academically or socially; acting out dreaded situations to practice different ways of coping; being open and honest about a fear of harm to self or loved ones.

3. Phobias are obsessive, persistent, and unrealistic fears that disrupt or distort normal behavior. They may be caused by an adverse experience with the feared object (e.g., being bitten by a dog), having a role model (usually a parent) who is markedly afraid of an object, or hearing about a bad outcome with the feared object.

a. Older children and adults generally recognize that their fear is irrational. However, even the thought of exposure to the feared object (e.g., an escalator) brings on anxiety.

b. A preoccupation with and anticipatory anxiety regarding the expectancy of an encounter with the feared object is present. Usually the child or adult tries to avoid these encounters by any means available.

c. Cajoling and ordering someone to encounter the phobic situation are of no use.

d. Common phobias in childhood and adolescence include animals, toilets (especially public ones), public speaking in class, and social situations.

e. Medications are of little use in simple phobias; psychotherapy, especially desensitization and imaging, is much more successful.

4

COMMON BEHAVIORAL PROBLEMS

4. Panic attacks differ from phobias. A panic attack is unexpected and not triggered by situations in which the person is the center of attention.

a. Panic attacks are accompanied by at least four of the following symptoms:
    (1) Shortness of breath or a sensation of smothering
    (2) Dizziness or faintness
    (3) Palpitations or a fast heart rate
    (4) Trembling or shaking
    (5) Sweating
    (6) Choking
    (7) Nausea or abdominal distress
    (8) Depersonalization or derealization
    (9) Numbness or tingling
    (10) Flushes or chills
    (11) Chest pain or discomfort
    (12) Fear of dying
    (13) Fear of going crazy or losing control

b. Diagnostic criteria for a panic attack are four attacks within a 4-week period or one or more attacks followed by 1 month of persistent fear that another will occur.

c. The most common panic reaction is in association with agoraphobia, which is the fear of being in places or situations from which escape might be difficult or embarrassing or in which help might not be available if another panic attack occurs.

d. Although tricyclic antidepressants are used in adults, their efficacy in children and adolescents is less established. Consultation with a mental health professional is needed.

H. GROWING PAINS

1. Growing pains are intermittent limb pains unrelated to the joints; such pains occur late in the day or at night and may be sufficiently intense to wake a child.

2. The pain is unaccompanied by fever, constitutional symptoms, redness, or swelling. If the pain is in the legs (as it usually is), the gait remains normal. Older children generally describe the pain as crampy, especially when it occurs in the muscles of the thighs or calves.

3. There can be symptom-free periods of weeks or months.

4. Growing pains are most likely to begin between ages 3 and 5 years or between ages 8 and 12 years. Girls are more likely to be affected than are boys.

5. The etiology of growing pains is unknown; everything from emotional causes, overuse, inadequate sleep, the weather, and other obscure reasons has been postulated. At one point, a discrepancy in the rate of bone growth vs. tendon/ligament/muscle growth (placing undue traction on these structures) was postulated, but there is no proof for this hypothesis.

6. The history is classic for pains that occur only at night, with a paucity of daytime symptoms and no limitation of activity. The PE and laboratory studies are normal.
7. The differential diagnosis includes hypermobility syndrome (joint laxity in very active children), intermittent nocturnal leg cramps, patellofemoral pain syndrome (patellar pain in adolescent girls), osteoid osteoma, and somatization syndrome in which the disability is out of proportion to physical findings.
8. There is a benign course; children do "grow out of it." Some investigators have reported that a leg muscle-stretching regimen may successfully decrease symptoms in children who are having frequent episodes.

I. HABITS

1. Many children have habits such as hair twisting or biting, nail chewing, pencil chewing, and nose picking. Although parents may be offended by such habits, they are not done intentionally and in most cases resolve. These habits often are associated with stress, deep concentration, or falling asleep.
2. Other children exhibit stereotypic behaviors such as body rocking, head rolling, or head banging. These behaviors may also be associated with stress or falling asleep. For most children the rhythmic nature of these stereotypies (with the possible exception of head banging) gives some pleasure and may help relieve tension. Head banging is common in temperamentally intense children and often responds to increased holding, rhythmic activation, or medication such as hydroxyzine. If the head banging leads to injury or if there are other behavioral problems, consultation with a mental health professional is necessary.
3. Habits are not to be confused with tic disorders (see Chapter 14), which are nonrhythmic and do not seem to give the child the degree of pleasure that habits give.
4. The prognosis for habit resolution is good as the child matures.

J. MUNCHAUSEN SYNDROME BY PROXY (POLLE SYNDROME)

1. Munchausen syndrome by proxy (Polle syndrome) is a condition in which parents or guardians purposely and needlessly subject their children, generally of age 6 years or under, to painful and sometimes life-threatening procedures and treatments. There is fabrication of illness and fraudulent reports of chronic or recurring symptoms.
2. The usual perpetrator is a mother, often with some medical background, who appears concerned about her child and is often friendly with and solicitous of the medical staff. She appears calm even when the child is ill. She is the "only one" for whom the child will comply and seldom leaves the bedside. There is often a pathologic symbiotic relationship between mother and child.

4

COMMON BEHAVIORAL PROBLEMS

3. Polle syndrome may represent the mother's efforts to keep her child completely dependent on her or may be an attempt to improve a poor relationship between the parents as they both focus on the child. Typically the father is aloof.
4. The child experiences unexplained, prolonged, or extraordinary illnesses, the signs and symptoms of which are witnessed only by the perpetrator and do not make sense clinically. Some children experience life-threatening events. These "illnesses" evoke extensive and painful diagnostic work-ups that are negative and treatments that are ineffective, costly, and sometimes painful.
5. Examples of Polle syndrome include placing the mother's or the child's own blood (from a disconnected IV line) in the child's vomitus, diaper, or ostomy bag; administering poisons, drugs, or abnormal electrolyte solutions; substituting maternal urine for the child's; injecting contaminated materials; and phlebotomizing the child by disconnecting an IV line (which leads to profound anemia).
6. On suspicion of this syndrome, all unnecessary tests and procedures must cease. In addition, the following should occur:
a. The child should be separated from the mother to see if symptoms occur in her absence.
b. A psychosocial history of the family should be obtained.
c. The temporal relationship between the mother's presence and the signs and symptoms of the child's illness should be verified.
d. Pertinent specimens, both when the mother has been present and when she has been absent, should be obtained.
e. Signs of the illness should be repeatedly checked and verified.
f. Video monitoring should be considered.
g. Psychiatric input is essential.
h. Child protective services may be needed.
7. The prognosis for children with Polle syndrome is guarded because there is significant morbidity and mortality. Children may experience long-term immaturity, separation problems, irritability, aggressiveness, and deception in presenting their own histories.

K. NIGHTMARES/NIGHT TERRORS/SLEEPWALKING/ NIGHT WAKING

1. Nightmares
a. Dreams occur in all persons and are the way the mind processes the events of the day or life. Dreams occur most often in the early morning hours before awakening.
b. Toddlers have nightmares about separation issues, preschool-age children about monsters (threat to well-being), and school-age children about dangers and death.
c. The occurrence of nightmares is strongly influenced by a child's viewing of violence either in real life (parental fighting at home, violence in the neighborhood) or in fantasy (television, videos, movies). Most young

children cannot distinguish fantasy from reality, thus making anything plausible in their minds.

d. Parents should be counseled to calm the child after a nightmare, to permit him or her to talk about it whenever ready to do so, and to limit the amount of violence that a child views either in real life or in fantasy.

e. If nightmares persist, worsen, or interfere with a child's normal functioning, consultation with a mental health professional is needed.

2. Night terrors

a. Night terrors represent an inherited disorder and affect 2% of all children.

b. Terrors consist of dream periods (10 to 30 minutes in duration) from which a child cannot be fully awakened. They generally begin during the first 90 minutes of sleep and can occur in clusters during the same night or on subsequent nights, sometimes for weeks. Even though the child's eyes are open, he or she does not appear to recognize familiar people or objects. The child is frightened and agitated and might scream or talk incoherently. The episode ends on its own in calm sleep. Afterward, the child has no memory of the event.

c. Parents should be counseled to refrain from waking a child in the midst of a night terror. They should speak to the child calmly and softly and should hold him or her if doing so does not cause further agitation. Parents should not shake or shout at the child in an effort to "snap him or her out of it"; such actions serve only to agitate the child further.

d. A cycle of night terrors can be interrupted by waking the child a half hour after he or she falls asleep each night.

e. Night terrors generally cease by 12 years of age.

3. Sleepwalking

a. Sleepwalking is an inherited disorder and is seen in 15% of all children.

b. The sleepwalker has open eyes but a blank look and has coordination that is clumsier than usual. He or she may make repeated stereotypic movements such as buttoning and unbuttoning clothes or turning the light on and off. The episode lasts 5 to 20 minutes, during which time he or she cannot be awakened.

c. Parents should be counseled to gently lead the child back to bed and to protect him or her from injury during the episode.

d. Children should be evaluated further if there are tonic-clonic movements during an episode, or if episodes last longer than 30 minutes, occur during the second half of the night, occur at least two times a week after attempting on seven occasions to awaken the child 15 minutes before the episode begins, or if there are daytime fears or a large amount of family stress.

4. Night waking/crying/feeding

a. Most young infants awaken at night for a feeding or for a brief episode of crying. By 6 months of age, 50% of children sleep from midnight to 5 AM without awakening; by 12 months of age, 90% do.

4

COMMON BEHAVIORAL PROBLEMS

b. Regardless of the reason, night waking is a problem when it is habitual, prolonged, more for the child's entertainment than for necessity, and interferes with parental functioning.

c. Some children have difficulty falling asleep and fight bedtime but sleep through the night once they are asleep; other children go to bed easily and sleep through the night but awaken early in the morning.

d. If a child is an early riser, he or she probably is getting sufficient sleep. Forcing the child to "sleep" more does not work. Techniques to help a child sleep later include delaying bedtime by an hour and eliminating a nap. Children who continue to rise early despite these measures may simply need less sleep. Older children can be instructed to remain in their room until 6 AM (or whatever time is comfortable for parents) and not call out or come into their parents' room until this time. Until this time, these children can play quietly or look at books. Infants should be kept in their crib until 6 AM (or whatever time is comfortable for parents) with a few favorite toys. If the infant cries, the parent can visit the crib but should not remove the infant from the crib. The lights should be off.

e. Different tactics must be tried if a child fights bedtime, repeatedly comes out of his or her room, or calls to a parent to come (or screams if preverbal).

    (1) Children should fall asleep in their own bed or crib. It is frightening for some children to fall asleep in one room and later awaken in another (dark) room. Being placed in the crib while awake or going to bed awake teaches children how to fall asleep on their own both at bedtime and during night waking episodes.

    (2) Many children are afraid of the darkness in their room. If so, a night-light helps. The parent should ensure that the night-light does not cast scary shadows, which can compound a child's fear.

    (3) Parents should attempt to make the hour or so before bedtime less stimulating so that children gradually unwind. Unfortunately, this situation often does not happen because parents who have been away all day use the middle to late evening hours to play actively with their children or to watch television or videos with them. Parents must adjust their habits if children are too "wound up" to go to bed.

    (4) Children's needs (e.g., bathroom visit, water, hugs) should be provided before they go to bed.

    (5) Children should be reminded that nighttime is when everyone sleeps—even most animals and birds. A child's fears should be acknowledged, but the parent needs to remain firm about the purpose of the night.

    (6) If a child is still in a crib, he or she needs to be left in it when he or she cries. The parent can visit at intervals and speak softly to the child, but removing the child from the crib should be avoided on most if not all visits.

(7) If an older child will not stay in bed, the parent can permit him or her to quietly play or look at books in his or her room. However, the child is to remain in his or her room and not disturb others. If the child comes out, he or she should be put back in his or her room without talking to him or her.

(8) Children who repeatedly leave their room and enter the parents' room are a challenge. Although some writers advise locking such children in their room (or locking the parents' door), others worry that such a drastic step creates even more fear and separation anxiety. Parents should insist on their need for rest just as such children insist on their need for continued companionship. Beneath the surface of this behavior may lurk psychological or psychosocial issues that need to be addressed and worked out for both the parents and the children. Severe problems may require the services of a mental health professional.

f. Many of the previous suggestions are also applicable to night wakers/criers/feeders. These suggestions include placing the infant in the crib awake, making brief visits to the crib to reassure the infant without providing entertainment and without removing him or her from the crib, and eliminating long daytime naps. Providing a cherished object as the infant's companion during sleep may be useful.

L. OBSESSIVE-COMPULSIVE DISORDER (OCD)

1. OCD is marked by repetitive actions that the patient knows are "crazy." The patient may insist on performing certain rituals, such as repetitive hand washing, before going out or going to bed, or uttering certain words before beginning a task.

2. Other patients with OCD have obsessive thoughts that often concern a fear of harm, illness, death, doing wrong or having done wrong, and contamination.

3. The hallmark of OCD is the patient's understanding that the repetitive actions are "crazy" and the repetitive thoughts irrational. This knowledge is in contrast to other psychological disorders in which the patient is unaware of his or her actions or thinks they are completely rational.

4. Treatment for OCD includes behavior modification, drug therapy, and psychotherapy. Helpful drugs are those that block serotonin reuptake. Other chemicals such as norepinephrine, dopamine, and certain hormones may also play a role in this disorder. PET scan studies of patients with OCD show increased metabolic activity in the frontal lobes and basal ganglia. Although drugs (clomipramine, fluoxetine, and fluvoxamine) have been used in OCD, other treatment modalities also may be useful. Treatment for OCD is best carried out by a mental health professional, usually a child psychiatrist or child psychologist.

4

COMMON BEHAVIORAL PROBLEMS

M. POSTTRAUMATIC STRESS DISORDER (PTSD)

1. PTSD is marked by a history of exposure to one or more adverse events that would be markedly distressing to nearly everyone, a trauma that is persistently reexperienced, a desire by the individual to avoid stimuli associated with the trauma, a psychological numbing of general responsiveness, and an increased state of arousal.

2. Initially, PTSD was described among adults who were exposed to combat, concentration camps, bombings, rapes, or other savage attacks. However, PTSD has been described among children, especially those who have been abused. Such children have difficulty sleeping, nightmares, anxiety, agitation, hypervigilance, and hypersensitivity.

3. PTSD in children can follow one episode or repeated episodes of abuse, sexual abuse, and witnessed violence, especially if inflicted on loved ones. The presence of more than one of these episodes increases the risk of PTSD, especially if the traumatic event was long-standing. There may be genetic, gender, perinatal, familial, and early childhood factors that are not yet clear.

4. Treatment for PTSD is best carried out by a mental health professional, usually a child psychiatrist or child psychologist.

N. "SPOILED" CHILD SYNDROME (UNDERCONTROLLING PARENTING)

1. A "spoiled" child is one who is excessively self-centered and immature. This condition results from parental failure to enforce age-appropriate limits. Such a child has a lack of consideration for others, a need to have his or her own way, difficulty in delaying gratification, and temper outbursts. A spoiled child is intrusive, obstructive, manipulative, and negative.

2. Children are not necessarily spoiled by doting parents if parents temper their indulgence with age-appropriate limits and clear expectations.

3. Behaviors not indicative of spoiling include the crying spells of young infants, the natural curiosity of toddlers, and the self-assertion of the toddler or 2-year-old who says "no."

4. Children who might be classified as spoiled include trained night feeders and trained night criers (both of whom are seeking attention), children with frequent temper tantrums, and children who demand everything they see in a store, demand constant amusement and attention, or demand that their every need be met immediately.

5. Parents should be counseled to provide age-appropriate limits for their children, to insist that their children cooperate with important rules, and not to give in to tantrums. Children should learn to entertain themselves, to wait their turn (or delay their gratification), and to respect their parents' rights and wishes. Success is more likely if parents and other adults in the home agree on these issues. Further evaluation may be needed if a child does not improve after several months of age-appropriate expectations and limit setting.

O. STUTTERING

1. The term *stuttering* is applied to the repetition of sounds and syllables. This condition occurs in 4% of the population at some time in their lives, and its prevalence is approximately 1% at any given time. There is a male predominance of 3.5:1.

2. Although there may be an inherited predisposition to stuttering, environmental stresses and a child's coping skills also play a role. The likelihood of repetitions and hesitations in speech is increased by anxieties, illness, fatigue, and attempts to speak rapidly. Although these incidents occur with all children, a subgroup never outgrow them. In such cases, the speech pattern worsens, which increases the child's frustration (and, hence, stress) and makes it more likely that the child will stutter. This is particularly true if a parent constantly corrects or shames the child. If left untreated, children who stutter may become reluctant to speak, socially disadvantaged, and eager to avoid situations in which they must communicate.

3. Because stuttering, especially in the early phase, is an intermittent condition, do not be fooled by a child who is reported to stutter but does not do so in your presence.

4. Children between 2 and 5 years of age normally experience hesitations and repetitions in their speech, especially when they are excited and try to talk rapidly. Signs that normal speech *dis*fluencies are becoming *dys*fluencies include part-word repetition (rather than an entire word); multiple rather than single repetitions of the problematic syllable; irregular, rapid, abrupt, or jerky repetitions; a high frequency of *dys*fluency in the speech; and marked facial grimaces while speaking.

5. When the items enumerated in Point 4 are accompanied by stress, frustration, a fear of failure or social situations, and high parental expectations or punitive attitudes, there is a high likelihood that a child will become a chronic stutterer.

6. Children who seem likely to become or who are already chronic stutterers should be referred to a speech pathologist to maximize the chances of a good outcome.

7. Children at low risk to become chronic stutterers are those who have speech *dis*fluencies without tension or embarrassment, very intermittent stuttering, stuttering that occurs most often when excited, and parents who are not overly concerned.

8. In such low-risk cases, a parent can help a stuttering child by encouraging conversation, speaking more slowly and in a more relaxed manner and thus acting as a role model, maintaining a calmness around the house to reduce any sense of hurry that a child might have, giving the child individual and calm attention each day so that the child does not need to compete with siblings, building self-esteem by appropriate praise and recognition of accomplishments, ceasing to correct or criticize speech, and ceasing to force the child to repeat what

he or she has said. These guidelines are to be followed by parents, siblings, and other adults with whom the child comes into contact. To avoid a self-fulfilling prophecy, a parent should not label the child as a stutterer. Interruptions of others' speech should be forbidden in the home, no matter who is speaking and who is interrupting.

P. SUBSTANCE ABUSE (also see Chapter 12)

1. Recognizing the adolescent substance abuser
   a. More than 50% of teenagers have some experience with an illicit drug by the time they are high-school seniors. The majority have some experience with alcohol and other drugs. Many experience adverse consequences, and some progress to dependence.
   b. Substance abuse is underidentified by health professionals. Adolescents rarely seek medical help for chemical dependency as a primary or secondary complaint. The clinical signs and symptoms of dependency are often not appreciated unless a thorough history with specific questions is conducted. The signs and symptoms of withdrawal are unusual in individuals who use drugs in an episodic fashion. However, acute overdoses and adverse reactions are a major problem. Every adolescent who seeks care, regardless of the chief complaint, should be asked about alcohol and drug abuse.
   c. Risk factors for substance abuse
      (1) Family history of alcoholism and other drug use
      (2) History of family conflict or verbal, physical, or sexual abuse
      (3) Antisocial behavior (conduct disorders), rebelliousness
      (4) Academic underachievement
      (5) Developmental disabilities
      (6) Low self-esteem, alienation
      (7) Friends who use drugs
      (8) Early first use of drugs
   d. The classic picture includes personality change, poor family interactions, deteriorating school performance, and withdrawal from positive environmental factors (e.g., church, sports, extracurricular activities).
   e. Often a progression from beer or wine and tobacco to liquor to marijuana to cocaine or heroin occurs. Multiple drug use is the rule for the majority of substance-abusing adolescents.
   f. Consider substance abuse in the adolescent who has any of the following:
      (1) Behavior that is unexplained or out of the ordinary (e.g., depression, emotional change)
      (2) Fatigue, nonspecific symptoms, or psychosomatic complaints
      (3) Injuries related to a fall, fighting, motor vehicle accident, or near-drowning
      (4) Attempted suicide. Half to two thirds of young individuals who commit suicide have a history of substance abuse (usually multiple drugs over many years)

g. Drug screening may be helpful but is only one part of a comprehensive clinical assessment. Indications include the following:
   (1) Psychiatric symptoms
   (2) Runaways, delinquents
   (3) Mental-status or performance changes
   (4) Acute-onset behavior changes
   (5) Recurrent accidents
   (6) Unexplained somatic symptoms
   (7) Monitoring of abstinence in a known abuser
2. General approach to the patient with an acute drug abuse reaction
a. Establish an airway and support ventilation (if indicated).
b. Start IV and support cardiac output, as needed.
c. If patient is obtunded, give IV or IM naloxone 2.0 mg/dose q2-3min × 3-4 prn.
d. Hypoglycemia should be considered in any adolescent with obtundation or seizures and confirmed whenever possible by rapid bedside testing. If hypoglycemia is suspected, treat immediately (before laboratory confirmation) with 50% dextrose, 25 to 50 ml IV.
e. Patients who remain obtunded or comatose despite these interventions should be examined for internal injuries, including head and neck trauma.
f. Extreme agitation in an acutely intoxicated adolescent can threaten patient safety and interfere with appropriate therapy. In this situation, IV diazepam 0.1 to 0.3 mg/kg or midazolam 0.05 to 0.1 mg/kg can be given.
g. Attempt gastric decontamination with activated charcoal 50 to 100 g bolus orally or via NG tube (see Chapter 12).
h. Initial evaluation
   (1) Talk with the patient, friends, parents, associates, and paramedics. Was the usage recreational, episodic, experimental, or habitual? Was the overuse intentional or accidental?
   (2) Complete PE: Closely monitor vital signs, check for associated trauma, and establish neurologic flow sheet and Glasgow Coma Scale score.
   (3) Check patient's clothing for clues to the ingested substance; identify any recovered substances; use the local poison control center.
i. Obtain urine and blood for toxicology screens; it is important to know what the screen does and does not detect.
j. Depending on the initial work-up, obtain CBC, ABGs, electrolytes, blood glucose, BUN, creatinine, LFTs, serum ketones, U/A, and ECG. Measure serum acetaminophen levels in all patients with intentional overdoses, regardless of drug class, to permit early treatment with NAC if serum levels are in the toxic range.
k. Need to evaluate for STDs and HIV infection (if indicated).
l. Provide reassurance and psychological support; restraint and force should be avoided if at all possible.

COMMON BEHAVIORAL PROBLEMS

4

m. Any patient with drug-induced cardiorespiratory compromise, seizures, or extreme agitation requires hospitalization.

3. Specific acute drug abuse reactions

a. Alcohol

(1) Clinical manifestations

(a) Mental status: Aggressive, belligerent behavior; impaired mental functioning; sleepiness; slurred speech.

(b) PE: Ataxia, incoordination, hypertension, hypotension, hypothermia, respiratory depression, arrhythmias, tachycardia. Look for signs of associated trauma and aspiration. CNS effects are proportional to the concentration of alcohol in the blood.

(c) Withdrawal syndrome: Anxiety, insomnia, irritability. Severe withdrawal (convulsions, delirium, hallucinations) is rarely seen in adolescents.

(2) Treatment: Supportive care and correction of metabolic abnormalities (hypoglycemia, acidosis). Hypoglycemia is a particular consideration for diabetic patients.

b. Anticholinergics: Atropine, belladonna, benztropine, henbane, jimsonweed seed, procyclidine, propantheline bromide, scopolamine, trihexyphenidyl

(1) Clinical manifestations

(a) Mental status: Amnesia, body image alterations, clouded sensorium, coma, confusion, convulsions, disorientation, drowsiness, restlessness, violent behavior, visual hallucinations

(b) PE: Dilated pupils, dry skin, flushed skin, hyperthermia, tachycardia, decreased bowel sounds, urinary retention

(c) Withdrawal syndrome: GI and musculoskeletal symptoms

(2) Treatment: Supportive care

c. Cannabis group: Marijuana, hashish, THC, hash oil, sinsemilla

(1) Clinical manifestations

(a) Mental status: Anxiety and anorexia, then increased appetite, confusion, delirium, depersonalization, dreamlike state, fantasy state, euphoria, excitement, hallucinations, panic reactions, paranoia, time-space distortions.

(b) PE: Ataxia, dry hacking cough, injected conjunctivae, laryngitis, pharyngitis, postural hypotension, tachycardia.

(c) Withdrawal syndrome: Anorexia, anxiety, depression, insomnia, irritability, nausea, restlessness. Acute withdrawal reactions are rare.

(2) Treatment: No specific treatment is indicated. Diazepam may be used for severe anxiety or panic reactions.

d. CNS depressants ("downers"): Barbiturates, benzodiazepines, chloral hydrate, glutethimide, meprobamate, methaqualone, methyprylon, paraldehyde, and others

(1) Clinical manifestations
    (a) Mental status: Coma, confusion, delirium, disorientation, drowsiness, slurred speech
    (b) PE: Ataxia, convulsions (methaqualone), hyporeflexia, hypotension, hypothermia, hypotonia, incoordination, nystagmus, pulmonary edema, respiratory depression
    (c) Withdrawal syndrome: Agitation, anxiety, arrhythmias, convulsions, delirium, disorientation, fever, hallucinations, hyperreflexia, hypertension, insomnia, irritability, sweating, tremors, weakness, cardiovascular collapse
(2) Treatment: Supportive care, maintenance of airway and ventilation, BP support, alkalinization of urine

Note: Acute withdrawal can be life threatening. The drug dosage may need to be tapered, or phenobarbital or pentobarbital may need to be substituted and the dosage gradually decreased.

e. CNS stimulants ("uppers"): Amphetamine, amphetamine-like antiobesity drugs, Bromo-DMA, caffeine, dextroamphetamine, dimethylpropione, MDA, methylphenidate, phenmetrazine, phenylpropanolamine
  (1) Clinical manifestations
    (a) Mental status: Agitation, anxiety, coma, decreased appetite, decreased sleep, delirium, hallucinations, hyperactivity, hyperacute or confused sensorium, impulsivity, paranoid ideation, restlessness
    (b) PE: Arrhythmias, blurred vision, convulsions, dilated pupils, dry mouth, hyperreflexia, hypertension, hyperthermia, hyperventilation, sweating, tachycardia, tremors
    (c) Withdrawal syndrome: Abdominal pain, anxiety, chills, depression, exhaustion, muscle aches, sleep disturbances, tremors, voracious appetite
  (2) Treatment: Supportive care; "talking the patient down"; haloperidol for aggressiveness, agitation, and hallucinations; diazepam for control of agitation and seizures; forced diuresis. After patient has "crashed," a mild antidepressant (e.g., nortriptyline) can be given.

f. Cocaine
  (1) Clinical manifestations
    (a) Mental status (see CNS stimulants): Agitation, coma, hallucinations, increased concentration, mood elevation, panic, paranoia, psychosis.
    (b) PE: Arrhythmia, convulsions, diaphoresis, dilated pupils, epistaxis, hyperpnea, hyperreflexia, hypertension, hyperthermia, myocardial infarction, myoclonus, respiratory failure, sweating, stroke, tachycardia, tremor. Epiglottitis has been reported secondary to smoking cocaine.
    (c) Withdrawal syndrome: Depression, irritability.

4

COMMON BEHAVIORAL PROBLEMS

      (2) Treatment: Support of ventilation, IV propranolol or nitroprusside for cardiotoxicity, IM haloperidol 2 to 5 mg q1-8h prn (max 10 to 30 mg) until psychotic behavior improves; IV diazepam for seizures; fans/evaporative cooling for hyperthermia. Observation in a coronary care unit may be indicated for serial monitoring of ECGs and cardiac enzymes.

  g. Hallucinogens: DMT, LSD, MDA, mescaline, morning glory seeds, nutmeg, psilocybin
     (1) Clinical manifestations
       (a) Mental status: Amnesia, anxiety, confusion, convulsions, delusions, depersonalization, depression, drooling, euphoria, hallucinations, hyperactivity, inappropriate affect, mutism, panic, paranoia, psychosis, synesthesias, time and visual distortions, violent behavior
       (b) PE: Ataxia, dilated pupils, flushed face, hyperreflexia, hypertension, hyperthermia, nystagmus, tachycardia, tremors
       (c) Withdrawal syndrome: None
     (2) Treatment: Supportive care; psychological support ("talking the patient down" in quiet area); mild tranquilizer for extreme anxiety; IM haloperidol for severe agitation; IV diazepam for sedation; fans/evaporative cooling for hyperthermia. *Avoid antipsychotic drugs.*

  h. Opioids: Codeine, fentanyl, heroin, hydromorphone, meperidine, methadone, morphine, opium, pentazocine, propoxyphene, sufentanil
     (1) Clinical manifestations
       (a) Mental status: Coma, euphoria, stupor
       (b) PE: Constricted pupils, convulsions, hyporeflexia, hypotension, hypothermia, hypoventilation, pulmonary edema
       (c) Withdrawal syndrome: Abdominal cramps, anxiety, diarrhea, dilated pupils, gooseflesh, lacrimation, muscle jerks, tachycardia, tremulousness, vomiting, yawning
     (2) Treatment: IV or IM naloxone 2.0 mg/dose q2-3min × 3-4 prn; positive end-expiratory pressure for pulmonary edema. Clonidine can be used to minimize the discomfort of opiate detoxification.

  i. Phencyclidine
     (1) Clinical manifestations
       (a) Mental status: Amnesia, anxiety, catalepsy, coma, convulsions, excitement, hallucinations, hyperactivity, impulsiveness, mutism, open-eyed coma, self-destructive or violent behavior, staring spells, stupor, psychosis.
       (b) PE: Ataxia, diaphoresis, drooling, arrhythmia, flushing, hypertension, hyperthermia, hyporeflexia, myoclonus, nystagmus, tachycardia. Always evaluate the patient carefully for signs of trauma.
       (c) Withdrawal syndrome: None.

    (2) Treatment: Psychological support; observation in a quiet area (do not "talk down"); IV diazepam for sedation and convulsions; haloperidol 2 to 5 mg/dose q1-8h prn (max 10 to 30 mg) for severe agitation until improved; forced diuresis; protection from harm; propranolol for arrhythmias. Admission for psychological evaluation often is required.

j. Volatile substances: Aliphatic and aromatic hydrocarbons (gasoline, butane, propane, toluene, benzene, xylene), halogenated hydrocarbons (freons, halothane, trichloroethylene), aliphatic nitrites (amyl, *m*-butyl, and isobutyl nitrite), nitrous oxide (see Chapter 12 for a discussion of hydrocarbon pneumonitis)

    Inhalants are often the first consciousness-altering substances used by children. They are popular because of the rapid onset of action, the quality and pattern of the "high," low cost, easy availability, convenient packaging, and the fact that possession is not illegal in most states.

    (1) Clinical manifestations

        (a) Mental status: Confusion, disorientation, dizziness, euphoria, hallucinations, headache, impulsive behavior, psychosis, somnolence, stupor

        (b) PE: Arrhythmias, ataxia, convulsions, coughing, drooling, hyporeflexia, hypotension, peripheral neuropathy, sneezing, tachycardia

        (c) Withdrawal syndrome: None

Note: Some volatile agents may be associated with acute renal failure, DIC, hemolytic anemia, hypokalemia, methemoglobinemia, and renal tubular acidosis.

    (2) Treatment: Support, maintenance of adequate ventilation

k. Occult cocaine exposure

    (1) Among young children who come to urban emergency rooms, 3% to 5% have evidence of unsuspected passive cocaine exposure on a urine toxicology screen.

    (2) Exposure may be secondary to accidental ingestion, passive inhalation of freebase cocaine vapors, or intentional administration.

    (3) Cocaine intoxication should be considered in the evaluation of infants and young children with new-onset generalized or focal seizures, arrhythmias, or hypertension.

Q. SUICIDE ATTEMPTS

1. Suicide ranks as one of the leading causes of death in adolescents.

2. Suicide attempts (parasuicides) outnumber completed suicides by 50:1 to 200:1. The male-female suicide ratio is 3:1.

3. Both suicides and suicide attempts can increase after media reports of a real or fictional suicide victim. Clustering of suicides has occurred in certain communities.

4

COMMON BEHAVIORAL PROBLEMS

4. Completed suicide attempts are more common in male patients; violent measures such as firearms are often used.

5. Suicide attempts are more common in females; ingestions (self-poisoning) are often used.

6. Adolescents with chronic conditions can attempt suicide by self-poisoning through overdoses of their own medications, OTC medications that they are using, or by neglecting to take necessary medications (e.g., insulin).

7. Although an acute event may trigger the suicide act, the following predisposing factors are common:

a. Parental loss, broken home, or other interpersonal loss

b. Depression (tearfulness vs. a raging "acting-out") or other major psychiatric disorder

c. Feelings of anger, rejection, social isolation, or expendability

d. Few friends/social supports

e. Failure socially or scholastically

f. Association with other troubled youths

g. Previous history of suicide gestures (very important!), especially if high potential of success

h. Physical illness

i. History of substance abuse, pregnancy, STD, or psychosocial problems not previously listed

j. History of prior abuse

k. Family history of alcoholism, psychiatric disorder, or suicide

l. Exposure to suicide (personally or via the media, especially if the person who took his or her life was admired)

m. Easy availability of firearms or drugs in the home

8. When a child or adolescent demonstrates suicidal behavior, take it very seriously!

9. Important historical information includes the following:

a. Method used (e.g., type and number of pills, weapon and time used)

b. Whether the victim announced the act

c. Whether victim expresses a wish to die, feels hopeless, has a desire to try again (determine if patient has access to method and a plan), or shows remorse about the attempt

d. The precipitating incident before the present attempt

e. Whether the patient has a history of suicide attempts, depression, aggression/acting out, drug/alcohol abuse, psychiatric illness

f. Whether there is a family history of psychiatric illness or suicide

g. The patient's interpersonal relationships with parents, siblings, and friends

h. The patient's functioning in school

i. The patient's social support systems

10. A complete PE is mandatory, with particular emphasis on skin (needle tracks, marks of inflicted injury), neurologic, and psychiatric assessments.

11. Different treatments are necessary depending on the method of the attempt (e.g., suturing lacerations, gastric decontamination for ingestions, hyperbaric O_2 for CO poisoning).

12. An adolescent who has distanced himself or herself from family and friends, disposed of valued possessions, talked about death or suicide, expressed hopelessness about the future, left a suicide note, or has attempted violent suicide (firearms, hanging, CO exposure) is at extremely high risk for a successful suicide in the future. Individual and family psychotherapy is necessary.

13. Involvement by social work and psychiatry as soon as possible is mandatory.

14. Interviews with family members should be conducted.

15. Admission to either a medical or a psychiatric unit is advisable. If the adolescent shows a high lethality index, keep him or her in a safe and secure environment under one-to-one supervision. If the adolescent refuses voluntary admission, initiate procedures for involuntary hospitalization.

R. TEMPER TANTRUMS

1. Approximately 14% of 1-year-olds, 20% of 2- to 3-year-olds, and 11% of 4-year-olds have temper tantrums. In addition, 5% of 5- to 17-year-olds are reported to have an explosive temper.

2. Tantrums occur when emotions exceed a child's ability to control them, which leads to frustration, rage, or fear. Therefore, preverbal toddlers have the most difficulty expressing their emotions except through tantrums. Tantrums decrease once a child is better able to express his or her feelings and is better equipped to understand spoken parental commands and explanations.

3. In trying to master the environment and the self, children experience a blow to their self-image after a tantrum. This is especially true when children lose a battle of wills with their parents. Parents should understand that their handling of the tantrum partly determines the occurrence of future tantrums.

4. Parents should be counseled to use distraction when frustration begins to rise, to present acceptable choices, and to minimize the need to say "no" by keeping children away from potentially explosive situations or tempting environments. Parents should pick their battles carefully. They should not leave younger children alone in the midst of a tantrum and should hold them if that will quickly calm them. Older children should be instructed to go to their room until they calm down. Parents should remain calm, not label the child as "bad," and permit the child to start afresh when the tantrum is over.

5. Many tantrums respond better to being ignored than to any direct intervention. Children have tantrums to attract attention; when the tantrums fail to produce the desired effect, many children abandon them. In addition, positive reinforcement works well. Giving the child

attention when he or she is doing something right (as opposed to when he or she is doing something wrong) is much more effective than giving belittling or negative messages.

6. Problem tantrums may suggest serious underlying problems in the child or parent and include the following:
a. Age less than 1 year or older than 4 years
b. Tantrums that occur in school
c. Tantrums associated with aggression or violent behavior
d. Associated disturbances in eating, sleep, play, and other activities
e. Flirtatiousness or heightened modesty (R/O sexual abuse)
f. Parental sadness, anger, or helplessness about the situation
g. Parental inability to say positive things about the child

7. Factors contributing to problem tantrums include the following:
a. Parental overcontrol (thwarting a child's autonomy)
b. Parental undercontrol (frightening lack of limits)
c. Parental depression or lack of support
d. Parental substance abuse
e. Domestic violence toward adults or children
f. Temperament mismatch between parent and child
g. Dysfunctional family
h. Unrealistic environmental restrictions
i. Child with poor adaptability or an intense temperament
j. Child with language defects or learning problems
k. Child with a hearing loss
l. Child with ADD/ADHD
m. Child under the influence of medications
n. Child seeking secondary gain from an unresponsive environment

Note: Points *h* through *n* increase the likelihood that the child will be frustrated and act out of frustration.

8. Suggested therapies for problem tantrums include those mentioned in Points 4 and 5, behavior modification, time-outs, and extinction techniques. These therapies should be provided with a large dose of positive reinforcement and with empathy directed toward both the parent and child. The parent must understand that not all battles will be eliminated; the parent must also come to terms with the child's degree of development (what can be expected of him or her and what cannot). In severe cases, referral to a mental health professional is necessary.

S. THUMB-SUCKING

1. The sucking reflex is one of the strongest reflexes that infants have; it is normal for them to suck their thumbs.
2. Many children suck their thumbs well beyond infancy. For some it is simply a habit, whereas for others it is evidence of a behavioral problem.
3. Thumb-sucking occurs in 45% of 3- to 4½-year-olds, 14% of 5-year-olds, and 6% of 6-year-olds. There is a female predominance.

4. Although thumb-sucking can cause dental malocclusion if it persists into middle childhood, it does not do so in infancy or early childhood. After 6 years of age, thumb-sucking has been associated with flared maxillary incisors, crossbite, open bite, an alteration in the shape of the roof of the mouth, a gap between the upper front teeth, and a flared upper lip.
5. Several aversive methods have been touted as treatments for thumb-sucking but have limited success and are cruel. Placing bitter substances on the thumb to make it less likely that the child will want to put the thumb in his or her mouth works only when the substance is on the thumb. This method cannot be used 24 hours a day, which limits its success. Applying an elastic bandage to the arm (middle arm to forearm) so that there is resistance when the child bends the arm is also not recommended as it can be done only when the child does not need his or her arms to play, write, or perform other activities. Another technique involves insisting that the child suck all 10 fingers sequentially for an equal amount of time whenever the thumb is sucked, but this technique works only when the child is monitored for compliance. A dental appliance can be used for older children who are experiencing malocclusion and for whom other techniques have been unsuccessful. Hypnosis is useful in motivated older children.
6. Most children stop sucking their thumbs when motivated to do so. Motivation often comes from peer pressure rather than from any aversive technique that a parent has tried. Children who suck their thumbs are less popular than other children, which makes the habit less appealing to a child interested in having friends.

T. VULNERABILITY

1. Early child health problems might significantly affect parental perceptions of child health. Such perceptions can linger and affect subsequent child development.
2. In the vulnerable child syndrome as originally described, severe health problems in infancy leave certain parents with a sense that their child is uniquely vulnerable for future serious medical conditions and needs added protection. Such beliefs might lead to a pathologic parent-child relationship.
3. Vulnerable child syndrome has been described after a number of conditions, including a complicated pregnancy, prematurity, birth problems, neonatal jaundice, meningitis, cancer, and even the diagnosis of an innocent heart murmur, which is a so-called nondisease.
4. The syndrome has been associated with the development of separation and discipline problems, overprotectiveness, parental obsessions about the child's health, sleep disturbances, hyperactivity (out-of-control child), and an increased use of medical services.
5. Because the parent believes that the child received a reprieve from death, there is a fear that the child will not be as fortunate the next

COMMON BEHAVIORAL PROBLEMS

time. The parent's impression of the child's health is easily picked up by the child, which leads the child to have a distorted image of his or her own health.

6. A patient approach to the parent and child is necessary. It may take several visits to learn about the "near brush with death" (real or imagined) in the child or the parent or about the death of another child, relative, or fetus.

7. The parent should be reassured that his or her child is healthy. The medical provider can empathize with parental concerns but can also point out that the parents' reactions contribute to the child's behavior. Parents can learn to set age-appropriate limits and sleeping practices for the child, reduce overprotectiveness, and see illnesses more realistically.

8. A psychological or psychiatric referral is needed if such counseling is not effective, if the parent is depressed or seriously anxious, or if the child is out of control.

9. For most families, the prognosis is good.

10. To prevent the development or persistence of the vulnerable child syndrome, medical providers should avoid hyperbole when describing either a child's condition or any "heroic" efforts to treat him or her.

U. BIBLIOGRAPHY

Aggressiveness
Alessi N, Wittekindt J: Childhood aggressive behavior, *Pediatr Ann* 18:94, 1989.
Gottlieb S, Friedman S: Conduct disorders in children and adolescents, *Pediatr Rev* 12:218, 1991.
Strasburger V, Grossman D: How many more columbines? What can pediatricians do about school and media violence? *Pediatr Ann* 30:87, 2001.

Autism
Bauer S: Autism and the pervasive developmental disorders. I. *Pediatr Rev* 16:130, 1995.
Bauer S: Autism and the pervasive developmental disorders. II. *Pediatr Rev* 16:130, 1995.

Colic and Crying
Fleisher D: Coping with colic, *Contemp Pediatr* 15:144, 1998.
Garrison M, Christakis D: A systematic review of treatments for infant colic, *Pediatrics* 106:184, 2000.

Conversion Reactions/Psychosomatic Disease
Hodgman C: Conversion and somatization in pediatrics, *Pediatr Rev* 16:29, 1995.
Poikolainen K, Kanerva R, Lonnqvist J: Life events and other risk factors for somatic symptoms in adolescence, *Pediatrics* 96:59, 1995.

Depression
Brown-Jones L, Orr D: Enlisting parents as allies against depression, *Contemp Pediatr* 13:67, 1996.
Sherry S, Jellinek M: The many guises of depression, *Contemp Pediatr* 13:63, 1996.
Shoaf T, Emslie G, Mayes T: Childhood depression—diagnosis and treatment strategies in general pediatrics, *Pediatr Ann* 30:130, 2001.
Zwaigenbaum L, Szatmari P, Boyle M et al: Highly somatizing young adolescents and the risk of depression, *Pediatrics* 103:1203, 1999.

Eating Disorders
Bulimia/Anorexia Nervosa
Harper G: Eating disorders in adolescents, *Pediatr Rev* 15:72, 1994.

4

Dieting/Obesity
Kreipe R, Dukarm C: Eating disorders in adolescents and older children, *Pediatr Rev* 20:410, 1999.

Fears/Phobias/Anxiety
Schowalter J: Fears and phobias, *Pediatr Rev* 15:384, 1994.

Shrand J, Jellinek M: Psychopharmacology in mood and anxiety disorders, *Contemp Pediatr* 12:21, 1995.

Williams T, Hodgman C: Medication for the management of anxiety disorders in children and adolescents, *Pediatr Ann* 30:146, 2001.

Growing Pains
Sizer I: Are those limb pains "growing" pains? *Contemp Pediatr* 6:143, 1989.

Munchausen Syndrome by Proxy (Polle Syndrome)
Donald T, Jureidini J: Munchausen syndrome by proxy, *Arch Pediatr Adolesc Med* 150:753, 1996.

Libow J: Child and adolescent illness falsification, *Pediatrics* 105:336, 2000.

Southall D, Plunkett M, Banks M et al: Covert video recordings of life-threatening child abuse, *Pediatrics* 100:735, 1997.

Nightmares/Night Terrors/Sleepwalking/Night Waking
Blader J, Koplewicz H, Abikoff H et al: Sleep problems of elementary school children, *Arch Pediatr Adolesc Med* 151:473, 1997.

Blum N, Carey W: Sleep problems among infants and young children, *Pediatr Rev* 17:87, 1996.

Laberge L, Tremblay R, Vitaro F et al: Development of parasomnias from childhood to early adolescence, *Pediatrics* 106:67, 2000.

Wise M: Parasomnias in children, *Pediatr Ann* 26:427, 1997.

Obsessive-Compulsive Disorder
Leonard H, Freeman J, Garcia A et al: Obsessive-compulsive disorder and related conditions, *Pediatr Ann* 30:154, 2001.

Sivedo S, Rapoport J: Bad news and good news about obsessive-compulsive disorder, *Contemp Pediatr* 6:130, 1989.

Post-Traumatic Stress Disorder
DeVries A, Kassam-Adams N, Cnaan A et al: Looking beyond the physical—posttraumatic stress disorder in children and parents after pediatric traffic injury, *Pediatrics* 104:1293, 1999.

McCloskey L, Southwick K: Psychosocial problems in refugee children exposed to war, *Pediatrics* 97:394, 1996.

Stuber M, Kazak A, Meeske K et al: Predictors of posttraumatic stress symptoms in childhood cancer survivors, *Pediatrics* 100:958, 1997.

Spoiled Child Syndrome
McIntosh B: Spoiled child syndrome, *Pediatrics* 83:108, 1989.

Schmitt B: Preventing spoiled children, *Contemp Pediatr* 9:44, 1992.

Stuttering
Guitar B: Is it stuttering or just normal language development? *Contemp Pediatr* 5:109, 1988.

Guitar B: Stuttering and stammering, *Pediatr Rev* 7:163, 1985.

Substance Abuse
American Academy of Pediatrics: A guide to acute medical management of intoxication in adolescents, *Adolesc Health Update* 6:1, 1994.

Suicide Attempts
AAP Committee on Adolescence, Suicide and suicide attempts in adolescents, *Pediatrics* 105:871, 2000.

Brent D: Depression and suicide in children and adolescents, *Pediatr Rev* 14:380, 1993.

Kjelsberg E, Winther M, Dahl AA: Overdose deaths in young substance abusers: accidents or hidden suicides, *Acta Psychiatr Scand* 91:236, 1995.

Woods E, Lin Y, Middleman A et al: The association of suicide attempts in adolescence, *Pediatrics* 99:791, 1997.

COMMON BEHAVIORAL PROBLEMS

Temper Tantrums

Needleman R et al: Temper tantrums: when to worry, *Contemp Pediatr* 6:12, 1989.

Thumb-Sucking

Friman F, McPherson KM, Warzak WJ et al: Influence of thumb-sucking on peer social acceptance in first-grade children, *Pediatrics* 91:784, 1993.

Heitlen S: Curing thumb-sucking by the book, *Contemp Pediatr* 5:95, 1988.

Vulnerability

Leslie L, Boyce WT: The vulnerable child, *Pediatr Rev* 17:323, 1996.

DERMATOLOGY

See Fig. 5-1 for a pattern diagnosis.

SPECIFIC CONDITIONS
A. ACNE

1. Acne results from obstruction of the pilosebaceous unit, enlargement of sebaceous glands, increased sebum production, proliferation of *Propionibacterium acnes,* and secondary inflammatory changes. Acne appears most commonly on the patient's face, chest, and back. Acne usually begins 1 to 2 years before the onset of puberty. In girls, early development of comedonal acne in the preteen years is predictive of later, more severe disease. A history of severe acne in a first-degree relative is a marker for potentially serious disease.
2. Lesions progress from closed comedones (whiteheads) to open comedones (blackheads) or pustules to inflammatory papules to nodules and cysts to atrophic and hypertrophic scars.
3. History: Other medical problems; medications; treatments tried; cosmetics, hair greases; occupational exposures (i.e., grease); menstrual history and hormonal therapy.
4. PE: Assess distribution, morphology, and severity of lesions. The course can be monitored by using a grading system or by obtaining serial photographs.
5. Laboratory evaluation: Not usually helpful. Endocrine evaluation is indicated for patients with signs of androgen excess (hirsutism, irregular menses) to R/O adrenal or ovarian disease and severe or persistent disease. Girls with nodulocystic disease may be at increased risk for polycystic ovarian disease.

Note: Acneiform eruption may occur secondary to systemic steroid therapy, anticonvulsants, INH, androgens. In drug-induced acne, the lesions tend to be uniform (closed comedones only). Closed comedones on the forehead and temples may occur secondary to the use of oil-based hair and scalp preparations.

6. Treatment needs to be individualized depending on the patient's gender, severity of disease, type and distribution of lesions, and therapeutic response.
a. Mild to moderate comedonal or inflammatory acne
   (1) Benzoyl peroxide
      (a) Begin by applying a thin coat of 2.5% to 5.0% gel or lotion qod, qd, or bid to all acne-prone areas. Titrate the concentration against therapeutic and irritant effects.
      (b) May initially cause dryness, redness, and peeling of the skin.

5

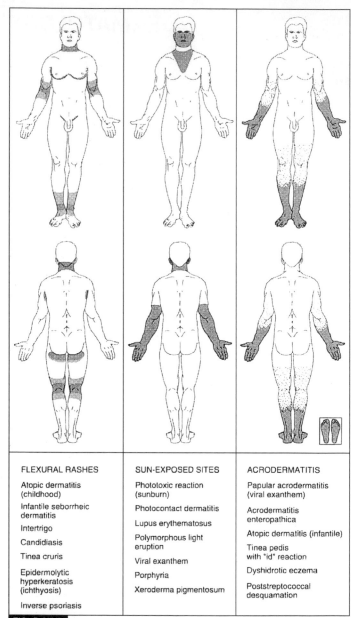

FLEXURAL RASHES	SUN-EXPOSED SITES	ACRODERMATITIS
Atopic dermatitis (childhood)	Phototoxic reaction (sunburn)	Papular acrodermatitis (viral exanthem)
Infantile seborrheic dermatitis	Photocontact dermatitis	Acrodermatitis enteropathica
Intertrigo	Lupus erythematosus	Atopic dermatitis (infantile)
Candidiasis	Polymorphous light eruption	Tinea pedis with "id" reaction
Tinea cruris	Viral exanthem	Dyshidrotic eczema
Epidermolytic hyperkeratosis (ichthyosis)	Porphyria	Poststreptococcal desquamation
Inverse psoriasis	Xeroderma pigmentosum	

FIG. 5-1

Pattern distribution of dermatologic conditions. (From Cohen B: *Atlas of pediatric dermatology,* London, 1993, Mosby.)

5

DERMATOLOGY

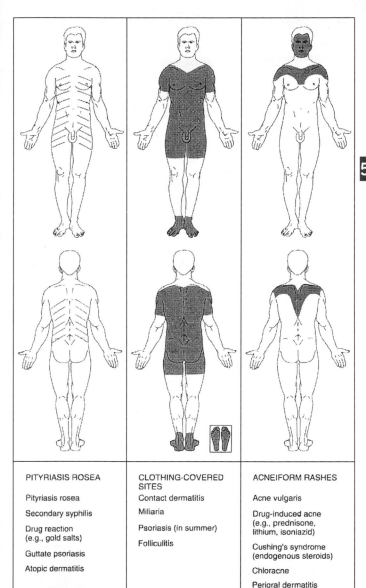

PITYRIASIS ROSEA	CLOTHING-COVERED SITES	ACNEIFORM RASHES
Pityriasis rosea	Contact dermatitis	Acne vulgaris
Secondary syphilis	Miliaria	Drug-induced acne (e.g., prednisone, lithium, isoniazid)
Drug reaction (e.g., gold salts)	Psoriasis (in summer)	Cushing's syndrome (endogenous steroids)
Guttate psoriasis	Folliculitis	Chloracne
Atopic dermatitis		Perioral dermatitis

FIG. 5-1—cont'd

For legend see opposite page.

    (2) Retinoids
       (a) Tretinoin, Retin A
          (i) Apply 0.025% cream, 0.01% gel, or 0.1% microgel every other night; after several weeks, increase to nightly application. The skin should be washed and allowed to dry for 30 minutes before tretinoin is applied.
          (ii) May cause irritation, redness, or dryness, and may lead to hypopigmentation. Irritation can be minimized by applying a moisturizer in the morning or by spacing applications to every second or third night.
          (iii) May be photosensitizing; a noncomedogenic sunscreen should be used.
          (iv) Because benzoyl peroxide inactivates tretinoin, these products should not be applied simultaneously, but benzoyl peroxide can be applied in the morning and tretinoin at night.
       (b) Adapalene (Differin) 0.1% gel may be less irritating than Retin A. It is applied at bedtime immediately after washing.
       (c) Tazarotene 0.1% gel is as effective as tretinoin and can be used on an alternate day regimen. It may cause local skin irritation.
    (3) Topical antibiotics
       (a) Erythromycin solution, gel, or ointment applied qd or bid.
       (b) Clindamycin 1% solution, gel, or lotion applied qd or bid.
       (c) These can be used alone or in combination with benzoyl peroxide. There are preparations that combine 5% benzoyl peroxide with 3% erythromycin (Benzamycin) and 5% benzoyl peroxide with 1% clindamycin, both of which are more effective than the individual drugs.
       (d) They are well tolerated but may cause dry skin and local irritation.
    (4) Other useful agents for mild to moderate comedonal or inflammatory acne include the following:
       (a) Tretinoin in a time-released delivery system (Retin A Micro, 0.1% gel) may be less irritating than other Tretinoin preparations.
       (b) Azelaic acid 20% (Azelex cream) has antimicrobial and comedeolytic activity. It is moisturizing, is not photosensitizing, and is thus a good choice for patients with dry or fair skin. However, it can be irritating. It can be applied twice daily or once in the morning in combination with a topical retinoid at night.
  b. Systemic antibiotics are indicated for moderate to severe papulopustular inflammatory acne, especially for patients with propensity to scarring, patients unresponsive to or unable to tolerate

topical medication, or patients whose acne involves the back, shoulders, and trunk.

(1) Tetracycline: 500 mg bid; tapered to maintenance dosage of 250 mg qd. Do *not* administer to pregnant women or children under 12 years of age. Side effects need to be monitored.

(2) Erythromycin: 500 mg bid tapered to maintenance dose of 250 mg qd-bid. Consider enteric-coated formulations to minimize gastritis.

(3) Doxycycline, 50 to 100 mg qd-bid.

(4) Minocycline, 50 to 100 mg qd-bid for patients unresponsive to tetracycline or erythromycin.

(5) A period of 4 to 6 weeks may be required to note a clinical response. Intensify topical medications as systemic therapy is tapered. Dosage should be tapered gradually over 2 to 4 months to the lowest dose required to maintain acne control.

(6) Use of oral antibiotics may diminish the efficacy of oral contraceptives.

c. Accutane (isotretinoin): Oral systemic analog of vitamin A indicated for patients with severe, recalcitrant, nodulocystic acne that is unresponsive to conventional treatment and especially for patients with a propensity to scarring. It should be used in consultation with a dermatologist.

(1) Dosage is 0.5 to 1 mg/kg/d ÷ bid, with adjustments based on efficacy and side effects; the usual duration of treatment is 4 to 5 months. If the patient does not achieve an adequate response, wait 2 to 4 months and then retreat.

(2) Because of teratogenic effects, a negative pregnancy test must be obtained before and within 2 weeks of initiating treatment and repeated at initiation of therapy at the beginning of the next menstrual period. Contraception must be used from 1 month before to 1 month after therapy. Informed consent should be obtained.

(3) Monitor for side effects (e.g., dry eyes, chapped lips, epistaxis, pruritus, arthralgias, myalgias, headache, alopecia, scaling on the palms and soles, an inability to wear contact lenses, pseudotumor cerebri). There is evidence that use of Accutane may be associated with depression and suicide attempts.

(4) Follow lipid profiles (increased triglycerides, decreased LDL and HDL), LFTs (increased enzymes),and obtain a pregnancy test monthly during therapy.

d. Other therapies (in consultation with a dermatologist)

(1) Triphasic oral contraceptive combining estrogen (ethinyl estradiol) with a progestin agent (Norgestimate) with low androgenicity for girls older than 16 years of age who are unresponsive to antibiotics and not candidates for Accutane. In girls who show

5

DERMATOLOGY

worsening of acne in association with menstrual cycles, a triphasic oral contraceptive should be considered before starting Accutane.

(2) Low-dose dexamethasone or prednisone for patients with evidence of androgen excess; may also be used in combination with oral estrogen.

(3) Intralesional corticosteroid injection of individual cystic lesions.

(4) Comedo extraction.

(5) Dermabrasion, chemical peels, and laser resurfacing for old scars.

(6) In treating acne, patient education is crucial. Points to stress include the following:

   (a) Treatment is a long-term process; response to therapy may take 6 to 8 weeks.

   (b) Traumatizing the lesions may prolong resolution and increase the likelihood of scarring.

   (c) There is no known relationship to diet or dirt. Excessive scrubbing can exacerbate acne; affected areas should be washed gently and patted dry.

   (d) Oil-based cosmetics and moisturizers may worsen acne; only those labeled noncomedogenic or nonacnegenic should be used.

   (e) There may be premenstrual flare-ups as a result of androgenic effects of progesterone.

B. ATOPIC DERMATITIS (ECZEMA)

1. Characterized by chronic or relapsing pruritic dermatitis distributed on the face and extensor surfaces in infants and young children and involving flexural surfaces in older children and adolescents. Some 60% of cases have onset by 1 year and 80% to 90% by 5 years. There are three phases:

a. Acute: Intensely pruritic papules and papulovesicles with serous exudate on a background of erythema.

b. Subacute: Scaling and plaques on a background of erythema.

c. Chronic: Thickened skin with lichenification.

2. The usual cycle is *itch* to *scratch* to *rash.* Paroxysmal and severe pruritus (often accentuated at night) is the hallmark of eczema. If there is no pruritus, the condition is not eczema.

3. Commonly associated findings include dry skin, keratosis pilaris (chicken-skin appearance), increased linear palmar markings, cheilitis of the upper lip, pityriasis alba, atopic pleats, and ichthyosis vulgaris.

4. Eczema often occurs in the setting of a personal or family history of atopy. Peripheral eosinophilia may exist and tends to correlate with disease severity; serum IgE levels are elevated in up to 80% of cases.

5. Triggers include excessive bathing and hand washing, occlusive clothing (especially wool), infections, sweating, and stress; the possible role of food allergy (e.g., eggs, milk, seafood, nuts, wheat, soy) is controversial.

6. Eczema may be seen in systemic disorders (e.g., Wiskott-Aldrich Syndrome, severe combined immunodeficiency syndrome).

7. Differential diagnosis

a. Seborrhea (the condition most often confused with eczema during infancy, but no pruritus or scratching/rubbing with seborrhea)

b. Scabies

c. Irritant and allergic contact dermatitis

d. Psoriasis

e. Tinea capitis

8. Treatment

a. Educate the family and patient that eczema is a chronic, recurring disorder that cannot be cured but can be controlled with conscientious therapy. The condition usually decreases in severity (and may disappear) with age.

b. Acute phase

(1) With weeping lesions, use wet compresses (cotton cloth) soaked in aluminum acetate solution (Burow's solution, Domeboro 1 packet/quart cool water). Apply 10 to 20 minutes, 4 to 6 times daily × 2 to 3 days. Plain cool water may also be used as a compress.

(2) Local steroids: Apply 1% hydrocortisone ointment bid for maintenance therapy of mild dermatitis of the face and intertriginous areas. An alternative is to add 2% hydrocortisone to Lubriderm or Eucerin. A more potent steroid such as triamcinolone 0.1% or even fluocinonide (Lidex) 0.05% may be needed to control flare-ups (e.g., Lidex bid × 4 to 5 days). *Do not use fluorinated steroids on the face or intertriginous areas.*

(3) Topical tacrolimus ointment (a nonsteroidal immunomodulator) applied sparingly bid is effective for both acute and chronic lesions. It may be associated with skin irritation and a transient burning sensation. It is not associated with atrophy and may be used on the face and in skin creases.

Note: **A short course of an oral corticosteroid may be effective for a severe, acute flare-up but systemic corticosteroids have no role in chronic management.**

(4) Emollients are best for dry, scaling, or fissured eruptions; apply petrolatum, Eucerin cream, or Aquaphor, 3 to 4 times daily (best applied after bath).

(5) Baths: Aveeno (oatmeal) bath. Use ½ cup per half tub of tepid water × 15 minutes. Hot baths, scented soaps, and bubble baths are contraindicated. Cleanse bacteria-prone areas with an unscented soap cleanser or nonsoap (Cetaphil). Always apply emollient after bathing.

Note: **Honey-crusting of lesions and extensive serous weeping indicates secondary infection (usually *S. aureus* organisms); treat with oral cephalexin or another antistaphylococcal antibiotic.**

    (6)   Antihistamines: Daytime use is not helpful, but diphenhydramine (25 mg) or hydroxyzine (Vistaril, Atarax) 1 to 2 mg/kg may be used hs for sedation until condition is controlled.

c. Chronic management: The goal is hydration of the skin and relief of itching.

    (1)   Avoid irritants (e.g., wool clothing, soaps, excessive bathing, dust mites, excessive sweating). Wear soft cotton clothing and open-weave, loose-fitting garments. Use allergen-free (e.g., Tide Free) detergent.

    (2)   Use a brief, tepid "drip-dry" bath without soaps (except in the groin, anal, and axillary areas) followed by the application of a lubricant. Do not rub or scrub skin with sponges, nylon puffs, or similar products.

        (a) If soap must be used, use a mild nonscented soap (e.g., Dove, Tone, Neutrogena).

        (b) With the skin still wet, apply a lubricant (e.g., petrolatum, Lubriderm, Eucerin, Keri lotion, Aquaphor) liberally and prn. Drip-dry or pat skin gently with a towel.

    (3)   Steroids: Cover involved areas adequately bid.

        (a) Use a low- or medium-potency steroid (1% hydrocortisone) for long-term use because of the danger of atrophy, hypopigmentation, and systemic absorption.

        (b) Attempt to wean the patient from steroids as soon as possible through the liberal use of lubricants several times each day.

    (4)   Bedtime administration of hydroxyzine is sometimes useful for itch relief. Make sure the fingernails are cut short.

    (5)   Skin testing and/or immunotherapy are not usually helpful or indicated.

    (6)   Severe, intractable eczema may lead to dysfunctional interaction between patient and family, which is best managed by addressing family psychodynamics.

C. CONTACT DERMATITIS

1. Contact dermatitis involves the acute onset of an intensely pruritic papulovesicular rash in patches or streaks that are usually localized to the site of antigen contact. In severe cases, autoeczematization or widespread lesions distant from the site of contact may appear. Contact dermatitis can be confused with insect bites, impetigo, scabies, herpes zoster, and eczema. Any dermatitis localized to one area of skin (e.g., earlobes, eyelids, subumbilical area, dorsum of feet) is suggestive of contact dermatitis. It is rare in young children but becomes more frequent with increasing age.

2. Diagnosis:

a. Base diagnosis on appearance/location of rash and history of allergen exposure.

b. Epicutaneous patch testing using prepackaged, standardized patch test kits can be helpful, but kits are not available for most plant antigens.

3. Contact dermatitis may be allergic or irritant (secondary to toxic chemicals); common causes include the following:

a. Poison ivy/oak/sumac; usually occur as linear streaks commonly on face, extremities, and scrotum

b. Shoe-leather (potassium dichromate) allergy; occurs on sides and dorsum of feet with sparing of interdigital areas and soles; can be confirmed by patch testing

c. Nickel allergy secondary to poor-quality jewelry (earlobes), belt buckles or metal fasteners (periumbilical), eyeglass frames

d. Topical medications (neomycin)

e. Wool alcohol (lanolin)

4. Treatment

a. Avoid further contact with allergen.

b. Initiate a 10- to 14-day course of a topical fluorinated steroid preparation; be cautious with quantity and frequency of application because of the risk of irritation.

c. An oral antihistamine may be useful to control itching.

d. If lesions are on the face or genitals, are widespread, or are accompanied by edema (especially with poison ivy), a 10- to 14-day course of oral prednisone (1 mg/kg/d, max 60 mg) followed by a taper is indicated.

Note: Poison ivy is not just a summertime problem.

D. DIAPER RASH

1. Some infants have sensitive skin in the diaper area that is predisposed to diaper dermatitis. Diaper rash represents a geographic condition secondary to the warm, humid, tropical climate.

2. General guidelines

a. The most important therapy for any type of diaper rash involves avoiding continuous moisture and excessive heat. Change diapers frequently. Avoid plastic pants and occlusive diapers. Keep skin dry (superabsorbent disposable diapers may help) and air dry the diaper area as much as possible.

b. Cleanse the diaper area with warm water at each diaper change. If soap is necessary, use a mild one (Dove, Neutrogena, Aveeno, Cetaphil).

c. Frequently apply a protective ointment with a petrolatum or zinc oxide base (e.g., A&D ointment, Desitin, zinc oxide ointment).

d. If pyoderma develops, use wet compresses and an oral antibiotic (e.g., cephalexin) for streptococcus and staphylococcus coverage. Do not use topical antibiotics because they are very sensitizing.

3. Primary irritant dermatitis results from prolonged contact with urine and feces and their irritating chemicals and enzymes. It is

5

DERMATOLOGY

characterized by erythema, scaling, shallow ulcerations, thickening of the skin, and possibly vesicles. It is accentuated on convex areas with sparing of the creases. The peak incidence is between 9 and 12 months of age.

a. Provide treatment as stated under Point 2.

b. If skin is inflamed, initiate a brief course of steroid (1% hydrocortisone) application with each diaper change × 3 to 5 days. Avoid fluorinated high-potency steroids.

c. Of the diaper rashes that last >4 days, 80% are colonized with *Candida* organisms even before the classic signs of monilial rash appear. Treatment includes topical application of nystatin, clotrimazole, or miconazole cream with each diaper change along with a tapering course of 1% steroid ointment bid. Avoid combination products.

4. Monilial rash *(Candida albicans):* Fiery red, papular lesions with peripheral scaling at times; may also be pustular. Folds and genitals are involved, and satellite lesions are present. It is often difficult to find yeast on KOH. Look for thrush in mouth and perianal lesions.

a. Provide treatment as stated under Point 2.

b. Use topical nystatin, clotrimazole, or miconazole. Treatment may be required for as long as 3 weeks.

c. Use oral nystatin for thrush, perianal candidiasis, or chronic/recurrent diaper dermatitis.

5. If diaper dermatitis does not respond to usual therapies, think of other diagnoses such as psoriasis, seborrhea, acrodermatitis enteropathica (zinc deficiency), biotin deficiency, and atopic contact dermatitis.

E. ERYTHEMA MULTIFORME (EM)

1. Clinical features

a. Symmetric distribution of lesions evolving through multiple morphologic stages; erythematous macules, papules, plaques, vesicles, and target (iris) lesions (doughnut-shaped with an erythematous outer border, an inner pale ring, and a purple center). Lesions occur in crops and evolve over days, not hours (hives evolve over hours, not days and usually are not symmetric in distribution).

b. In patients with minor variant EM, lesions tend to occur over the face, dorsum of hands and feet, palms and soles, and extensor surfaces of extremities. The lesions may spread to the trunk and may be associated with burning and itching. There may be shallow mucosal ulcers and lesions, and photoaccentuation is common.

c. Systemic manifestations include fever, malaise, and myalgias.

d. Stevens-Johnson syndrome (SJS) and toxic epidermal necrolysis (TEN): Severe systemic disorders in which there is a prodrome of fever, malaise, myalgias, headache, and diarrhea followed by a sudden onset of high fever, toxicity, skin eruption (EM), and inflammatory bullous lesions on two or more mucous membranes (oral mucosa, lips, bulbar conjunctiva, and anogenital area). The skin lesions tend to be more monoform, and there may not be neat target lesions.

2. Etiology
a. Most cases of EM are triggered by viral (especially herpes simplex), mycoplasma, bacterial, fungal, and protozoal infection. The most common trigger for recurrent EM is HSV infection.
b. SJS and TEN are usually precipitated by oral medications (anticonvulsants, antibiotics, NSAIDs) but may also be seen in association with malignancies and connective tissue disorders.
3. Management: Work-up should aim at finding the underlying cause.
a. EM minor: Usually mild and self-limited; complete healing in 3 to 4 weeks
   (1) Oral antihistamines
   (2) Moist compresses
   (3) Colloidal oatmeal baths
b. Stevens-Johnson syndrome
   (1) Hospitalization with barrier isolation
   (2) Fluid and electrolyte support
   (3) Treatment of secondary bacterial infection
   (4) Moist compresses to bullae, colloidal baths
   (5) For mucosal lesions, frequent mouthwashes (diphenhydramine [Benadryl]/Maalox)
   (6) There is no good evidence that systemic corticosteroids are effective, but they are occasionally used in patients experiencing toxicity
   (7) Obtain an ophthalmology consult. Patients are prone to corneal ulcers, keratitis, uveitis, and panophthalmitis. Eye lesions of HSV infection may mimic EM.

Note: Topical acyclovir is not effective in *treating* herpes-associated EM, but long-term, maintenance oral acyclovir is effective in *preventing* herpes-associated EM.

F. IMPETIGO

1. Etiology
a. Bullous lesions: *Staphylococcus aureus*
b. Nonbullous, crusted, honey-combed lesions: *S. aureus* ± GABHS
c. A high percentage of *S. aureus* isolates are resistant to penicillin, and 5% to 15% are resistant to erythromycin
2. Treatment
a. For superficial, localized lesions, topical mupirocin cream (Bactroban) applied tid × 7 to 10 days is the treatment of choice. Bacterial resistance and side effects (transient pruritus and stinging) are rare. Better compliance is achieved with topical treatment than with systemic therapy.

5

DERMATOLOGY

b. For patients with widespread lesions, lymphadenopathy, fever, or lesions around the mouth, treat with a course of oral cephalosporin, amoxicillin-clavulanate or erythromycin × 7 to 10 days or azithromycin × 5 days. Penicillin is no longer considered adequate treatment for impetigo.

c. Gently cleanse skin; trim nails.

Note: Impetigo is highly contagious; check other family members and treat accordingly.

G. PEDICULOSIS

Pediculosis may involve the scalp, pubic area, eyelashes, and body; each type is caused by a specific louse.

1. Pediculosis capitis (head lice)

a. Scalp pruritus with erythema, excoriations, and crusts; secondary infection is common. Live lice, eggs, and nits may be seen on the hair shaft.

b. Head lice are spread by hair-to-hair contact, clothing, brushes, and hair apparel. The home and classroom are major sources of infestation. Infestation affects girls more than boys and whites more than blacks (negligible incidence in blacks in North America).

c. Treatment

   (1) Wash hair with regular shampoo and apply 1% permethrin cream rinse (Nix) or pyrethrin (RID, A-200) or apply 0.5% malathione lotion overnight and then wash off. With either treatment, repeat in 1 week and reexamine for visible lice or viable nits. Nits that are seen at least 10 mm from the scalp can be considered nonviable.

   (2) For resistant cases, apply 1% permethrin cream rinse every 4 days × 3 to 4 cycles along with a 3- to 4-week course of sulfamethoxazole-trimethoprim.

   (3) Soak combs and hair apparel in alcohol for 1 hour. Bedding and clothing should be machine washed in hot water and/or stored in a sealed container for 2 to 3 weeks.

   (4) After shampooing the hair, remove nits with a fine-tooth comb.

   (5) Examine other family members; notify the school. Among children with nits alone, only 15% to 20% will become infested. They should not be excluded from school but should have repeat examinations to exclude the presence of crawling lice.

2. Pediculosis pubis

a. This condition may involve the pubic and perianal areas, thighs, axillae, beard, mustache, and eyelashes; it causes intense pruritus.

b. It is sexually transmitted in adolescents. Look for other sexually transmitted diseases.

c. In children, *Pediculus pubis* may infest eyelids and may be a marker of sexual abuse.

Note: PCR enables identification of host DNA from lice via their blood meal, thereby providing information in cases of rape and child abuse.

d. Treatment
  (1) Shampoo the pubic area for 4 minutes with 1% lindane (Kwell) shampoo *or* apply pyrethrin lotion (RID, A-200) for 10 to 20 minutes; repeat in 1 week.
  (2) Treat all sexual partners.
  (3) For eyelid infestation, apply petrolatum 3 to 5 times daily to asphyxiate the lice and nits.

3. Pediculosis corporis (body lice)
a. Related to poor hygiene. Uncommon in the United States but is a problem in homeless populations.
b. Erythematous papules on covered areas (trunk, axillae, groin) of body and severe pruritus (nocturnal exacerbation).
c. Diagnosis is based on finding live lice or eggs in the seams of clothing, especially axillae and waistline.
d. Treatment involves bathing and machine washing of infected clothing. A topical pediculoside (1% permethrin, 1% lindane) is indicated in epidemic situations.

5

DERMATOLOGY

H. SCABIES

1. Scabies is caused by the mite *Sarcoptes scabiei;* the mode of transmission is usually skin-to-skin, but it may (rarely) be picked up from bedding, clothes, and similar objects.

2. Scabies is characterized by pruritic papules, vesicles, pustules, nodules, and linear burrows. Secondary bacterial infection is common. Severe pruritus, especially at night, may precede skin lesions. Highest prevalence is in children older than 2 years of age.

3. In older children and adults, areas of involvement are the webs of fingers, axillae, flexures of the arms and wrists, belt line, and areas around the umbilicus, nipples, genitals, and lower buttocks. In infants, the palms, soles, head, neck, and intergluteal folds may be involved.

4. Differential diagnosis: Atopic dermatitis, contact dermatitis, drug reaction, insect bites, lichen planus, papular urticaria, acropustulosis.

Note: The diagnosis of scabies is highly likely in a child older than 5 years of age referred because of a first-time episode of atopic dermatitis.

5. Diagnosis: The burrow can be identified as a 4-mm oval or linear papule with a vesicle or pustule at one end. Lesions should be scraped with a mineral oil–coated scalpel blade and the debris placed on a slide and covered. Under low power, look for mites, ova, or fecal pellets. However, the yield with this procedure is low; diagnosis is usually based on the clinical appearance and response to treatment.

Note: In a family infestation, burrows are most commonly found in infants and young children.

6. Treatment

a. Permethrin cream 5% (Elimite) is the drug of choice. Apply from the neck down at bedtime and wash off in the morning. In infants and young children, the head should also be treated. For severe cases, repeat in 1 week.

b. An alternate treatment is lindane lotion 1% (Kwell). Apply to cool, dry skin at bedtime and wash off after 6 to 8 hours. The treatment should be repeated in 1 week. This treatment is not recommended for young infants.

c. For severe cases and for patients with HIV infection, Stromectol (ivermectin) 200 mcg/kg as a single dose and then repeated in 10 days can be very effective. It is not recommended for use in children under age 5 years.

Note: Pruritus may persist for 4 to 6 weeks after adequate treatment, especially in children younger than 2 years of age. Additional treatment is warranted only if mites are demonstrated. Antihistamines and topical steroids may help.

d. Family members should be treated, even if asymptomatic. Permethrin is not approved for use during pregnancy; check with obstetrician.

e. Clothing and bed linens should be machine washed in hot water (60° C).

f. Use oral antihistamine for pruritus.

I. SEBORRHEIC DERMATITIS

1. Seborrheic dermatitis is characterized by erythematous, dry, scaling, crusting lesions with or without a greasy, yellowish appearance.

a. It occurs in areas rich in sebaceous glands (face, scalp, perineum, postauricular, and intertriginous areas).

b. Affected areas are sharply demarcated from uninvolved skin. It is common in infancy (appearing between 2 and 10 weeks of age); it usually resolves by 1 year of age, but a small percentage may go on to adult seborrheic dermatitis.

c. Scalp lesions (cradle cap) consist of a greasy, salmon-colored, scaly dermatitis.

d. This condition may be confused with eczema (less itching with seborrhea).

e. In older children, psoriasis should also be considered in the differential diagnosis.

2. Treatment

a. Use 1% hydrocortisone cream for dermatitis (not cradle cap).

b. Keep diaper area dry.

c. For severe cradle cap, apply baby oil to scalp × 15 minutes, then gently wash with a shampoo containing salicylic acid and sulfur (Sebulex) or zinc pyrithione (Head and Shoulders). The scales should not be vigorously scraped off the scalp, but wiped off as they loosen.

d. Must often treat for candidal superinfection.

J. TINEA (DERMATOPHYTE INFECTIONS)

1. Two organisms (*Trichophyton tonsorans* [95%] and *Microsporum canis* [5%]) cause most tinea infections in the United States. Therapy is the same regardless of the organism but differs with the site and extent of infection (topical therapy for localized skin infection in nonhair-bearing areas; systemic therapy for widespread skin infection and infection of the scalp, hair, or nails).

a. Clinical appearance: Expanding raised margins, erythema, and scaling. Scalp infection may be associated with alopecia and visible broken hair stubble; may create a "salt and pepper" appearance with short residual hairs poking above the scalp surface as black dots. May present as seborrheic dermatitis.

b. Diagnostic procedures
   (1) Wood lamp: Fluorescence is seen with skin lesions of tinea versicolor and with *Microsporum* scalp infections. However, *Trichophyton* skin and scalp infections do not fluoresce.
   (2) Obtain a KOH preparation of scales, nail scrapings, or epilated hairs. Look for spores in hair or hyphae.
   (3) Send a culture in uncertain cases and in all cases in which oral medication will be used. For scalp infection, gently rub a sterile toothbrush or vigorously rub a moistened sterile cotton tip applicator over scalp areas of erythema, scale, alopecia, or any combination of these conditions, and then inoculate onto fungal (e.g., Mycosel) culture medium.

2. Tinea corporis (body, "ringworm"), tinea cruris (genitocrural area, "jock itch"), tinea pedis (foot, "athlete's foot")

a. Treatment: Use topical clotrimazole (Lotrimin), miconazole, ketoconazole, or other imidazole until completely clear, then 1 to 2 weeks longer. When lesions are multiple and widespread, oral therapy with griseofulvin is indicated.

b. Erythrasma (caused by *Corynebacterium minutissimum*) is commonly confused with tinea cruris.
   (1) Erythrasma is not as inflamed as jock itch and appears as reddish brown, scaly patches in the intertriginous areas. Lesions fluoresce coral red under the Wood lamp.
   (2) Treat with oral erythromycin 30 to 50 mg/kg/d × 7 days. It may take weeks to completely resolve.

3. Tinea capitis (scalp and hair)

a. Treatment: Use ultra micronized griseofulvin 20 mg/kg/d administered qd.
   (1) Give with whole milk or other foods containing fat to ensure optimal absorption.
   (2) At least 8 weeks of griseofulvin are required for scalp and extensive skin infections.
   (3) Oral ketoconazole is not as effective as griseofulvin and should be used only if there is intolerance to griseofulvin. Liver function should be monitored.

5

DERMATOLOGY

       (4)   Adjunct therapy includes antiseborrheic shampoo (selenium
              sulfide) q2-3d.
  b.   It is not necessary to conduct laboratory tests.
  c.   Transmission
       (1)   Infection is very common in school-age children, especially in
              inner cities.
       (2)   Infection may be spread from fallen hair, hair brushes, combs,
              and hats.
       (3)   Some 30% of asymptomatic adult contacts of children with tinea
              capitis have positive cultures. The asymptomatic carrier state can
              persist for 6 to 8 months.
       (4)   It is impractical to keep children with tinea scalp infection out of
              the classroom because shedding of spores can occur for many
              months despite therapy.
4. Kerion: Circumscribed erythematous, boggy, tender scalp mass with
       multiple pustules on surface. There may be a low-grade fever and
       local adenopathy, which represents an immune response to the
       dermatophyte and should be treated with griseofulvin as previously
       described.
  a.   In some instances, there may be secondary bacterial infection, in which
       case an antibiotic is also required.
  b.   Steroids are helpful for severe inflammation. Start prednisone at a
       dosage of 1 mg/kg/d and taper over a 10- to 14-day course.
5. Tinea unguium (nails): The most difficult tinea infection to treat.
       Treatment requires itraconazole, fluconazole, or terbinafine.
**Note: Although not yet approved by the FDA for the treatment of tinea
infections in children, a number of oral agents have been shown to be
effective and to have a good safety profile:**
       • Fluconazole (Diflucan) 5 to 6 mg/kg/day × 4 to 6 weeks
       • Itraconazole (Sporanox) 3 mg/kg/day (liquid) or 5 mg/kg/day (capsule)
         up to 100 mg/day × 4 weeks
       • Terbinafine (Lamisil)
            <20 kg : 62.5 mg/day × 2 to 4 weeks
            20-40 kg : 125 mg/day × 2 to 4 weeks
            >40 kg : 250 mg/day × 2 to 4 weeks
6. Tinea versicolor: Technically a yeast infection. It is characterized by
       superficial light tan, red, or white scaly macules appearing usually on
       the neck, upper part of the back, chest, and proximal arms. Lesions are
       darker than surrounding skin in nonexposed areas and lighter on
       tanned or black skin.
  a.   Diagnosis: A KOH preparation from scale scrapings shows the
       characteristic grapelike clusters of spores and the curved hyphae of
       tinea versicolor.
  b.   Treatment: Use selenium sulfide solution (Selsun shampoo [OTC]) or
       propylene glycol 20% to 40%. Oral itraconazole or possibly
       ketoconazole can be used for resistant cases.

K. URTICARIA

1. Intensely pruritic, evanescent wheal and erythema reactions
a. Lesions are usually circular and well circumscribed but can be of variable size and pattern.
b. Angioedema (deep dermal or subcutaneous) consists of transient localized areas of nondependent edema.
c. Lesions may be localized or generalized. Rarely, lesions may be associated with swelling of the tongue, hypopharynx, or larynx.
2. Multiple causes, but often not identified
a. Drugs: Penicillin, aspirin, NSAIDs
b. Food: Milk, peanuts, shellfish, egg whites, nuts, food additives
c. Insect bites
d. Infection: Bacterial, viral (Epstein-Barr virus, hepatitis), fungal, parasitic
e. Physical: Heat, cold, exercise, mechanical pressure
f. Direct skin contact: Medication, chemicals, animal dander
g. With chronic (>6 weeks) urticaria, think of lymphoma (very rare), collagen disease, or psychogenic disease. Consider a work-up if symptoms suggest that a systemic condition is present. Keeping a symptom diary may be helpful for the family. Skin tests are helpful only if food, a food additive, or penicillin is the suspected allergen.
3. Treatment
a. Acute urticaria
   (1) Antihistamines
       (a) Hydroxyzine (Atarax, Vistaril) 0.5 to 1.0 mg/kg/dose q4-6h IM; 0.5 to 1.0 mg/kg q6-8h PO
       (b) Cyproheptadine (Periactin) 2 to 4 mg q8-12h or diphenhydramine (Benadryl) 1.25 mg/kg q6h
   (2) If urticaria is severe, a short course of oral prednisone may be used but is rarely necessary.
   (3) Topical steroids are of no benefit.

Note: Patients with recurrent acute episodes should keep an EpiPen kit (0.15 to 0.30 mg epinephrine self-injector) handy.

b. Chronic urticaria
   (1) Try to identify and avoid allergens; identification is possible in only 20% to 30% of cases.
   (2) Nonsedating antihistamine may be helpful.
   (3) Steroids are not indicated.

L. VIRAL RASHES

1. Gianotti-Crosti syndrome (papular acrodermatitis of childhood)
a. Symmetric distribution of multiple nonpruritic, 5- to 10-mm, pinkish-red papules over the face, arms, legs, buttocks, palms, and soles. Lesions often first appear over the elbows and knees. The lesions fade slowly over 4 to 10 weeks with mild desquamation. There may be

5

DERMATOLOGY

generalized lymphadenopathy, low-grade fever, mild constitutional symptoms, and hepatomegaly.

b. In some parts of the world (not the United States), Gianotti-Crosti syndrome may be associated with hepatitis B infection.

c. No treatment is required.

2. Herpes simplex

a. Cold sores: Grouped vesicles on an erythematous base. They are most common on the mucocutaneous border of the lips (usually localized to one side) but may occur anywhere on the body. The usual culprit is HSV type 1.

b. Primary gingivostomatitis: Small vesicles on the gingiva, tongue, buccal mucosa, and lips. After the vesicle breaks, a ragged shallow ulcer with an erythematous base remains and is often covered by a yellowish crust. Episodes are often accompanied by fever, adenopathy, and irritability and may last 7 to 10 days.

c. The diagnosis can be confirmed by a Tzanck preparation or viral culture, but such tests are rarely necessary.

d. In general, treatment is symptomatic.

(1) Use a mouthwash with diphenhydramine (5 ml) or sodium bicarbonate (2.5 ml in 250 ml of warm water). Viscous lidocaine (Xylocaine) should be avoided (risk of seizures or arrhythmias secondary to mucosal absorption).

(2) Cold, nonacidic fluids.

(3) Cool compresses.

(4) In recurrent disease, the initiation of oral acyclovir or valacyclovir at the time of prodromal skin tingling may abort the episode. Long-term suppressive therapy with acyclovir may be indicated in a child with recurrent widespread eruptions. Acyclovir is also indicated in a child with immune suppression.

e. Herpetic whitlow: Painful clustered vesicles and crusted lesions of the fingers. This condition may be seen at the time of primary oral herpes infection and is often confused with paronychia. It is common in medical personnel. It may spread after inappropriate incision and drainage. It is often recurrent.

Note: Herpes genital infections are uncommon in prepubertal children. Such infections should always raise the suspicion of sexual abuse, but most cases are probably not sexually transmitted.

M. WARTS

1. Common warts: Usually found on dorsum of the hands and fingers. They are caused by HPV infection. Local trauma promotes inoculation of the virus, and treatment is as follows:

a. Benign neglect: Most warts (two or three) involute over a 2-year period. However, warts that do not resolve often spread to other areas. Isolated warts can be watched, but multiple lesions should be treated.

b. Keratolytics (Duofilm—lactic acid and salicylic acid in flexible collodion): Apply each evening; soak for 5 minutes before application, then cover with adhesive tape. Remove in morning. Reapply Duofilm the next evening. Continue until the wart clears. If the lesions become sore, use tape only and temporarily discontinue the keratolytic.

c. If Duofilm is unsuccessful, refer to a dermatologist for "CCCCC" (cutting, cautery, carbon dioxide laser, chemical, or cold [liquid nitrogen]).

d. Rub wart with a potato cut in half, which is then thrown over the right shoulder in the lee of a tree and buried where it lands (Tunnessen, 1985). This must be done at midnight in the light of a full moon!

e. Other unconventional therapies include oral cimetidine and topical sensitization.

2. Subungual and periungual warts: Common in children who bite nails or pick at hangnails. May occasionally be covered by intact healthy skin. Treatment is as follows:

a. Wrap involved finger with common adhesive tape longitudinally and then circumferentially. Tape is removed for 12 hours every 6½ days and then reapplied. This procedure sounds like voodoo but often works after 3 to 4 weeks.

b. If this procedure does not work, refer to a dermatologist for CCCCC.

3. Plantar warts: Large size may be hidden by a collarette of apparently normal skin. Treatment is as follows:

a. Pare away superficial thickened skin over the wart. Apply a piece of 40% salicylic acid plaster and cover with tape. Remove the acid plaster every 2 to 3 days, pare the area, and reapply the plaster. Repeat the procedure until the wart has cleared.

b. If treatment is unsuccessful, refer to a dermatologist.

4. Anogenital warts (condyloma acuminatum)

a. Caused by HPV. In adults, several types have been associated with premalignant and malignant cervical carcinoma.

b. Nonsexual transmission may be the most common mode of transmission in children younger than 3 years, but in older children, sexual contact is the usual source of transmission. The presence of anogenital warts should prompt an investigation for sexual abuse.

c. Children who have genital warts should be screened for other STDs.

d. Refer to a dermatologist or gynecologist for treatment with podophylotoxin (podofilox). Destructive therapies such as cryotherapy, excision, laser ablation, or electrocautery should be reserved for symptomatic lesions. In 10% to 20% of patients there may be spontaneous resolution over 3 to 4 months.

Note: Patients with immunodeficiency states (AIDS, transplants) may develop multiple, resistant warts. Injection of *Candida* antigen has been successful in some cases.

5

DERMATOLOGY

N. BIBLIOGRAPHY

Acne

Hurwitz S: Acne vulgaris: pathogenesis and management, *Pediatr Rev* 15:47, 1994.

Krowchuk DP: Managing acne in adolescents, *Pediatr Dermatol* 47:841, 2000.

Sidbury R, Paller AS: The diagnosis and management of acne, *Pediatr Ann* 29:17, 2000.

Strauss JS, Rapini RP, Shalita AR et al: Isotretinoin therapy for acne: results of a multicenter dose-response study, *J Am Acad Dermatol* 10:490, 1984.

Usatine RP, Quan MA: Pearls in the management of acne, *Primary Care* 27:289, 2000.

Atopic Dermatitis

Beltrani VS: The clinical spectrum of atopic dermatitis, *J Allergy Clin Immunol* 104:S87, 1999.

Hanifen JM: Atopic dermatitis, *Pediatr Clin North Am* 38:763, 1991.

Hurwitz S: Eczematous eruptions in childhood, *Pediatr Rev* 3:23, 1981.

Koblenzer PJ: Parental issues in the treatment of chronic infantile eczema, *Dermatol Clin* 14:423, 1996.

Kristal L, Klein PA: Atopic dermatitis in infants and children, *Pediatr Clin North Am* 47:877, 2000.

Krowchuk D: Practical aspects of the diagnosis and management of atopic dermatitis, *Pediatr Ann* 16:57, 1987.

Paller A, Eichenfield LF, Leung DY et al: A 12-week study of tacrolimus ointment for the treatment of atopic dermatitis in pediatric patients, *J Am Acad Dermatol* 44:547, 2001.

Contact Dermatitis

Hogan PA, Weston WL: Allergic contact dermatitis in children, *Pediatr Rev* 14:240, 1993.

Tunnessen WW Jr: Poison ivy, oak and sumac: the three witches of summer, *Contemp Pediatr* 2:24, 1985.

Weston WL, Bruckner A: Allergic contact dermatitis, *Pediatri Clin North Am* 47:897, 2000.

Diaper Rash

Berg RW: Etiology and pathophysiology of diaper dermatitis, *Arch Dermatol* 3:75, 1988.

Boiko S: Treatment of diaper dermatitis, *Dermatol Clin* 17:235, 1999.

Kazaks EL, Lane AT: Diaper dermatitis, *Pediatr Clin North Am* 47:909, 2000.

Singalavanija S: Diaper dermatitis, *Pediatr Rev* 16:142, 1995.

Erythema Multiforme

Esterly NB: Special symposium: corticosteroids for erythema multiforme? *Pediatr Dermatol* 6:229, 1989.

Ginsberg CM: Stevens-Johnson syndrome in children, *Pediatr Infect Dis J* 1:155, 1982.

Hurwitz S: Erythema multiforme: a review of its characteristics, diagnostic criteria and management, *Pediatr Rev* 11:217, 1990.

Lemak MA, Duvic M, Bean SF: Oral acyclovir for the prevention of herpes-associated erythema multiforme, *J Am Acad Dermatol* 15:50, 1986.

Williams REA, Lever R: Very low-dose acyclovir can be effective as prophylaxis for postherpetic erythema multiforme, *Br J Dermatol* 124:111, 1991.

Impetigo

Demidovich CW, Wittler RR, Ruff ME et al: Impetigo: current etiology and comparison of penicillin, erythromycin and cephalexin therapies, *Am J Dis Child* 144:1313, 1990.

Leyden JJ: A review of mupirocin ointment in the treatment of impetigo, *Clin Pediatr* 31:549, 1992.

Lookingbill DP: Impetigo, *Pediatr Rev* 7:177, 1985.

Scabies and Pediculosis

Angel TA, Nigro J, Levy ML: Infestations in the pediatric patient, *Pediatr Clin North Am* 47:921, 2000.

Carson DS, Tribble PW, Weart CW: Pyrethins combined with piperonyl butoxide (RID) vs. 1% permethrin (NIX) in the treatment of head lice, *Am J Dis Child* 142:768, 1988.

Chosidow O: Scabies and pediculosis, *Lancet* 355:819, 2000.

Hogan DJ, Schachner L, Tanglertsampan C: Diagnosis and treatment of childhood scabies and pediculosis, *Pediatr Clin North Am* 38:941, 1991.

Meinking TL, Entzel P, Villar ME: Comparative efficacy of treatments for pediculosis capitis infestations: update 2000, *Arch Dermatol* 137:287, 2000.

Pruksachatkunakorn C, Duarte AM, Schachner L: Scabies: how to find and stop the itch, *Postgrad Med* 91:263, 1992.

Williams LK, Reichert A, MacKenzie WR et al: Lice, nits, and school policy, *Pediatrics* 107:1011, 2001.

Seborrheic Dermatitis

Allen HB, Honig PJ: Scaling scalp diseases in children, *Clin Pediatr* 22:374, 1983.

Mimouni K, Mukamel M, Zeharia A et al: Prognosis of infantile seborrheic dermatitis, *J Pediatr* 127:744, 1995.

Williams ML: Differential diagnosis of seborrheic dermatitis, *Pediatr Rev* 7:204, 1986.

Tinea

Aly R: Ecology, epidemiology and diagnosis of tinea capitis, *Pediatr Infect Dis J* 18:180, 1999.

Frieden IJ: Diagnosis and management of tinea capitis, *Pediatr Ann* 16:39, 1987.

Friedlander SF: The evolving role of itraconazole, fluconazole and terbinafine in the treatment of tinea capitis, *Pediatr Infec Dis J* 18:205, 1999.

Friedlander SF, Pickering B, Cunningham BB et al: Use of the cotton swab method in diagnosing tinea capitis, *Pediatrics* 104:276, 1999.

Honig PJ: Tinea capitis: recommendations for school attendance, *Pediatr Infect Dis J* 18:211, 1999.

Tanz RR, Hebert AA, Esterly NB: Treating tinea capitis: should ketoconazole replace griseofulvin? *J Pediatr* 112:987, 1988.

Viral Rashes

Spear KL, Winkelman RK: Gianotti-Crosti syndrome: a review of ten cases not associated with hepatitis B, *Arch Dermatol* 120:891, 1984.

Warts

Cohen BA, Honig P, Androphy E: Anogenital warts in children: clinical and virologic evaluation for sexual abuse, *Arch Dermatol* 126:1575, 1990.

Darville T: Genital warts, *Pediatr Rev* 20:271, 1999.

Gellis SS: Warts and molluscum contagiosum in children, *Pediatr Ann* 16:69, 1987.

Hengge UR, Esser S, Schultewolter T et al: Self-administered topical 5% imiquimod for treatment of common warts and molluscum contagiosum, *Br J Dermatol* 143:1026, 2000.

Plasencia JM: Cutaneous warts: diagnosis and treatment, *Primary Care* 27:423, 2000.

5

DERMATOLOGY

ENDOCRINOLOGY

A. DIABETES

1. Diabetes mellitus is a chronic metabolic disorder in which there is hyperglycemia that is generally secondary to insulin deficiency or, less commonly, to insulin antagonism.

2. There are two major types of primary diabetes: insulin-dependent (type I, IDDM) and noninsulin-dependent (type II, NIDDM).

a. In IDDM, the insulin-producing capacity of the pancreas is severely limited as a result of the loss of β-cell function.

b. In NIDDM, which is occurring more frequently in children than previously, insulin resistance is often found because of obesity or insulin receptor abnormalities.

3. Secondary diabetes may occur when there is insulin antagonism (excess glucocorticoid, hyperthyroidism, pheochromocytoma, growth hormone excess), unavailable glucose (glycogen storage disease), or the use of certain drugs (thiazide diuretics).

4. Important historical information includes the presence of weight loss, polydypsia, polyphagia, polyuria (especially nocturia or nocturnal enuresis), general health (physical and emotional), school performance, and a family history of diabetes.

5. Unless there has been weight loss or there is marked obesity (NIDDM), results of the PE usually are normal, except when the patient is in diabetic ketoacidosis (see Section B).

6. Laboratory tests include assessment of fasting blood glucose concentrations (suggestive: fasting level >120 mg/dL) or 2-hour postprandial concentrations (>180 mg/dL) on two separate occasions. Consider measuring ketones, HCO_3, and Hb A_{1C}; an elevated glucose level and positive ketones points to type I DM. Consider a glucose tolerance test if elevated glucose concentrations are discovered coincidentally during a well-child or acute-illness visit. In this test, the child is given 1.75 g/kg (max 75 g) of glucose in an oral solution after a 3-day preparation during which the child should take in at least 50% of calories as carbohydrates. Glucose concentrations are measured at baseline and at 30, 60, 120, 180, and 240 minutes.

7. Treatment

a. Insulin: The child newly diagnosed with diabetes usually requires 0.5 to 1.5 U/kg/d of insulin; adolescents may have increased requirements. Insulin requirements are lower during the "honeymoon" or remission period; therefore individual monitoring is always essential. Insulin can be given by SQ injection, insulin "pens," or insulin pump.

    (1) Control is usually achieved with two daily doses of insulin; approximately two thirds of the daily dose is usually given in the morning, and one third is given in the late afternoon before dinner.

(2) The doses are usually split as one-third regular (rapid- [lispro] or short-acting) insulin and two-thirds intermediate in the morning, and half regular and half intermediate in the evening, although there may be individual variations to these regimens. Both types are drawn into the same syringe and injected SQ.

(3) The target range for premeal glycemia is 70 to 150 mg/dL.

(4) If hyperglycemia is present between breakfast and lunch, the amount of morning regular insulin may be increased. If hyperglycemia is present later in the day, the amount of morning intermediate insulin may be increased.

(5) Insulin dosages >1.5 to 2 U/kg/d might worsen diabetic control and produce widely variable blood glucose values. Rebound hyperglycemia following hypoglycemia (Somogyi phenomenon) results from the release of counterregulatory hormones (catecholamines, cortisol, glucagon, growth hormone) in response to hypoglycemia.

(6) Increases or decreases in insulin dosage should be on the order of 10% at a time.

(7) Blood glucose concentrations are assessed via glucose meters or strips before meals, before snacks, at bedtime, and, if evening intermediate-acting insulin is used, in the middle of the night. Fasting and preprandial blood glucose levels in the 70 to 150 mg/dL range and middle-of-the-night values above 65 to 70 mg/dL indicate good control. To avoid nocturnal hypoglycemia, never aim for a serum glucose level that is too low.

(8) Additional insulin may be needed during times of medical, surgical, or emotional stress.

(9) Measuring Hb A_{1C} levels approximately every 3 months gives a picture of the quality of glucose control during the previous 3 to 4 months. Acceptable values depend on each laboratory's normal range. Most labs report a normal range up to 7%.

(10) Urinary ketones can be monitored periodically, especially if blood glucose levels are above 250 to 300 mg/dL or if the child is sick.

(11) Blood lipids should be assessed.

(12) TSH should be measured as the most sensitive indicator of hypothyroidism secondary to a possible concomitant autoimmune thyroiditis (occurs approximately 10% of the time).

b. Diet: A child with diabetes requires the proper calories and nutrients to control his or her disease and to promote adequate growth.

(1) Before puberty, total intake usually approximates 1000 calories + (100 calories × age in years).

(2) The diet should be composed of approximately 50% to 55% carbohydrates (starches rather than simple sugars), 25% to 30% fat (polyunsaturated, vegetable sources), and approximately 20% to 25% protein.

(3) Traditional wisdom held that 20% of the calories should be consumed at breakfast, 20% at lunch, 30% at dinner, and 30% divided into three snacks, but these percentages depend on each individual's activity level. A newer approach is to distribute carbohydrate consumption throughout the day based on the family's eating pattern and the child's habits and preferences. Meals should be timed on a regular basis.

c. Exercise: The child with diabetes needs adequate exercise. He or she should always carry a simple sugar in case he or she becomes hypoglycemic during exercise. If this condition occurs repeatedly, the diet should be adjusted or the insulin dose decreased.

d. Hypoglycemia: The symptoms of hypoglycemia result from catecholamine release (trembling, sweating, tachycardia) and from cerebral glucopenia (sleepiness, confusion, mood changes, seizures, coma).

   (1) Causes include excess insulin, decreased oral intake, and exercise without a concomitant increase in calories.

   (2) The child and family should be educated in depth about hypoglycemic episodes. If alert, the child with hypoglycemia may ingest a carbohydrate snack to stop the attack. Instant glucose or cake icing can be applied between the teeth and cheek in children who are vomiting or unable to eat on their own.

   (3) Particularly worrisome is nocturnal hypoglycemia. To avoid this entity, the patient should eat a large snack if blood glucose is <100 to 120 mg/dL before going to bed. Blood glucose should be greater than 100 to 120 mg/dL before retiring at night. Blood glucose may need to be checked at midnight and at 3 AM.

   (4) The child who is having seizures, is stuporous, or is vomiting intractably should receive IV glucose and/or 0.1 mg/kg glucagon (max 1 g) IM.

e. Psychological support is needed for both patients and parents to assist in coping with the impact of a chronic condition on their daily lives.

f. Diabetes should *always* be managed in conjunction with an endocrinologist and diabetes management team.

B. DIABETIC KETOACIDOSIS

1. DKA is a state of metabolic derangement in which the patient is acidotic, has an elevated serum glucose level, and has serum ketones present; the acidosis is secondary to the ketosis. DKA occurs at times of physical or emotional stress, infectious illness, and noncompliance with insulin therapy. The first presentation of new-onset diabetes is often DKA.

2. Important historical information includes whether the patient is known to have diabetes, the usual (and most recent) insulin dose, diet in the previous 24 hours, and whether the child is physically or emotionally ill or stressed (and the symptoms thereof).

6

ENDOCRINOLOGY

3. The PE of the patient with DKA often reveals him or her to be weak, sleepy, lethargic, or frankly comatose. The patient may be severely dehydrated. If awake, the patient may have diffuse abdominal pain, nausea, or vomiting. There may be a fruity odor (ketosis) to the breath, and Kussmaul's respirations may be present.

4. For a patient in whom DKA is suspected, the following baseline studies should be performed immediately:

a. Dextrostix/Chemstrip/Glucometer: Glucose elevated
b. Serum glucose: Elevated
c. Serum acetone: Positive
d. Venous pH: Low
e. Serum CO_2: Low
f. Serum BUN: Normal or high
g. Serum PO_4: Low
h. Serum K: Usually normal or high
i. Serum Ca: Low to normal
j. Serum osmolality: Elevated
k. Urine glucose/ketones: Present
l. WBC: Usually elevated due to counterregulatory hormones; if a left shift, think infection
m. ECG: Normal unless hypo- or hyperkalemia

5. DKA constitutes a medical emergency. Begin treatment immediately.

a. Fluids
   (1) Assess hydration; the patient with DKA *will* be dehydrated. May assume a 10% dehydration status.
   (2) Administer normal saline (or Ringer's) solution at 10 to 20 ml/kg/h × 1 to 2 hours; some endocrinologists would limit the infusion to 1 hour, unless the patient is in shock. If the patient is in shock, administer rapidly 20 cc/kg NS and repeat until hemodynamically stable. In children whose serum osmolality is high, a normal saline infusion is continued until serum osmolality decreases toward normal.
   (3) Administer half-normal saline solution to replace the deficit plus maintenance and ongoing losses over 24 hours.
       (a) Half of the deficit is replaced in the first 8 to 12 hours, and the other half over the subsequent 14 to 36 hours. Use half-normal saline for deficit replacement, calculated as 10 ml/kg for each 1% dehydration. Subtract the amount of fluid given in the first 1 to 2 hours from the total amount of fluid to be replaced.
       (b) Daily maintenance fluids should be given evenly over the following 24 hours. Infants younger than 6 months of age should receive 0.2% or 0.33% NaCl after the initial fluid resuscitation. Always remember to subtract fluids received in any other infusions from the total fluids. Fluids can be given before insulin administration.

Note: To minimize the risk of cerebral edema, be careful not to administer fluids too quickly. The total fluid volume should not exceed $4L/m^2/24h$.

b. Insulin

(1) Administer regular insulin 0.1 U/kg/h by drip *after* the blood glucose level is known. Some endocrinologists recommend administering 1 hour of IV fluid before giving any insulin. If the patient is less than 3 years of age or has a blood glucose level >1000 mg/dL, administer insulin 0.05 to 0.1 U/kg/h immediately.

(2) Follow with a regular insulin drip of 0.1 U/kg/h piggybacked into the IV line (e.g., 50 U insulin/250 ml saline solution). An insulin drip is preferable to repeated boluses to maintain finer control of the serum glucose level.

    (a) The goal is to decrease acidosis by 0.03 pH units/h and the glucose by 100 mg/dL/h. If acidosis does not improve within 2 hours, the IV insulin rate may be increased to 0.15 to 0.20 U/kg/h.

Note: To maintain potency, insulin infusates should be discarded every 6 hours and are preferably administered through a constant infusion pump. Never delay starting an insulin drip because the patient has had a recent dose of insulin.

c. Glucose

(1) Measure Dextrostix/Chemstrip/glucometer qh.

(2) Measure serum glucose q3-4h (more frequently early in therapy).

(3) Rate of glucose fall should be 75 to 100 mg/dL/h. A drop that is too rapid may precipitate CNS dysfunction. Mannitol should always be easily accessible in case of the development of cerebral edema.

    (a) If glucose falls <50 mg/dL/h, consider increasing the insulin rate.

    (b) If glucose falls >100 mg/dL/h, continue insulin drip (0.1 U/kg/h) and add dextrose to the IV.

(4) When serum glucose approaches 250 to 300 mg/dL, add $D_5\frac{1}{2}$ NS to the IV, even if early in therapy.

(5) When serum glucose is <200 to 250 mg/dL and if ketonemia is still present, continue insulin drip and add more IV glucose until ketosis is cleared.

d. Acidosis

(1) Administer bicarbonate *only if* pH <7.0, serum HCO_3 <5 mEq/L. The dosage is 1 mEq/kg $NaHCO_3$ IV over 2 hours *or* added to the first bottle of half-normal saline solution. Administer only enough bicarbonate to raise the pH to a maximum of 7.10.

(2) Follow venous pH and HCO_3 30 minutes after the infusion and then q2-4h.

e. Serum ketones

(1) Consider initially measuring serum ketones along with serum glucose.

(2) β-Hydroxybutyrate is not measured by Acetest tablets, but as therapy progresses it converts to a measurable ketone, acetoacetate. This phenomenon can give the false impression that ketosis is worsening.

Note: Even though ABG results are now available rapidly, serum ketones are still very helpful in monitoring the patient with DKA.

f. Electrolytes

(1) Follow serum electrolytes q3-4h.

(2) Phosphate

(a) Phosphate is depleted in DKA and is further depleted with therapy.

(b) Replace with potassium phosphate (see the following point).

(c) After 8 to 12 hours of treatment with potassium phosphate, there is risk of hypocalcemia developing; must monitor serum Ca! Best to change to KCl by 12 hours into therapy.

(3) Potassium

(a) K is depleted in DKA even though serum K can be "normal," high, or low.

(b) ECG can be used to identify signs of hypokalemia.

(c) Withhold K at the beginning of therapy if the serum K level is elevated or if the patient is anuric.

(d) Administer maintenance plus deficit K over 24 hours. If serum K is >6.0, do not give K. If serum K is 5.0 to 6.0, administer 20 mEq/l K; if serum K is 4.0 to 5.0, give 30 mEq/l K; if serum K is 3.0 to 4.0, give 40 mEq/l K; and if K is <3.0, give 40 to 60 mEq/l. Replace K, half as KAc and half as KPO_4. Depending on the dose infused, patients may require cardiac monitoring while receiving K.

(4) Sodium

(a) There is a close relationship between serum sodium and serum glucose: Na rises by 1.6 mEq/L for every 100 mg/dL fall in serum glucose. If the serum Na is <130 mEq/L, give NS; if Na is >130 mEq/L, give ½ NS.

g. Monitor vital signs, fluid intake, and output.

h. The patient in DKA requires a consultation from an endocrinologist.

C. HYPOGLYCEMIA

1. Hypoglycemia is defined by a low serum glucose concentration (premature infant ≤25 mg/dL; term infant 1 to 3 days old ≤35 mg/dL; infant ≤40 mg/dL; children ≤50 mg/dL).

2. Hypoglycemia may result from prolonged or excessive insulin secretion or from disturbances in gluconeogenesis or glycogenolysis, which occur when there are excessive body needs (e.g., sick premature infants).

3. Symptoms of hypoglycemia are caused by catecholamine release (tachycardia, diaphoresis, flushing, anxiety, weakness, hunger) and by cerebral glucopenia (confusion, behavior changes, stupor, seizures, coma).

a. If severe and prolonged, hypoglycemia may cause brain damage.

b. In the neonate, symptoms include jitteriness, pallor, diaphoresis, hypothermia, weakness, poor feeding, apathy, seizures, and apnea/tachypnea.

4. Important historical information includes the presence of the aforementioned symptoms, their timing and frequency, the possibility of drug or toxin ingestion, the patient's growth and general health, and a family history of similar episodes.

5. The PE should be complete.

6. Causes of hypoglycemia

a. Neonatal hypoglycemia: Secondary to hepatic enzyme immaturity, reduced hepatic glycogen stores resulting from in-utero malnutrition, sepsis, severe systemic illness, hyperinsulinism resulting from maternal diabetes, or hyperplasia/increased secretion (nesidioblastosis) of β cells or islet cells

b. Postprandial hypoglycemia: Postprandial hypersecretion of insulin or heightened tissue response to normal insulin levels

c. Fasting (hyperinsulinism)

d. Deficiency of hormones regulating serum glucose levels: Growth hormone, ACTH/cortisol, catecholamines, thyroid hormone, glucagon

e. Defective liver enzymes that control gluconeogenesis/glycogenolysis: Glycogen storage disease, galactosemia, maple syrup–urine disease, fructose metabolism disorders, fatty acid degradation defects

f. Adrenal disease: Insufficiency, congenital adrenal hypoplasia

g. Hepatic disease: Insults resulting from tumors, leukemia, hepatitis, toxins

h. Ketotic hypoglycemia: Thought to be secondary to endogenous gluconeogenic amino acids (notably alanine). Attacks occur in the morning; are associated with stress, fasting, or infection; and respond rapidly to glucose administration. Such children are normal between attacks.

i. Early stages of NIDDM: Erratic insulin secretion, exercise-induced hypoglycemia, insulin overdose

j. Miscellaneous: Drugs (e.g., insulin, alcohol, salicylates, oral hypoglycemic agents, propranolol), kwashiorkor, Reye's syndrome

7. Laboratory tests are dictated by the findings of the history and PE. A 5-hour glucose tolerance test and glucagon tolerance test, which challenges the liver's glycogenolysis potential, may be useful, especially if the child has no reactive symptoms. A workup for hyperinsulinism, hormonal deficiencies, and metabolic defects is very important.

8. Short-term treatment of hypoglycemia includes PO or IV glucose administration.

6

ENDOCRINOLOGY

a. If the child is alert, he or she should be encouraged to eat 10 to 20 g fast-acting carbohydrate (carbohydrate solutions, juices, gel, tablets); after 10 to 20 minutes, this dosage can be repeated. If the child is incapable of taking oral fluids, he or she should receive IV glucose (10% to 25% dextrose solution at 2 to 4 ml/kg).

b. Glucagon (0.025 to 0.1 mg/kg/dose not to exceed 1 mg/dose) may also terminate the hypoglycemic attack but is useful only in children with hyperinsulinemia. Blood glucose and insulin levels should be followed.

c. Long-term management is tailored to the underlying disorder causing the attacks. Children with ketotic hypoglycemia should be fed frequently; those with hormonal deficiencies may respond to exogenous replacement; those with enzyme deficiencies should receive the appropriate diet; those with hyperinsulinism may improve with diazoxide, although a subtotal pancreatectomy is necessary is some cases.

9. Both patients and parents require psychological support to assist them in coping with the impact of this condition on their lives.

10. The patient with hypoglycemia should be managed by an endocrinologist.

D. HYPERTHYROIDISM

1. Hyperthyroidism results from the excessive secretion of thyroid hormone.

a. There is a neonatal variant of hyperthyroidism (usually secondary to maternal hyperthyroidism or Graves disease) and the more common acquired type. A diffuse goiter is generally present. Hyperthyroidism usually is considered a manifestation of an autoimmune disease.

b. The sex ratio is equal in the congenital variant; in the acquired variant, the female-to-male ratio is 5:1.

2. Important historical information includes the child's appetite (usually voracious with weight loss or little or no weight gain), mental state (restless, irritable, hyperactive, anxious), presence of tremors, proptosis (uncommon in children), excessive sweating, and increased stool frequency, as well as loose stools. The older patient may complain of palpitations.

3. The PE should be complete, with particular attention given to behavior (usually hyperexcitable or irritable), weight (usually poor weight gain), vital signs (elevated HR and widened pulse pressure), ocular signs (proptosis), cardiac assessment (decompensation may occur, especially in infants), abdominal examination (presence of enlarged liver or spleen), and thyroid (size, appearance, consistency, presence of a bruit).

4. In thyroid "storm" (malignant hyperthyroidism, which is rare in pediatric patients), the patient may have hyperthermia, tachycardia, delirium, or coma; such an episode may be fatal.

5. Laboratory tests include measurement of thyroxine (T_4), free T_4, and triiodothyronine (T_3) by RIA; both T_3 and T_4, as well as T_3 resin uptake and free T_4, are elevated. Antithyroglobulin and TSH receptor-stimulating antibodies may be present.

6. Treatment modalities include surgical and medical approaches, but surgery usually is performed *only* if medical therapy is unsuccessful or not feasible.

a. Medical therapy of congenital hyperthyroidism consists of Lugol's solution (1 gt q8h) and propylthiouracil (5 to 10 mg/kg/d ÷ q8h). Propranolol (0.5 to 2.0 mg/kg/d PO ÷ q6h) might also be needed to control tachycardia.

b. Parenteral fluids, digoxin, and propranolol may be necessary if the infant is ill (especially cardiac decompensation).

c. Medical therapy for acquired hyperthyroidism consists of propylthiouracil (5 to 10 mg/kg/d ÷ q8h; max 300 mg/d) or methimazole (initial dose: 0.5 to 0.7 mg/kg/d ÷ q8h; max 30 mg/d); the drug dosage is carefully titrated to the child's response as excess medication can precipitate hypothyroidism. Propranolol might also be needed (see dose above). The CBC should be followed to look for agranulocytosis. Treatment continues for at least 1 to 2 years and should be tapered slowly before discontinuation. Some endocrinologists recommend radioiodine or surgery for certain patients.

d. Hyperthyroidism should be managed in conjunction with an endocrinologist.

6

ENDOCRINOLOGY

E. HYPOTHYROIDISM

1. Hypothyroidism results from deficient production of thyroid hormones. There is a congenital variant and an acquired type.

2. Congenital form (cretinism): Early (first weeks of life) signs/symptoms include prolonged neonatal jaundice, poor appetite and suck (large tongue), choking or dyspnea with feeding, constipation, infrequent cry, sluggishness, hypothermia, and bradycardia.

a. If the condition remains uncorrected for the first 3 to 6 months of life, the infant is likely to display linear growth retardation, large fontanelles, hypertelorism with periorbital puffiness, a flat nose, a gaping mouth with a protruding and enlarged tongue, a hoarse cry, a short neck, sparse hair, hypotonicity, and apathy.

b. If untreated, mental development is permanently retarded. If not treated within the first month of life, an effect on IQ can be seen; this effect worsens as length of time to treatment increases.

3. Acquired form: The patient may have apathy, dry skin, hypothermia, and constipation.

a. Depending on age and the duration of symptoms, physical growth and development may be affected to a greater or lesser degree.

b. The thyroid gland may be enlarged or small.

c. In lymphocytic thyroiditis, the gland is nodular, firm, and nontender. In suppurative thyroiditis, which is a rare cause of hypothyroidism, the gland is tender, large, and warm, with redness of the overlying skin.

d. A bone age can provide an estimate of the time of onset of the hypothyroidism.

4. Causes of hypothyroidism

a. Pituitary or hypothalamic disease (global)

b. Deficiency of TSH or TRH (usually associated with other hormonal abnormalities)

c. Thyroid gland dysgenesis: Absence, hypoplasia, ectopia

d. Thyroid gland dysfunction/enzyme deficiencies: Defects in iodide trapping, oxidation, or incorporation into hormones; defects in thyroglobulin synthesis, hormone production, storage, or release

e. Suppurative thyroiditis: Secondary to infection or trauma; rare cause of hypothyroidism

f. Autoimmune thyroiditis (Hashimoto's disease): Most common form of acquired hypothyroidism with female-to-male ratio of $4:1$ to $7:1$. The gland is infiltrated by lymphocytes and plasma cells. At least half of all affected patients have antithyroid antibodies. Familial clustering occurs. This condition is associated with other autoimmune diseases, Down syndrome, and Turner syndrome.

g. Lack of dietary iodine (rare)

h. S/P subtotal thyroidectomy

i. Antithyroid (i.e., RAI) medication overdose

j. Maternal ingestion of iodides or antithyroid medications during pregnancy

5. The history and PE should elicit signs and symptoms as listed under Points 2 and 3.

6. Laboratory tests include measurement of T_4 (low or borderline), T_3 resin uptake (low), and TSH (high if defect in thyroid, low if defect in pituitary or hypothalamus).

7. Neonatal screening identifies the majority of patients with congenital hypothyroidism.

8. Treatment of congenital hypothyroidism must be extremely prompt if mental retardation is to be avoided.

a. Because a good portion of T_3 is derived from T_4, the patient with hypothyroidism may be treated with oral sodium-l-thyroxine (neonates: initially 10 to 15 mcg/kg/d; 0 to 3 months: 8 to 12 mcg/kg/d; 3 to 6 months: 7 to 10 mcg/kg/d; 6 to 12 months: 6 to 8 mcg/kg/d; 1 to 3 years: 4 to 6 mcg/kg/d; 3 to 10 years: 3 to 5 mcg/kg/d; 10 to 20 years: 2 to 4 mcg/kg/d).

b. The patient with suppurative thyroiditis merits I&D of the gland, with appropriate antibiotic therapy.

c. Patients with hypothyroidism should be managed in conjunction with an endocrinologist.

F. SHORT STATURE

1. In infants, short stature may be associated with an overall failure to thrive. In older children and adolescents, short stature may be an isolated finding.

2. Short stature may result from growth failure or marked deceleration of growth so that the individual "falls" from his or her prior height percentile.

3. Important historical information includes prenatal and birth histories, growth pattern, presence of chronic disease, long-term medication use, developmental milestones, and the heights and pubertal patterns of parents and siblings.

4. A thorough PE is mandatory; however, most individuals with short stature have an otherwise normal examination.

5. The causes of short stature are numerous.

a. Genetic or familial (heights of relatives are useful)

b. Constitutional delay: Normal growth in early infancy with deceleration of growth by late infancy, early toddlerhood, or early childhood years; puberty, height, and bone age delayed by 2 to 4 years; adult height usually normal

c. Small for gestational age

d. Malnutrition or malabsorption (lack of calories for growth)

e. Chronic debilitating disease, especially inflammatory bowel disease and HIV infection

f. Emotional deprivation (hypothalamic suppression?)

g. Medications such as glucocorticoids, methylphenidate (Ritalin), pemoline (Cylert), and dextroamphetamine (Dexedrine)

h. Endogenous cortisol excess (Cushing's syndrome): Other associated signs are moon facies, hirsutism, buffalo hump, striae, hypertension, fatigue, voice deepening, obesity, and amenorrhea

i. Cartilage or skeletal dysplasia (short extremities with normal-size head and trunk)

j. Turner syndrome (genotype 45, XO, and mosaic forms, such as 45XO/46XX): Other associated signs are webbed neck, small jaw, prominent ears, epicanthal folds, low posterior hairline, a broad chest, and cardiac defects

k. Pituitary dysgenesis/dysfunction: Growth may be normal initially, but by 1 to 2 years of age, growth is usually retarded and the body habitus is infantile. Other signs of pituitary dysfunction may be evident.

l. Hypothyroidism

m. Miscellaneous: Hypoparathyroidism, pseudohypoparathyroidism, and rickets

6. Laboratory tests are dictated by the history and PE. Bone age should be assessed.

7. Treatment includes reassurance when the workup is negative and height velocity is normal; the provision of adequate calories for growth

6

ENDOCRINOLOGY

and the proper control of chronic illnesses are mandatory. Growth hormone and/or thyroid hormone is used in *appropriate* individuals and *always* in consultation with an endocrinologist.

G. GYNECOMASTIA

1. Gynecomastia in the male adolescent refers to unilateral or bilateral breast enlargement and is usually a result of a transient estrogen/testosterone imbalance.

a. Gynecomastia usually begins at Tanner stage II or III, lasts for several months, and gradually disappears within 1 to 2 years.

b. The most common finding is a small, tender, round subareolar mass between 2 and 3 cm in diameter. The mass is not fixed, and there is no overlying skin dimpling.

c. Massive gynecomastia may indicate a major endocrine abnormality, perhaps in association with other abnormalities of sexual maturation, and deserves referral to an endocrinologist.

2. Important historical information includes the duration of breast enlargement, breast symptoms, and pubertal progression.

3. A complete PE usually reveals only the breast enlargement, with the remainder of the examination being normal. However, the testes must be palpated because gynecomastia may be a first sign of a testicular tumor or Klinefelter's syndrome.

4. Common causes of gynecomastia

a. Normal variant: Adolescent gynecomastia

b. Pseudogynecomastia: "Swelling" not a result of breast tissue but a result of obesity or increased muscle mass

c. Klinefelter's syndrome: Karyotype, XXY

d. Drug use: Estrogen, chorionic gonadotropin, steroid, tricyclic antidepressant, methadone, marijuana, amphetamine, digitalis, cimetidine

e. Testicular tumor, liver cancer

5. Treatment consists of reassuring the patient; in most cases discontinuation of causative medications may help. Surgical correction may be required.

H. PREMATURE THELARCHE

1. Premature thelarche is isolated early breast development in girls. It might (rarely) result from exogenous estrogen (not "true" premature thelarche) or from a slight increase in endogenous estrogen release.

2. The condition usually appears in girls between 1 and 4 years of age. Breast buds of 2 to 4 cm are evident without nipple or areola involvement. The child may complain of breast tenderness, and one breast may be more involved than the other. No linear growth acceleration is noted.

3. Important historical information includes the growth pattern and the use of medications or creams containing estrogen.

4. The PE should be complete. Note the appearance and size of the breasts, the appearance of the vaginal mucosa, and whether genital hair is present. A rectal examination should be done to detect any ovarian or uterine enlargement.
5. Laboratory tests
a. Laboratory tests *may* include a bone-age assessment (normal in premature thelarche), a vaginal smear for estrogen effect, a pelvic ultrasound (to R/O organ enlargement, masses), and serum concentrations of LH, FSH, and estradiol-17β.
b. In many cases no laboratory tests are indicated.
6. Treatment consists of close follow-up to detect other signs of puberty, discontinuation of any estrogen preparation (if used), and reassurance. Breast development may regress or stay the same. The onset of puberty usually occurs at the normal age. Follow-up is extremely important.

I. PREMATURE ADRENARCHE

1. Premature adrenarche is the isolated appearance of sexual hair (with or without axillary hair) before 8 years of age in girls and 9 years of age in boys without estrogen effects or other androgenic signs.
2. The condition probably results from increased hormonal production by the adrenal gland. Urinary 17-ketosteroid levels are generally slightly elevated for the patient's age.
3. Important historical information includes that obtained for precocious puberty (see Section J).
4. A complete PE is mandatory, including a careful genital examination. Breast enlargement is usually absent; no estrogen effects are evident. Virilization is absent. Growth velocity and clitoral size should be normal.
5. Laboratory tests include bone-age assessment (usually normal or only slightly advanced), vaginal smear (should be prepubertal pattern), and serum androgen levels. It is not unusual for dihydroepiandrosterone sulfate (DHEA) to be elevated.
6. The patient and family should be reassured. The patient should be carefully followed to note any progression of development, especially height or bone-age acceleration. If virilization occurs, adrenal hypersecretion or an ovarian or adrenal tumor should be suspected.

J. PRECOCIOUS PUBERTY

1. Precocious puberty is present when pubertal development begins before 8 years of age in girls and 9 years of age in boys.
a. Isosexual precocious puberty refers to development appropriate to gender, whereas heterosexual precocious puberty refers to development appropriate to the opposite sex.
2. Important historical information includes the following:
a. Prenatal and birth histories
b. Age of attainment of developmental milestones
c. Growth pattern

6

ENDOCRINOLOGY

d. The presence of chronic medical conditions; long-term use of medications

e. A history of encephalitis, seizures, head trauma, hydrocephalus, headaches, visual symptoms, behavior changes, abdominal pain, or genitourinary symptoms

f. A family history of neurofibromatosis, tuberous sclerosis, or McCune-Albright syndrome

g. If the patient is a boy, information on the ages of pubertal attainment of the father and brothers is necessary

h. If the patient is a girl, the age of menarche for sisters, mother, and grandmothers should be elicited

3. The PE must be complete. Emphasis should be placed on the neurologic examination, the ophthalmologic evaluation (fundoscopic and visual fields assessment), and the genital examination (Tanner staging of pubic hair, genitals, and breasts). A rectal examination should be performed in girls to exclude the possibility of an ovarian mass.

4. Causes of precocious puberty

a. Idiopathic (central): Premature activation of the hypothalamic-pituitary axis for unknown reasons. 80% of girls and <50% of boys with precocious puberty have this diagnosis. The diagnosis is confirmed by demonstrating pubertal levels of LH after the IV or SQ administration of GnRH.

b. Central pituitary/hypothalamic disease: Postinjury, hemorrhage, tumor, hydrocephalus, postinfectious

c. Neurofibromatosis, tuberous sclerosis, McCune-Albright (café au lait spots, fibrous dysplasia, bone cysts)

d. Gonadotropin-secreting tumors: Teratoma, hepatoblastoma, chorioepithelioma

e. Ovarian tumors: Granulosa cell tumor, arrhenoblastoma, lipid cell tumor, thecoma, dysgerminoma, cyst

f. Testicular tumors: Leydig's cell tumor, seminoma

g. Adrenal tumor or hyperplasia

h. Exogenous estrogen therapy

i. Anabolic steroid therapy

j. Androgen therapy

k. Hypothyroidism (severe and prolonged)

5. Useful laboratory tests include the following:

a. Serum FSH, LH, estradiol, testosterone, TSH, thyroxine (T_4).

b. If a central cause is suspected, consider a GnRH stimulation test: Either a traditional multisample IV test or a newer single sample SQ test can give a reliable LH level

c. If a central cause is suspected, obtain a head MRI or CT scan to detect an intracranial lesion in the hypothalamus

d. Bone-age assessment: Advanced in precocious puberty; delayed in hypothyroidism

e.   Serum gonadotropins (as noted above): May be useful as a screen for puberty. However, low levels do not rule out central precocious puberty.

f.   Serum estradiol concentration (as noted above): Elevated to levels consistent with the stage of puberty

g.   Serum hCG concentration to exclude pregnancy or a gonadotropin-secreting tumor

h.   Serum dihydroepiandrosterone sulfate concentration as a measure of adrenal function

6.   If an ovarian tumor is suspected by PE or if serum gonadotropin levels are prepubertal, an abdominal ultrasound or CT/MRI scan should be obtained.

a.   Depending on the type of ovarian tumor, various hormones are elevated in the serum (e.g., estradiol with granulosa cell tumors, progesterone with thecomas).

b.   A vaginal smear to determine the amount of estrogen or progesterone effect may be useful.

7.   If adrenal pathology is suspected (e.g., heterosexual precocious puberty in a girl), an abdominal CT or MRI scan is useful.

8.   Treatment

a.   The first rule of treatment is to reassure and support the child. Parents should be encouraged to treat the child in an age-appropriate manner.

b.   Tumors should be removed, if possible, or otherwise treated medically.

c.   Congenital adrenal hyperplasia (the classic 21-OH deficiency type) is treated with maintenance glucocorticoid (hydrocortisone 20 to 25 mg/m²/d) therapy; increased doses of 2 to 3 times the daily amount are given at times of stress, including physical illness. Patients with classic 21-OH deficiency also require mineralcorticoid supplementation.

d.   In girls, idiopathic and several variants of central precocious puberty may be treated with a GnRH analog (*only* under an endocrinologist's direction).

K. DELAYED PUBERTY

1.   Delayed puberty is defined as a lack of pubertal development by age 14 years for males (testicular volume <4 ml) and 13 years for girls (lack of thelarche). Alternatively, delayed puberty may be present when pubertal changes have started but have not progressed over several years.

2.   Etiologies of pubertal delay include:

a.   Constitutional delay (ultimately normal development, family H/O pubertal delay, no organic abnormalities)

b.   Delay secondary to chronic conditions (varies by condition and associated severity, onset, duration)

c.   Gonadal failure (e.g., Turner's syndrome (females), Klinefelter's syndrome (males)

d.   CNS pathology

ENDOCRINOLOGY

6

      (1)   Congenital (e.g., pituitary defects/lesions, defects in the hypothalamic-pituitary pathways so that there is a lack of gonadotropin releasing hormone, deficiencies in LH or FSH, etc.)

      (2)   Acquired (e.g., tumors, CNS trauma, CNS infections, radiotherapy, etc.)

3.   Laboratory tests include

a.   Serum FSH, LH, estradiol, testosterone, TSH, thyroxine

b.   If a central cause is suspected, consider a GnRH stimulation test

c.   If a central cause is suspected, obtain a head MRI or CT scan

d.   Bone-age assessment

e.   Serum gonadotropins (as noted above)

f.   Serum estradiol-17β concentration (as noted above)

4.   If sex steroid secretion is deficient because of gonadal failure or gonadotropin deficiency, replace sex steroids.

5.   In boys who have psychological problems because of delayed puberty, a short course of injectable testosterone might be considered.

6.   *Always* manage these patients with a pediatric endocrinologist especially if replacement therapy is given.

L. BIBLIOGRAPHY

Diabetes

Kaufman F: Diabetes in children and adolescents, *Med Clin NA* 82:721, 1998.

Kaufman F, Halvorson M: New trends in managing type I diabetes, *Contemp Pediatr* 16:112, 1999.

Plotnik L: Insulin-dependent diabetes mellitus, *Pediatr Rev* 15:137, 1994.

Plotnik L, Henderson R: *Clinical management of the child and teenager with diabetes.* Baltimore: The Johns Hopkins University Press, 1996.

Silverstein J, Rosenbloom A: New developments in type I (insulin-dependent) diabetes, *Clin Pediatr* 39:257, 2000.

Diabetic Ketoacidosis

Brink SJ: Diabetic ketoacidosis, *Acta Paediatr Suppl* 427:14, 1999.

Hafeez W: Managing diabetic ketacidosis—a delicate balance, *Contemp Pediatr* 17:72, 2000.

Plotnick L: Insulin-dependent diabetes mellitus, *Pediatr Rev* 15:137, 1994.

Hypoglycemia

Chiarelli F, Verrotti A, Catino M et al: Hypoglycaemia in children with type I diabetes mellitus, *Acta Paediatr Suppl* 472:31, 1999.

Schatz D: Hypoglycemia in childhood diabetes, *Pediatr Ann* 23:289, 1994.

Hyperthyroidism

Gruters A: Treatment of Graves' disease in children and adolescents, *Horm Res* 49:255, 1998.

Polak M: Hyperthyroidism in early infancy, *Thyroid* 8:1171, 1998.

Rivkees S, Sklar C, Freemark M: The management of Graves' disease in children, with special emphasis on radioiodine treatment, *J Clin Endo & Metab* 83:3767, 1998.

Sills I: Hyperthyroidism, *Pediatr Rev* 15:417, 1994.

Hypothyroidism

Fisher D: Hypothyroidism, *Pediatr Rev* 15:227, 1994.

LaFranchi S: Congenital hypothyroidism—etiologies, diagnosis, and management, *Thyroid* 9:735, 1999.

Van Vliet G: Neonatal hypothyroidism—treatment and outcome, *Thyroid* 9:79, 1999.

Short Stature

LaFranchi S et al: Constitutional delay of growth, *Pediatrics* 81:82, 1991.

Gynecomastia

Neinstein LS: Gynecomastia. In *Adolescent health care,* ed 2, Baltimore, 1991, Urban & Schwarzenberg.

Premature Thelarche/Premature Adrenarche/Precocious Puberty/Delayed Puberty

Argenete J: Diagnosis of late puberty, *Horm Res* 51(suppl 3):95, 1999.

Blondell R, Foster M, Dave K: Disorders of puberty, *Amer Fam Physician* 60:209, 1999.

Brook CGD: Treatment of late puberty, *Horm Res* 51(suppl 3):101, 1999.

Eckert KL et al: A single-sample, subcutaneous gonadotropin-releasing hormone test for central precocious puberty, *Pediatrics* 97:517, 1996.

Kaplowitz P, Oberfield S: Reexamination of the age limit for defining when puberty is precocious in girls in the U.S., *Pediatrics* 104:936, 1999.

Klein K: Precocious puberty—Who has it? Who should be treated? *J Clin Endo & Metab* 84:411, 1999.

Laue L, Cutler G: Unusual presentation: precocious puberty, *Contemp Pediatr* 10:102, 1993.

Lee P: Laboratory monitoring of children with precocious puberty, *Arch Pediatr Adolesc Med* 148:369, 1994.

6

ENDOCRINOLOGY

FEVER

Fever is the cause of great consternation for parents and pediatricians alike. About fever, there are as many myths and misconceptions as there are truths. When managing fever, it is important to approach parental concerns from a scientific perspective. While some aspects of fever management remain controversial, many others can be addressed in a uniform manner.

A. DEFINITION

1. Fever is defined as a rectal temperature greater than 38° C.
2. Rectal temperature is approximately 0.6° C higher than oral temperature, 1.1° C higher than axillary temperature. These conversions are estimates, and can vary from child to child.

7

B. DETECTION

1. Experienced pediatricians generally agree that mothers can identify the presence of fever in many young children without the use of a thermometer. Similarly, a mother is also often correct when she says that her child does *not* have fever on the basis of subjective criteria.
2. Rectal temperature is the most reliable method of estimating true body (core) temperature. Aural temperature devices are *not* reliable in young infants. Liquid-crystal forehead temperature strips are *not* reliable in any setting. Temporal artery temperature measurement devices seem to have the most promise of reliability, but have not been adequately "field-tested" to date.
3. Fever may result from over-bundling a small infant. When this condition is suspected, the child should be unbundled and the temperature retaken in 15 to 30 minutes. The repeat temperature is likely a more accurate reflection of the infant's true temperature.

C. CONSEQUENCES

Fever is an important physiologic sign of illness. It can be a helpful indicator of the course of an illness and the response to therapy.

1. Response of fever to antipyretics, however, can be overvalued. While many parents and physicians believe that "unresponsiveness" of fever to administration of antipyretics is an indication of either etiology or seriousness of disease, neither has been proven to be true. Research indicates that disease process cannot be predicted by response or lack of response of fever to antipyretics.
2. Effects of fever include the following:
a. Increased HR, increased cardiac output
b. Enhanced response to infection
c. Malaise, discomfort, irritability
d. Increased insensible loss of water
e. Increased risk of seizures in young children

D. NOT ALL FEVERS NEED TREATMENT

1. Although most parents will request or expect chemical treatment of fever, not all fevers warrant treatment. Some clinical studies have indicated that children with fever recover from some infectious illnesses quicker than their counterparts whose temperatures have been modified with antipyretics. Nevertheless, it is reasonable to attempt to reduce fever in children for the following reasons:

a. To possibly reduce discomfort
b. To possibly reduce the risk of a febrile seizure
c. To possibly decrease energy expenditure in patients with cardiovascular compromise (e.g., CHD or sickle cell disease)

2. It is important to provide both comfort and proper advice. Many parents have serious concerns about fever and its potential harmful effects. Some simple and helpful comments can give parents a balanced perspective. Whenever possible, educate parents on the following points:

a. Their child's temperature "will not keep going up" if no treatment is given. Although temperatures above 41° C occur, they are rare.
b. A temperature <41° C does not cause damage to the child.
c. The responsiveness of fever to antipyretics does not indicate anything about either the cause of the fever or the severity of the child's illness.
d. The child's appearance and behavior are more important than the degree of fever.

E. TREATMENT

1. Place the child in a comfortable environment that will neither induce sweating nor shivering.
a. Remove *excess* clothing and blankets.
b. Adjust the room temperature to a *comfortable* range.
c. Hydrate the patient with cool oral liquids.
2. Chemicals (Antipyretics)
a. Acetaminophen is recommended at 15 mg/kg/dose, q4-6h. The usual adult single regular dose is 325 mg. The "extra strength" adult single dose is 500 mg. Be sure parents understand the difference in concentration of acetaminophen in drops vs. elixir (1 tsp elixir = 80, 120, 160, or 325 mg; 1 tsp drops = 240 or 500 mg). Acetaminophen preparations include the following:
   (1) Drops = 100 mg/ml
   (2) Elixir = 160 mg/5 ml
   (3) Chewable tablets = 80, 160 mg
   (4) Tablets = 325, 500, 650 mg
   (5) Suppositories = 80, 120, 325, 650 mg
b. Ibuprofen, a nonsteroidal antiinflammatory drug, at a dosage of 10 mg/kg q6-8h is as effective an antipyretic as acetaminophen.
c. Although an effective antipyretic, aspirin is generally not recommended for that use in children because of the concern of Reye's syndrome.

3. Other methods of fever reduction
a. Bathing (or sponge-bathing) is a method of fever reduction that is used by many parents and grandparents. This technique can help reduce fever. However, it is cumbersome and prone to errors in application. If parents or other family members desire to utilize bathing as an alternate or supplemental method of fever reduction, be certain to provide them with the following precautions:
   (1) Supervise the child one-on-one at all times during the process.
   (2) Use only plain water (do not add or substitute alcohol, since it will be readily absorbed).
   (3) Use tepid (comfortably warm) water to avoid shivering.
   (4) Never leave the child unattended in a container of water.

7

FEVER

F. EVALUATION OF THE FEBRILE INFANT <2 MONTHS OF AGE

Infants younger than 2 months of age are different in many regards from older infants and children. Their immune defenses are less competent, their communication skills rudimentary, and their exposures to infecting agents unique. For them, the signs and symptoms of serious bacterial infection (SBI) can be subtle and nonspecific. Approximately 10% to 13% of all infants with fever whose parents have sought the advice of a physician have bacterial diseases. The most common of those is isolated urinary tract infection. Bacteremia, bacterial meningitis, and other bacterial infections are less common. Given the limitations of current technology, it is incumbent upon the physician to approach fever in this age group with diligence and caution. Although different investigators debate some aspects of the approach to fever in young infants, most can agree on the following points:

1. The appearance of the infant is *not* a reliable predictor of SBI. While one should always assume that ill appearance indicates possible presence of serious disease, multiple studies have demonstrated that young infants with life-threatening infections, including bacterial meningitis, can appear entirely well.
2. Infants younger than 4 weeks of age are even more difficult to evaluate than those 4 to 8 weeks of age. Methods of identifying those who are at low risk for SBI are unreliable when applied to this younger population.
3. Infants who have a history of *documented* fever but are afebrile on presentation should receive a complete evaluation for possible SBI. For those who have a history of *tactile* temperature elevation, but are afebrile on presentation, there are no reliable data regarding incidence of SBI.
4. There are three different screening tools (Rochester, Boston, and Philadelphia) for detecting infants at low risk of SBI that have been prospectively studied. Each screen varies slightly from the other. The Rochester criteria are least inclusive, and the Philadelphia criteria most strict.

a. Rochester Criteria (for age <60 days):
   (1) General well appearance, no identifiable bacterial disease on examination
   (2) No previous or underlying disease; no perinatal complications
   (3) No treatment with antimicrobial agent
   (4) Peripheral WBC count: 5000 to 15,000; absolute band count: <1500
   (5) U/A: <10 WBC/hpf
   (6) Stool: <5 WBC/hpf (in infants with diarrhea)
b. Boston Criteria (for age 1 to 3 months):
   (1) General well appearance, no identifiable bacterial disease on examination
   (2) Peripheral WBC count: <20,000
   (3) U/A: <10 WBC/hpf
   (4) CSF: <10 WBC/mm^3
   (5) CXR: no infiltrate
c. Philadelphia Criteria (for age 29 to 56 days):
   (1) General well appearance, no identifiable bacterial disease on examination
   (2) Yale IOS (infant observation score: *Pediatrics* 1982; 70:802): <11
   (3) Peripheral WBC count: <15,000
   (4) BNR (band-to-neutrophil ratio: sum of immature segmented forms divided by sum of all segmented forms): <0.2
   (5) U/A: <10 WBC/hpf, and no bacteria seen on microscopic examination
   (6) CSF: <8 WBC/mm^3
   (7) CXR: no infiltrate

When applied to the indicated age ranges of infants who present with fever, the following values have been reported:

	Rochester	Boston*	Philadelphia*
Age ranged evaluated	<60 days	1-3 mo	29-56 days
SBI in "low risk" group	1.1%	5.4%	0.0%
Negative Predictive Value	98.9%	94.6%	100%
Sensitivity	92.4%	N/A	100%

5. U/A and urine culture
a. In febrile infants, the prevalence of UTI ranges from 4.0% to 7.5%.
b. The U/A may not accurately predict urine culture results; 20% to 50% of febrile infants with UTI do *not* have pyuria. A Gram's stain of urine

---

*Application of the Boston or Philadelphia tools to <1 month old infants results in higher rates of failure to detect SBI. Those tools should not be applied to infants younger than 1 month.

sediment may be a better screen. Thus, a urine culture should be obtained regardless of the results of the U/A.

c.   Urine should be collected by catheterization or suprapubic aspiration. Bag collections of urine are unreliable.

6.   Chest x-ray study

a.   Research has shown that infants who are symptom free with regard to their respiratory system, are unlikely to have an abnormal CXR.

b.   In order to qualify as symptom free, the infant's examination must reveal all of the following findings: RR <50/min, no rales, no rhonchi, no wheezes, no cough, no coryza, no grunting, no flaring, no retractions. In studies of infants who have positive CXRs, zero to 14% are respiratory "symptom free".

7.   Blood culture

a.   Up to 20% of positive blood cultures obtained from febrile infants are contaminated with nonpathogens.

b.   The length of time before blood cultures become positive helps distinguish "true" pathogens from contaminants; 97% of "true" pathogens result in a positive blood culture within 24 hours.

8.   Stool examination and culture

a.   A stool examination is of value only in infants with watery or bloody diarrhea. In such cases, stool should be examined for blood (hemoccult) and PMNs (methylene blue stain), and a culture should be sent for enteric pathogens.

b.   The best predictor of bacterial enteritis is the presence of blood in the stool. Most infants with bacterial enteritis also have high BNRs. Fewer than one third of infants with bacterial enteritis have PMNs present on stool smear.

9.   Lumbar puncture (LP)

a.   An LP is indicated for any child in whom the diagnosis of sepsis or meningitis is being considered on the basis of the history, observational assessment, or physical examination.

b.   The incidence of bacterial meningitis is quite low (~1%), and most infants with bacterial meningitis are ill appearing on presentation. Nevertheless, occasional infants with bacterial meningitis appear well, and have abnormal CSF as the only "positive" component of their fever workup.

c.   In neonates, it is important to consider obtaining CSF VDRL to rule out congenital syphilis.

10. Viral cultures

a.   The highest yield comes from the nasopharynx and stool.

b.   Among febrile infants <3 months of age, more than half have identified viral illnesses (RSV, enterovirus, influenza). In many cases those infections can be detected early enough to alter management.

c.   Many infants with documented viral illnesses (i.e., rotavirus, RSV, influenza) have substantial band counts on peripheral WBC examination.

d. A small number of infants with documented viral infection have concomitant bacterial disease.

11. C-reactive protein (CRP)

a. C-reactive protein is an acute phase reactant that has been shown to be present in higher concentrations in the serum of young children with bacterial disease. It has not been well studied in young infants with fever.

b. Current studies indicate that some febrile infants younger than 2 months of age have low serum concentrations of CRP, in spite of having documented bacterial disease.

G. MANAGEMENT OF THE FEBRILE INFANT <3 MONTHS OF AGE

1. Febrile neonates up to 1 month of age

a. All neonates <1 month of age who have fever, should have a full sepsis workup (including CBC, blood culture, LP, U/A, urine culture, and CXR). Because current methods of identification of those at low risk for bacterial disease are unreliable in this age group, all should be hospitalized for parenteral antibiotic therapy pending culture results.

b. For this age group, no studies have demonstrated efficacy or safety of alternative methods of management.

2. Febrile infants 1 to 2 months of age

a. All infants should have a full sepsis workup. Those who do not meet the low-risk criteria should be hospitalized and receive parenteral antibiotics pending culture results.

b. Depending on the screening tool used, for infants who meet the low-risk criteria, the probability of an SBI ranges from zero to approximately 5%. If the parents are reliable and prompt medical follow-up can be ensured, the infant can be managed as an outpatient. When Philadelphia criteria are utilized, low-risk patients can be followed without antibiotics as outpatients. Proponents of the Boston criteria recommend administration of IM ceftriaxone (50 mg/kg) to all infants who, by their criteria, are at low risk for SBI. Regardless of the screening tool used, all low-risk infants need additional check-ups 24 and 48 hours after their initial evaluation.

c. At the time of recheck:

(1) Infants whose CSF or blood culture is positive or who show clinical deterioration should be admitted for antibiotic therapy.

(2) Infants with positive urine cultures should be treated with an appropriate course of antibiotics and receive a follow-up radiographic evaluation.

3. Febrile infants 2 to 3 months of age

a. This age range represents a transition from higher risk to lower risk for bacterial disease. Few investigators have properly studied fever in infants between the ages of 2 and 6 months.

b. A practical approach to fever in this age group is to follow guidelines designed for 1- to 2-month-old infants for those closer to 2 months of age. For well-appearing infants closer to 3 months of age, less extensive routine workup can be performed. Even in those infants, however, their still-limited social skills, and relatively higher rates of bacterial disease demand prudence. It is reasonable to obtain a CBC (with differential), blood culture, urinalysis, and urine culture from all infants in this age range. CSF analysis and chest radiographs should also be obtained when clinically indicated.

H. FEVER IN THE CHILD 3 TO 36 MONTHS OF AGE

1. Fever in this age group is most often due to a viral illness. However, treatable conditions such as otitis, pneumonia, osteomyelitis, meningitis, UTI, and bacteremia need to be ruled out.
2. Occult bacteremia is present in approximately 2% to 4% of febrile children in this age group: 85% *S. pneumoniae,* 10% *Haemophilus influenzae* (lower since the widespread immunization of infants with HIB vaccine), and 3% *Neisseria meningitidis.*
3. Risk factors for bacteremia include the following:
a. Temperature >39° C
b. WBC >15,000 (as WBC rises, so does the risk of bacteremia; >20,000, 25% risk of bacteremia; >30,000, 40% risk of bacteremia)
c. ESR >30 mm/h
d. C-reactive protein concentration >7 mg/dL
e. Toxic appearance (most important)
f. Immunosuppression
4. Untreated bacteremia is associated with a 56% risk of persistent fever, a 21% risk of persistent bacteremia, and a 9% risk of meningitis. These rates vary by organism (for meningitis, *H. influenzae* 26%, *S. pneumoniae* 6%) and are significantly reduced by outpatient antibiotic therapy.
5. It is extremely rare for bacterial meningitis to be manifest solely as a febrile seizure in the absence of other findings (altered sensorium, toxic appearance, nuchal rigidity, abnormal neurologic examination) that would mandate an LP. The workup of a child who has had a febrile seizure and has fully recovered (e.g., returned to preseizure neurologic status) consists solely of the workup of the fever. Not all children with a fever and seizures(s) require an LP. However, an LP is indicated for any child with signs or symptoms of meningitis, and for infants <6 months of age who have had fever and seizure activity. An LP should also be strongly considered for children between 6 and 12 months of age who have had a febrile seizure.

I. EVALUATION AND MANAGEMENT OF THE FEBRILE CHILD 3 TO 36 MONTHS OF AGE

1. Clinical assessment by an experienced clinician is the *most important* component of evaluation of fever in children in this age range.
2. The WBC and differential count can be useful when attempting to determine the risk of bacteremia. Several algorithms have been

7

FEVER

developed that outline the evaluation and management of fever without apparent source in a previously healthy child. None are uniformly accepted or followed. If a patient is considered at high risk for bacteremia (temperature >39° C, WBC >15,000), it is reasonable to obtain a blood culture. Ill appearing children should also receive antibiotics pending culture results.

3. The usefulness of the serum C-reactive protein (CRP) concentration has not been clearly established. In a small sample of febrile children 1 to 36 months of age, SBI was much more likely when the serum CRP was >9 mg/dL (positive predictive value 67%), and very unlikely when serum CRP was <5 mg/dL (negative predictive value 98%). Also, serum CRP concentrations have been shown to be higher in children with Gram stain-negative bacterial meningitis when compared to those with viral meningitis.

4. The incidence of urinary tract infection in febrile infants and young children is as high or higher than that of bacteremia. Therefore, from boys younger than 6 months, and from girls younger than 6 years, U/A and urine culture should be obtained.

5. Close follow-up of children treated as outpatients is essential.

J. PETECHIAE AND FEVER

1. The presentation of fever and petechiae is rare when compared with the number of visits for fever without petechiae. Published reports indicate that the incidence of invasive bacterial infection in children with fever and petechial rash is between 1.9% and 20%. Data collected and published after widespread use of the *H. influenzae* vaccine indicate an incidence of 1.9%. Although the most common bacterium associated with fever and petechiae is *N. meningitidis,* others *(H. influenzae, S. pneumoniae, S. aureus, E. coli)* have also been identified. Children 2 years of age or younger are at the greatest risk for sporadic meningococcal disease. Outbreaks of meningococcal infections tend to occur in teenagers and young adults.

2. Children with fever and petechiae who are at low risk for invasive bacterial disease are those who are well appearing, have petechiae above the nipple line, and have a normal laboratory evaluation. Children with pharyngitis and a positive streptococcal antigen test are also at low risk. Children who are immunocompromised, were pretreated with antibiotics, have a documented exposure to meningococcus, or are brought for evaluation during a known epidemic of meningococcal disease need to be managed differently, and should *not* be considered at low risk for meningococcal disease.

3. The laboratory evaluation includes CBC (with differential), prothrombin time, and possibly CSF analysis. For those for whom the presentation of

meningitis might be subtle (i.e., infants and young children), analysis of CSF should be strongly considered.

4. Any child who is ill appearing or has an abnormal laboratory evaluation (an abnormal WBC, an increased band count, or an abnormal CSF examination result) should be hospitalized and empirically administered antibiotics pending culture results. Less aggressive management may be appropriate in the patient >3 years of age who fulfills the low-risk criteria noted above. Those managed as outpatients should receive explicit instructions to return for reevaluation if the child is becoming more ill, and should have arrangements made for follow-up within 24 hours.

5. The differential diagnosis includes streptococcal infection and respiratory virus infections.

7

FEVER

K. HEAT ILLNESS

1. Environmental and exertional heat illness results from excessive heat generation and storage. These occur when high ambient temperature prevents heat dissipation by radiation or convection, and cooling by sweat evaporation continues. There are three types of heat illness; heat cramps, heat exhaustion, and heat stroke. Heat stroke is the most serious of the three.

2. Clinical findings:

a. Heat cramps
    (1) Usually involves a highly conditioned and acclimatized subject.
    (2) Patients usually have adequate water but inadequate salt replacement, resulting in hyponatremia, hypochloremia, virtually absent urine sodium, and normal or slightly elevated BUN.
    (3) Symptoms usually consist of sudden onset of brief, intermittent, excruciating cramps in muscles following severe work stress. Cramps tend to occur during relaxation or during exposure to cold air or water.

b. Heat exhaustion
    (1) Usually involves a nonacclimatized patient working or exercising in a hot environment.
    (2) Patients usually have predominant water depletion, resulting in hemoconcentration, hypernatremia, hyperchloremia, and urinary concentration.
    (3) For patients with predominant water depletion, initial symptoms include progressive lethargy, intense thirst, inability to carry out normal functions, headache, vomiting, CNS dysfunction, hypotension, and tachycardia. Body temperature rarely exceeds 39° C.
    (4) Less often, patients have inadequate salt replacement, resulting in hyponatremia, hemoconcentration, and significantly diminished urine sodium.

(5) For patients with predominant salt depletion, initial symptoms include profound weakness, fatigue, frontal headache, anorexia, nausea, vomiting, diarrhea, and severe muscle cramps. Tachycardia and orthostatic hypotension can also occur.

(6) If unattended, heat exhaustion can progress to heat stroke.

c. Heat stroke

(1) Usually involves the very young or very old, including overdressed infants or infants in closed cars. Children engaged in activities involving extreme exertion (e.g., athletics), or children exposed to certain drugs (e.g., phenothiazines) are also at risk. Cases often occur during heat waves.

(2) Classic signs and symptoms include hyperpyrexia (41° C, or higher), hot and dry skin that is pink or ashen (depending on the circulatory state), and severe CNS dysfunction. Onset of CNS symptoms can be abrupt, for instance, with sudden loss of consciousness. However, virtually any neurologic abnormality can manifest as a premonitory finding. Sweating often ceases before the onset of heat stroke. Severe dehydration is not a necessary component of heat stroke, but can be present. Polyuria is sometimes noted. Acute tubular necrosis occurs in up to 35% of patients. Nontraumatic rhabdomyolysis and acute renal failure have been described.

(3) Electrolyte abnormalities can occur, especially in the nonacclimatized patient with inadequate salt replacement. Testing reveals elevated serum creatinine phosphokinase, potassium, and creatinine levels, and initial hypocalcemia. In acclimatized patients, sodium is conserved, but at the expense of severe potassium deficit. Urinalysis is Hematest-positive for blood, but without red blood cells. Red-gold granular casts are usually seen.

(4) Heat stroke is a life-threatening emergency. The extent of damage to the CNS is related to the time and extent of hyperpyrexia and the adequacy of circulation. Children able to maintain adequate cardiac output are most likely to survive.

(5) Complications of heat stroke include:
(a) Cardiovascular: ECG changes, hypotension, myocardial dysfunction
(b) Hematologic: DIC, fibrinolysis, thrombocytopenia
(c) Hepatic: Cholestasis, increased liver enzymes, jaundice (often delayed 1 to 3 days)
(d) Metabolic: Hypernatremia, hypoglycemia, hypocalcemia, hypokalemia, lactic acidosis
(e) Renal: Acute renal failure, myoglobinuria
(f) Neurologic: Coma, focal neurologic signs, seizures

3. Treatment

a. Heat cramps

   (1)   Cessation of exercise
   (2)   Rest in cool environment
   (3)   Oral fluid and electrolyte replacement
b.   Heat exhaustion
   (1)   Remove to a cool, well-ventilated environment; remove
         constrictive clothing.
   (2)   For those with predominant water depletion, encourage drinking
         cool liquids. No restrictions should be placed on dietary sodium.
         If weakness or level of consciousness preclude adequate oral
         intake, replace fluid losses with intravenous fluids as appropriate
         for hypernatremic dehydration.
   (3)   Those with predominant salt depletion who are able to drink
         relatively salty drinks should be encouraged to do so. Hypotonic
         fluids should be avoided until salt repletion has been initiated.
         For those who require it, intravenous rehydration with isotonic
         solutions is also effective. In especially severe cases (e.g.,
         intractible seizures or muscle cramps), hypertonic saline (5 ml/kg
         bolus of 3% saline, followed by 5 ml/kg over 4 to 6 hours) can be
         used.
c.   Heat stroke
   (1)   Treat heat stroke as a true emergency; transport the patient to the
         nearest emergency medical facility.
   (2)   During transport, remove all clothing and cool the patient with ice
         packs, if possible; provide supplemental oxygen, and monitor
         ECG and temperature.
   (3)   In the ED, several methods of active cooling can be employed.
         Although immersion in ice water might be a more efficient means
         of lowering temperature, it might complicate other support and
         monitoring. Peritoneal lavage with iced fluids is efficient, but
         invasive. In animal models, using fans to blow room air over
         subjects sprayed with cool (15° C) tap water is equally efficient.
   (4)   Temperature should be continuously monitored with a rectal
         probe. Active cooling should be discontinued when rectal
         temperature drops to 38.5° C or below.
   (5)   The need for cardiovascular support varies. Although severe
         dehydration and electrolyte disturbances are uncommon, these
         should be assessed and appropriately corrected. Children with
         flushed skin and adequate blood pressure might not require
         cardiovascular support. Such adult patients rarely have required
         more than 20 ml/kg over the first 24 hours. Alternatively, children
         with ashen skin, tachycardia, and hypotension are in
         decompensated shock, and in imminent danger of death. The
         degree of cardiovascular support for those children should be
         guided by continuous monitoring of arterial blood pressure and
         electrocardiogram.

7

FEVER

(6) Renal function should be carefully monitored, especially in children with documented hypotension or in whom vigorous exercise precipitated shock.

L. BIBLIOGRAPHY

Fever

Baker MD et al: Failure of infant observation scales in detecting serious illness in febrile, 4- to 8-week-old infants, *Pediatrics* 85:1040, 1990.

Baker MD et al: Outpatient management without antibiotics of fever in selected infants, *N Engl J Med* 329:1437, 1993.

Baker MD et al: The efficacy of routine outpatient management without antibiotics of fever in selected infants, *Pediatrics* 103:627, 1999.

Baker MD et al: Unpredictability of serious bacterial illness in febrile infants from birth to 1 month of age, *Arch Pediatr Adolesc Med* 153:508, 1999.

Baker RC et al: Fever and petechiae in children, *Pediatrics* 84:1051, 1989.

Banco L, Veltri D: Ability of mothers to subjectively assess the presence of fever in their children, *Am J Dis Child* 138:976, 1984.

Baraff LJ et al: Effect of antibiotic therapy and etiologic microorganism on the risk of bacterial meningitis in children with occult bacteremia, *Pediatrics* 92:140, 1993.

Baskin MN et al: Outpatient treatment of febrile infants 28 to 89 days of age with intramuscular ceftriaxone, *J Pediatr* 120:22, 1992.

Bass JW et al: Antimicrobial treatment of occult bacteremia: a multicenter cooperative study, *Pediatr Infect Dis J* 12:466, 1993.

Bramson RT et al: The futility of the chest radiograph in the febrile infant without respiratory symptoms, *Pediatrics* 92:524, 1993.

Crain EG, Gershel JC: Urinary tract infections in febrile infants younger than 8 weeks of age, *Pediatrics* 86:363, 1990.

Crocetti M et al: Fever phobia revisited: have parental misconceptions about fever changed in 20 years? *Pediatrics* 107:1241, 2001.

Dagan R et al: Epidemiology and laboratory diagnosis of infection with viral and bacterial pathogens in infants hospitalized for suspected sepsis, *J Pediatr* 115:351, 1989.

DiGuilio GR: Fever and petechiae, *Clin Ped Emerg Med* 1:132, 2000.

Fleisher GR et al: Intramuscular versus oral antibiotic therapy for the prevention of meningitis and other bacterial sequelae in young febrile children at risk for occult bacteremia, *J Pediatr* 124:504, 1994.

Hoberman A et al: Prevalence of urinary tract infection in febrile infants, *J Pediatr* 123:17, 1993.

Jaskiewicz JA et al: Febrile infants at low risk for serious bacterial infection, an appraisal of the Rochester criteria and implications for management, *Pediatrics* 94:390, 1994.

McCarthy CA et al: Outpatient management of selected infants younger than two months of age evaluated for possible sepsis, *Pediatr Infect Dis J* 9:385, 1990.

Muma BK et al: Comparison of rectal, axillary, and tympanic membrane temperatures in infants and young children, *Ann Emerg Med* 20:41, 1991.

Pulliam PN, Attia MW, Cronan KM: C-reactive protein in febrile children 1-36 months of age with clinically undetectable serious bacterial infection, *Pediatrics* 108:1275, 2001.

Schmitt BD: Fever phobia: misconceptions of parents about fevers, *Am J Dis Child* 123:204, 1972.

Sormunen P et al: C-reactive protein is useful in distinguishing Gram stain-negative bacterial meningitis from viral meningitis in children, *J Pediatr* 134:725, 1999.

Stephen M, Baraff LJ: Care of the febrile child: an annotated bibliography, *Am J Emerg Med* 9:281, 1991.

Heat Stress

Bacon C et al: Heat stroke in well-wrapped infants, *Lancet* 1:422, 1979.

Baum CR: Environmental and exertional heat stress, In Fleisher GR, Ludwig S, eds: *Textbook of Pediatric Emergency Medicine*, ed 4, Philadelphia: Lippincott Williams & Wilkins, 2000:951.

Robinson MD, Seward PN: Heat injury in children, *Pediatr Emerg Care* 3:114, 1987.

Rosenstein BJ: The twin perils of heat exhaustion and heat stroke, *Contemp Pediatr* 3:46, 1986.

Semenza JC et al: Heat-related deaths during the July 1995 heat wave in Chicago, *N Engl J Med* 335:84, 1996.

GASTROINTESTINAL DISORDERS

A. ABDOMINAL PAIN

1. Abdominal pain may be acute or chronic/recurrent (at least three episodes in 3 months). It may represent surgical, medical, and emotional conditions. Chronic/recurrent abdominal pain occurs in approximately 10% of children between 5 and 10 years of age; however, less than 10% of these cases have an organic basis (often genitourinary) for the pain.

2. The history should be tailored to the circumstances of the pain (acute vs. chronic/recurrent).

a. Where is the pain located? Does it radiate? Is it cramping, sharp, dull, constant, or intermittent?

b. Does the pain make the child cry or abandon his or her usual activities? Does it occur at particular times of the day or certain days of the week? Does the pain awaken the child from sleep? Is it present on awakening? What is its relation to meals?

c. How long does the pain last? Is the child totally well between episodes?

d. What are the events, factors, or medications (including prescriptions, OTC preparations, home remedies) that relieve the pain?

e. What is the child's diet? (Check especially for intake of lactose, fiber, and fruit juices.)

f. Does the child have any allergies or food intolerances? Which ones?

g. Is the child taking any medications? Which ones?

h. Does the child have a chronic medical condition? Which one?

i. Has the child ever had a diagnosed GI medical problem or GI surgery? Which one(s)?

j. Is the pain accompanied by anorexia, nausea, reflux, vomiting, bloating, flatulence, diarrhea, or constipation?

k. Are non-GI symptoms present (e.g., fever, oral ulcers, sore throat, rash, cough, headache, joint symptoms)?

l. Is there a history of trauma? Elaborate.

m. Do other family members have similar symptoms?

n. In the female adolescent, when did menses begin? Is there a history of vaginal discharge or bleeding?

o. Has there been a change in the child's environment (e.g., home, friends, school) or behavior (e.g., poor school performance, apathy, argumentativeness)?

3. A complete PE is essential, with special emphasis on the abdomen and rectal examination.

a. With the patient in the supine position, inspect the abdomen for evidence of trauma (e.g., bruises, lacerations), chronic medical conditions (café au lait spots, neurofibroma, ash-leaf spots, tuberous

111

sclerosis), rashes, petechiae, asymmetries, or distension. Does the patient have a scaphoid abdomen? Is a hernia present? Is reverse peristalsis evident?

b.   Palpation of the abdomen should be performed to elicit evidence of tenderness (including rebound), masses, or organomegaly. Are fluid waves present?

c.   Detection of tenderness may be difficult in a crying, frightened child; performing the examination with the child sitting on the parent's lap may sometimes lessen the child's fear. In addition, if a child reports that "everything hurts" but does not act accordingly, palpation with the stethoscope ("I'm going to listen to you now") may help sort out real areas (if any) of tenderness. The child in real pain will say, "Ow," flinch, jump, blink, dilate pupils, or tear if the stethoscope palpation is painful.

d.   Percussion of the abdomen is performed to determine the liver span, areas of dullness (shifting?), and overall tympanicity.

e.   Auscultation should be used to determine the presence and quality of bowel sounds in each quadrant (hypoactive, normal, hyperactive, tinkles, rushes).

f.   Try to elicit the presence of peritoneal signs (obturator, psoas).

g.   A rectal examination should be performed to detect masses, tenderness, hard stool, and other signs.

h.   If the patient is a female adolescent, a pelvic examination should be considered.

i.   To gain some insight into the degree of incapacitation or emotional overlay that may be present, patients with abdominal pain should be observed walking, climbing onto the examination table, getting down from the table, and interacting with both parents and staff.

4.   Selected causes of abdominal pain.

a.   Infectious: Viral GE, bacterial enteritis, food poisoning (especially *Staphylococcus aureus, Salmonella* organisms), *Clostridium difficile* infection, parasite infestation, hepatitis, pneumonia (basilar), urinary tract infection, group A streptococcal infection.

b.   Surgical: Obstruction, stenosis, malrotation, intussusception, Meckel's diverticulum, appendicitis, cholelithiasis, tumor. The diagnosis of appendicitis in young children is difficult to make before rupture. Pain is often periumbilical early in the course and only later moves to the RLQ. Anorexia and vomiting are often associated symptoms, whereas diarrhea is not.

c.   Medical: Peptic gastritis, reflux, esophagitis, cholecystitis, pancreatitis, renal calculi, constipation, ulcerative colitis, regional enteritis, Hirschsprung's disease, abdominal migraine, indigestion, allergic reactions to foods, medication use (especially macrolides), porphyria, lactase deficiency, irritable colon, sickle cell crisis.

d.   Trauma: Blows to the abdomen or back, falls (remember duodenal hematoma and pancreatic pseudocyst).

e.   Emotional: Depression, anxiety, school phobia, abuse.

5. Laboratory tests are dictated by the history and PE findings.

a. If an acute surgical condition is suspected, a CBC with differential, ESR, serum chemistry studies (electrolytes, BUN, creatinine, glucose), and type and crossmatch are indicated in conjunction with radiographic studies of the abdomen, a stool test for occult blood, and U/A.

b. The same studies may be indicated with blunt abdominal trauma. An ultrasound or CT study may be needed to locate the site and extent of hematomas and other conditions.

c. If pancreatitis is suspected or if there is diffuse abdominal pain, serum amylase and lipase levels should be obtained.

d. If renal stones are suspected, U/A and radiographic (or ultrasound) studies of the abdomen may be diagnostic.

e. When inflammatory bowel disease is being considered, a CBC with differential; ESR; stool for occult blood, culture, and *C. difficile* toxin; and flat and upright abdominal x-ray studies may be helpful initially. Sigmoidoscopy and biopsy confirm the diagnosis.

f. When gastroesophageal reflux/esophagitis is suspected, a stool examination for occult blood should be obtained; diagnosis of these entities is confirmed by endoscopy. Barium radiography evaluates anatomy; scintigraphy evaluates the role of delayed gastric emptying or aspiration; pH probe defines the temporal association of reflux events with symptoms; endoscopy (with or without biopsy) visually notes whether the esophagus, stomach, and duodenum are diseased. Results of a barium swallow may be normal if reflux is only intermittent. A barium swallow often shows reflux in young infants and should not be the only basis for a diagnosis of pathologic gastroesophageal reflux.

g. Lactase deficiency is diagnosed by an abnormal lactose breath hydrogen test.

h. When uncomplicated viral GE is suspected, no laboratory tests (except perhaps U/A) are mandatory. However, when a bacterial enteritis is suspected, a stool for occult blood, a methylene blue examination (to detect WBCs), and culture are indicated. A CBC with differential and blood culture should be performed if the child is ill.

i. If parasitic infestation is suspected, a fresh stool sample for *Giardia* antigen, ova, and parasites should be obtained.

j. The possibility of hepatitis necessitates U/A, stool examination, serum bilirubin, liver enzymes (ALT, AST, GGT), and serologic screen for hepatitis A, B, and C.

k. Group A streptococcus pharyngitis, urinary tract infection, and pelvic inflammatory disease require appropriate cultures.

l. The child with suspected emotion-related pain should undergo few studies: U/A (to R/O occult urinary tract infection); a stool for occult blood, stool culture, *Giardia* antigens and ova/parasites (to R/O occult infection); and *perhaps* a CBC with differential and ESR.

6. Treatment is directed at the underlying cause of the pain.

a. Surgical problems are treated accordingly.

b. Infections are treated with the appropriate antibiotic or antimicrobial.

c. Inflammatory bowel disease responds to proper diet, antiinflammatory medications, and aggressive nutrition intervention.

d. Individuals with a lactase deficiency benefit from a lactose-free diet or exogenous lactase replacement (available in tablets).

e. Patients with reflux esophagitis benefit from small, frequent meals rather than infrequent, large ones; sitting upright or sleeping at a 45-degree angle after eating; avoidance of late-evening meals; an H_2 blocker or proton pump inhibitor (see Section G); and properistaltic medication (e.g., metoclopramide, bethanechol).

f. Patients with ulcers benefit from eliminating foods that seem to exacerbate symptoms and from the use of antacids, H_2 blocker or proton pump inhibitor, and relaxation techniques (see Section K). The exclusion of *Helicobacter pylori* is indicated if symptoms persist or recur.

g. Children with emotion-related abdominal pain, as well as their parents, require patience and reassurance. Psychotherapy may be indicated in children with handicapping pain (missing school) whether or not it is organic.

B. ANAL FISSURE

1. An anal fissure is a break in the anal skin or rectal mucosa.

a. Such breaks are caused by passing (with straining) hard stools; external fissures suggest Crohn's disease or possible child abuse.

b. Blood is either on the outside of a hard stool or is mixed in a linear pattern in a looser stool.

c. Fissures are particularly common in infants.

d. The child is otherwise well but may cry before or during stooling.

e. A history of incomplete evacuation, constipation, or attempts to stimulate stooling may be obtained.

2. The PE is important. With the child in the supine position, the buttocks are spread to stretch the anus. The location of the fissure is compared to the position of the hands on a clock (e.g., "fissure at the 8-o'clock position"). A proctoscopic examination is performed to ascertain the presence of internal fissures. It is best to use a true proctoscope and not a test tube.

3. Treatment of anal fissures is simple; soften the stools (see Section D), keep the area as clean as possible, and apply petroleum jelly locally with each diaper change.

C. GASTROINTESTINAL BLEEDING

1. Bleeding can occur anywhere in the GI tract. Such bleeding may be acute or chronic, gross or microscopic, and manifested in vomitus (hematemesis) or stool or both. Hematemesis and melena (black stool resulting from blood) usually indicate a proximal GI site as the source of

bleeding. Hematochezia (bright red blood in stool) usually indicates bleeding in the distal small intestine or colon. However, if there is rapid GI transit time, the patient can have hematochezia after a proximal GI bleed.

2. Important historical information includes the following:
a. Onset and duration of the bleeding.
b. Color (bright red vs. dark red).
c. Rate (brisk vs. gradual).
d. Possible non-GI sources (e.g., epistaxis).
e. Presence of clots.
f. Description of any vomiting or diarrhea.
g. Child's condition and mental status (normal vs. semiconsciousness or shock).
h. Presence of pain (location, radiation).
i. Presence of previous GI bleeding, trauma (e.g., lye ingestion), surgery, or medical condition.
j. Presence of a chronic medical condition (e.g., hemosiderosis) or medication use (which?).
k. Hematologic problems.
l. The possibility of an ingestion (elaborate as to what, how much, and when).
m. Remember, many episodes of "red" vomitus or diarrhea are not secondary to bleeding but instead are the result of the ingestion of red fluids or foods. Therefore a dietary history of the previous 24 to 48 hours is necessary for all patients.

3. The PE should be complete, and particular attention should be given to the following:
a. Vital signs (look for evidence of shock, orthostatic changes, and other abnormal signs), capillary refill time.
b. Mental status (clues to pain, shock), spontaneous movements (clues to presence of peritonitis, surgical abdomen).
c. Skin: Petechiae, purpura, trauma.
d. Mouth and nose: Evidence of recent bleeding.
e. Abdomen: Distension, areas of tenderness, organomegaly, presence of masses or bruits, quality and location of bowel sounds.
f. Rectal examination: Fissures, hemorrhoids, trauma.
g. Is active bleeding occurring? From what orifice?

4. A CBC with differential, ESR, a platelet count, and coagulation studies should be performed unless the source of the bleeding is clearly from the oropharynx, epistaxis, an anal fissure, or hemorrhoids.
a. Urine should be examined for the presence of blood.
b. If the stool is bloody, a methylene blue stain and a stool culture should be performed.
c. A sepsis workup may need to be considered for certain patients, especially neonates.

8

GASTROINTESTINAL DISORDERS

d. A CXR may be indicated if the respiratory examination is abnormal.

e. If the child is actively bleeding, in shock, or has an acute surgical abdomen, other laboratory tests may be necessary (e.g., clotting studies, serum electrolytes, BUN, creatinine, type and crossmatch, imaging studies).

5. Causes of GI bleeding include the following:

a. Swallowed blood: Neonate postdelivery, infant nursing at cracked or bleeding nipple, epistaxis, oral or pharyngeal trauma; amount of bleeding may vary

b. Esophagitis/gastritis: Results from ingestion of a corrosive material, alcohol, iron or aspirin overdose; variable amount of bleeding, but may be massive

c. Esophageal varices: Secondary to portal hypertension; massive or chronic low-grade bleeding

d. Esophageal tear: Results from trauma or foreign body ingestion; variable bleeding (usually large)

e. Esophagitis: Results from hiatal hernia or gastroesophageal reflux; variable bleeding

f. Gastritis: Results from intractable vomiting (viral infection, ipecac use, anorexia nervosa, pyloric stenosis); small amount of bleeding

g. Hemorrhagic gastritis of the neonate: Result of sepsis, CNS disease, overwhelming systemic illness; massive bleeding

h. Gastric ulcer/duodenal ulcer: Midepigastric pain, vomiting; variable bleeding (may be massive)

i. Stress ulcer: Result of sepsis, CNS disease; large amount of bleeding

j. Gastric outlet obstruction (especially pyloric stenosis); small amount of bleeding

k. Enteritis: Result of infection with certain viruses, especially rotavirus, *Salmonella* and *Shigella* organisms, invasive *Escherichia coli, Campylobacter* organisms, and *C. difficile* overgrowth after antibiotic therapy; variable bleeding

l. Intestinal surgical disorders: Volvulus, obstruction, intussusception (currant jelly stools), Meckel's diverticulum, polyps, masses, perforation resulting from foreign-body ingestion; variable bleeding (usually large)

m. Intestinal hemangiomas; variable bleeding

n. Infantile milk allergy; variable bleeding

o. Hemosiderosis; may be massive bleeding

p. Medication related (e.g., steroids, NSAIDs); variable bleeding

q. Henoch-Schönlein purpura: Hemorrhagic rash, melena, abdominal pain, arthritis, hematuria; variable bleeding, may be marked

r. Hemolytic-uremic syndrome: Bloody diarrhea, renal failure, anemia, thrombocytopenia, CNS disturbances; may be massive bleeding

s. Ulcerative colitis: Bloody diarrhea, weight loss, abdominal pain, awakening during the night, arthritis, uveitis; variable bleeding

t. Regional enteritis: Bloody diarrhea, weight loss, abdominal pain, growth failure, perirectal disease, anemia, arthritis, fever; variable bleeding, may be marked

u. Anal fissure: Small amount of bleeding

v. Hemorrhoids: Small-to-moderate bleeding

w. Proctitis resulting from gonorrhea: Usually a small amount of bleeding

x. Hematologic disorders: Vitamin K deficiency in the neonate, aplastic anemia, leukemia, thrombocytopenia, hemophilia; may be massive bleeding

y. Sepsis, especially as a result of *Neisseria meningitidis*

6. The child with moderate-to-massive upper GI bleeding should be given nothing by mouth.

a. Any child having blood in emesis or stool and showing signs of tachycardia, orthostatic changes, prolonged capillary refill time, or altered level of consciousness should be emergently fluid resuscitated. Administer oxygen and give 15 to 20 cc/kg of isotonic fluid IV. Certain patients (those with active bleeding, those with thrombocytopenia, those with coagulation disorders) will require blood products also.

b. A nasogastric tube is inserted and gastric lavage is instituted using normal saline; lavage until the return is clear. Leave the tube in place (intermittent suction). If active bleeding continues, the child may need to go to the operating room. Diagnostic endoscopy often is indicated.

c. Surgical conditions should be corrected. Intussusception is treated by reduction with contrast or air enema, or by surgery (if nonsurgical correction is unsuccessful).

d. Infections should be treated with the appropriate antibiotic.

e. Iron ingestion is treated with fluids and electrolytes (and base if pH is less than 7.10) and IV deferoxamine if the serum iron is greater than 500 mcg/dL 2 to 4 hours after ingestion (see Chapter 12).

f. ASA ingestion is treated with lavage, activated charcoal, fluids, electrolytes, and base if pH is less than 7.10; dialysis may be necessary (see Chapter 12).

g. Uncomplicated Henoch-Schönlein purpura can be treated with steroids.

h. Patients with a milk allergy and hemosiderosis require the elimination of milk from their diets.

i. The management of ulcerative colitis, regional enteritis, anal fissure, hemolytic-uremic syndrome, and foreign-body ingestion is discussed elsewhere in this chapter.

j. Hemorrhoids are treated by keeping the stools soft and applying a topical anesthetic; recalcitrant cases may require proctoscopic evaluation, followed by surgical or laser therapy.

D. CONSTIPATION

1. Constipation is the condition in which the child fails to completely empty the colon with bowel movements. Stools are often hard, difficult

8

GASTROINTESTINAL DISORDERS

to pass, and infrequent. If severe, may be associated with rectal prolapse.

a. The usual cause of constipation is voluntary withholding and is commonly associated with a diet that is high in dairy products and complex carbohydrates or low in fiber and bulk.

b. Starvation or intractable vomiting may lead to infrequent stooling.

c. Resistance to toilet training and psychological problems may lead to constipation (with or without encopresis) in the absence of an organic condition.

d. Irritation of the anus (rashes, fissures) may cause avoidance of stooling.

e. Miscellaneous causes of constipation include Hirschsprung's disease, hypothyroidism, and certain medications, especially antidepressants.

2. Important historical information includes the following:

a. Onset, duration, and recurrences of the constipation. Most patients with Hirschsprung's disease have a history of abnormal stools beginning within the first month of life.

b. Patient's usual stool pattern and daily diet.

c. Age of successful toilet training (if applicable).

d. Presence of anorexia or vomiting.

e. Presence of diarrhea or fecal spotting that alternates with periods of constipation (Hirschsprung's disease, encopresis).

f. Presence of anal lesions, fissures, rashes.

g. Psychological difficulties.

h. Medication use (which ones?).

i. Hypothyroidism (see Chapter 6).

3. The PE is usually normal except for the presence of hard stool palpable in the lower abdomen or in the rectum. The anus and surrounding area should be examined for rashes, lesions, and fissures.

4. Most children with constipation require no laboratory tests. If hypothyroidism is suspected, T_4 and TSH determinations are indicated. A rectal mucosal biopsy confirms the diagnosis of Hirschsprung's disease.

5. Treatment

a. The child experiencing constipation with impaction must be managed initially with an enema (Fleet or Pediatric Fleet, depending on the child's age) to achieve complete evacuation.

b. The child with constipation without impaction does not require an initial enema.

c. The diet should be improved, which specifically involves increasing fluid intake, decreasing the amount of complex carbohydrates (especially junk food) and cheese, increasing the amount of fiber and bulk (leafy vegetables work well), and encouraging daily ingestion of undiluted apple juice or pineapple juice.

d. Stool softeners and stimulants should be reserved for children (not infants) in whom dietary measures are insufficient.

(1) Softeners include mineral oil (1 to 4 cc/kg qd or bid) and lactulose (1 to 2 cc/kg/dose qd or bid).

(2) Stimulants must be free of phenolphthalein.

e. The child is encouraged to develop (with behavior modification) a habit of regular toilet use.

f. Anal fissures that can be associated with constipation are discussed in Section C in this chapater and Chapter 13, Section A.

g. Battles over toilet training and emotional dysfunction require patience and counseling; emotional dysfunction may also require psychotherapy.

h. Hirschsprung's disease should be managed in consultation with a pediatric surgeon. Affected children also require emotional support.

E. DIARRHEA

1. Diarrhea is increased frequency and water content of stools.
2. The history should elicit the duration (chronic, acute, recurrent), frequency, amount, and consistency of the stools; compare with the patient's usual stooling pattern.

a. What are the characteristics of the stool (e.g., blood, mucus, black, pale, greasy, foul smelling)?

b. Determine the diet history, which may give clues to lactose intolerance, excessive juice intake, celiac disease, and food poisoning; also determine medication use (especially antibiotic) and travel history.

c. Is there fever, vomiting, anorexia, cramps, headache, rash, lethargy, or a decrease in urination?

d. Can the patient tolerate oral liquids?

e. Has there been a recent exposure to others with diarrhea or previous *Salmonella* infection, or to food handlers?

f. Is the child in day care? Are day-care contacts ill?

3. The PE should assess the child's vital signs, weight, appearance (toxic vs. well), degree of hydration, and perfusion.

a. Other possible foci of infection (ear, throat, lungs, urinary tract) should be checked.

b. Emphasize the abdominal examination, the skin examination (turgor, mucous membranes, purpura, exanthem), and the neurologic examination (alertness, activity, tone, seizures).

c. A rectal examination may be necessary if the diarrheal illness is more than mild.

4. Laboratory assessment of diarrhea includes the following:

a. Stool examination: Evaluate for blood, mucus, appearance, and consistency. Obtain a methylene blue stain of stool smear to look for PMNs. Obtain a culture for bacteria if organisms such as *Salmonella, Shigella,* and *Campylobacter* are suspected or if the child is febrile and appears toxic. Test stool for parasites (if warranted by history) and *Clostridium* toxin, if indicated.

b. Urine: Dipstick, specific gravity, microscopic; culture if indicated.

c. Blood: Obtain CBC, electrolytes, BUN; culture when indicated.

8

GASTROINTESTINAL DISORDERS

5. Causes

a. Acute diarrhea

  (1) Viral

    (a) Rotavirus

      (i) Common cause of acute diarrhea in infants; often preceded or accompanied by vomiting

      (ii) Occurs year-round but usually in winter

      (iii) Incubation 1 to 3 days; duration 5 to 8 days

      (iv) May have fever and vomiting

      (v) May have decreased HCO_3

      (vi) Diagnosis by ELISA

    (b) Enterovirus

      (i) Occurs usually in summer

      (ii) Diagnosis by ELISA

    (c) Adenovirus

      (i) Year-round occurrence

      (ii) Causes both GI and respiratory symptoms

      (iii) Diagnosis by ELISA

    (d) Norwalk virus

      (i) Epidemic

      (ii) Self-limited (24 to 48 hours); prominent emesis

      (iii) Diagnosis by reverse transcriptase PCR assay

  (2) Bacterial (accounts for 20% of acute GE)

    (a) *Shigella* organisms

      (i) Seasonal; peak July to September

      (ii) Peak incidence 1 to 5 years of age

      (iii) Invades gut wall; bloody, mucoid stools

      (iv) May be associated with febrile seizures

      (v) Vomiting not prominent

      (vi) PMNs in stool

      (vii) Bands in blood

      (viii) Treatment: Ampicillin (*not* amoxicillin) 75 to 100 mg/kg/d ÷ qid or TMP/SMZ 8 mg/kg/d (dose based on TMP) ÷ bid

    (b) *Salmonella* organisms

      (i) Any age, but higher incidence under 1 year of age.

      (ii) Invades gut wall; bloody, mucoid stools.

      (iii) Temperature elevation possible.

      (iv) Vomiting not prominent.

      (v) PMNs in stool.

      (vi) Incubation 6 to 48 hours; 2- to 5-day course.

      (vii) Organism may be shed in stool for months.

      (viii) Transient bacteremia in 20% to 40% of infants with *Salmonella* GE.

      (ix) No treatment necessary for uncomplicated GE. Antibiotic (usually ampicillin) indicated for infants under

3 months of age (increased incidence of complications), highly febrile patients (enteric fever picture), debilitated patients, patients with sickle cell disease or immune compromise, and day-care attendees.

(c) *E.coli*

    (i) Either invades mucosa (bloody stool) or produces an enterotoxin

    (ii) Patient (usually infant) may be very ill; requires IV antibiotics

(d) *Campylobacter* organisms

    (i) Invasive (blood and mucus); in neonates may cause bloody diarrhea without other clinical manifestations

    (ii) Severe abdominal cramps

    (iii) Vomiting/dehydration uncommon

    (iv) Highest incidence in summer

    (v) Usually resolves spontaneously, but if treatment is needed, use erythromycin 40 mg/kg/d ÷ qid

(e) *Yersinia enterocolitica*

    (i) Mucoid stools.

    (ii) PMNs often present in stools.

    (iii) Severe abdominal pain possible.

    (iv) Diarrhea may persist for 1 to 2 weeks.

    (v) Often mimics appendicitis.

    (vi) Treatment: Not usually indicated for infections confined to GI tract. If treatment is indicated, use TMP/SMZ 8 mg/kg/d ÷ bid × 5 days.

(3) Miscellaneous

    (a) Acute poisoning: Fe, Hg, Pb, fluoride.

    (b) Antibiotic-induced: Ampicillin in particular; pseudomembranous enterocolitis caused by *C. difficile* overgrowth after antibiotic use.

    (c) Hemolytic-uremic syndrome: Hemolysis, thrombocytopenia, melena, hematuria, renal failure; CNS symptoms such as seizures, behavior changes, coma, and shock; look for specific *E. coli* serotypes.

    (d) Toxic shock syndrome: Mediated by *S. aureus* toxin; has been associated with tampon use and with osteomyelitis, abscess, pneumonia, GU infection. Signs and symptoms include fever, diarrhea, hyperemic mucous membranes, generalized macular red rash, hypotension, and shock.

    (e) Intussusception: Paroxysms of pain, bloody diarrhea, currant jelly stools, and irritability *or* pale apathetic state.

b. Chronic diarrhea (infectious causes)

  (1) Amebiasis

    (a) Chronic diarrhea, lower abdominal pain, or perianal abscess

    (b) May be asymptomatic

8

GASTROINTESTINAL DISORDERS

        (c) Stool PMNs may be present
        (d) Recurrent fever may be present
        (e) Mucoid stool
        (f) Treatment: Iodoquinol 30 to 40 mg/kg/d ÷ tid × 20 days (maximum 2 g/d) or metronidazole 30 to 50 mg/kg/d ÷ tid × 10 days (maximum 750 mg/d)

    (2) Giardiasis
        (a) Chronic diarrhea or lower abdominal pain
        (b) May be asymptomatic or have frequent relapses
        (c) Treatment: Furazolidone 6 mg/kg/d PO divided q6h × 7 to 10 days or metronidazole 15 mg/kg/d PO ÷ tid × 5 to 10 days (maximum 750 mg/d).

    (3) *E. coli, Salmonella,* and *Yersinia* diarrhea may occasionally become persistent or recurrent.

  c. Chronic diarrhea (noninfectious causes)
    (1) Ulcerative colitis: Fever, abdominal pain, diarrhea (may be bloody), arthralgias, arthritis, growth failure
    (2) Regional enteritis: Fever, abdominal pain, arthritis, diarrhea (may be bloody), growth failure
    (3) Hirschsprung's disease: Constipation alternating with diarrhea or fecal spotting
    (4) Lactase deficiency
    (5) Metabolic/malabsorption diseases: Cystic fibrosis, disaccharidase deficiencies, celiac disease, and other conditions
    (6) Irritable colon
    (7) Encopresis
    (8) Food allergies
    (9) Excessive fructose intake

6. Treatment

Controversy exists regarding the most appropriate way to manage outpatient acute diarrhea. Some authorities recommend stopping lactose-containing products; others do not. The following recommendations are guidelines. The goal is to correct hydration and electrolyte imbalances and to maximize nutrition.

  a. Consider discontinuing lactose-containing formulas and milk. Older children may be able to tolerate a solid diet plus oral glucose-electrolyte solution. Breast-fed infants appear to tolerate a continuation of nursing. Children who continue regular formula or solids, as well as breast-fed infants who continue nursing, may have an initial slight increase in stooling but no prolongation of total duration of diarrhea. If the stool output is excessive, an infant may be managed with oral glucose-electrolyte solutions (see Point b) and advance to a lactose-free formula. If an infant is not or is only mildly dehydrated and is tolerating oral feedings, he or she may also be managed with a full-strength lactose-free formula (see the following discussion).

b. Oral glucose-electrolyte solutions (OGESs)
   (1) If an infant can take PO fluids and is mildly to moderately dehydrated (less than 8%), rehydration may proceed with an OGES. Rehydration with an OGES can be carried out even in patients with mild-to-moderate hyponatremia or hypernatremia. Some OGESs are low in Na concentration (30 mEq/L), which is usually not a problem with mild, self-limited diarrhea. Continue OGES × 12 to 36 hours.
   (2) The child with moderate-to-severe dehydration (more than 7% to 8%) *may* need admission for appropriate replacement of fluids and electrolytes; replacement may be PO, if tolerated, or IV.
c. Dehydration
   (1) If a child is severely dehydrated (10% or more), provide rapid volume expansion by IV Ringer's lactate or normal saline (20 ml/kg); give over 20 minutes and repeat as necessary until the child is hemodynamically stable. Calculate estimated deficits of water and electrolytes. Replace deficits over 4 to 8 hours. Give patient his or her maintenance and cover ongoing losses for that same period.
   (2) After this initial period, continue calculated maintenance and ongoing loss therapy. Patient may be given an OGES (see Table 8-1) after initial 4- to 8-hour therapy if tolerated. Continue × 12 to 36 hours.
   (3) Never treat diarrhea with half-strength Pedialyte or Lytren; those dilutions do not even supply *maintenance* electrolytes for someone *without* diarrhea.
   (4) Other commonly used "clear liquids" (e.g., apple juice, cola, ginger ale, Kool-Aid) are inadequate in electrolyte composition for rehydration or maintenance therapy; thus they should not be used as a mainstay of therapy except for very brief intervals or as "free-water" replacement.
   (5) Homemade solutions are fraught with all the hazards of errors in measuring and mixing, and their use should be discouraged.

8

GASTROINTESTINAL DISORDERS

TABLE 8-1

COMPOSITION OF SOLUTIONS AVAILABLE FOR ORAL THERAPY

	Lytren	Ricelyte (rice syrup solids)	Pedia-lyte	WHO std.	Resol	Rehy-dralyte
Na (mEq/L)	50	50	45	90	50	75
K (mEq/L)	25	25	20	20	20	20
Cl (mEq/L)	45	45	35	80	50	65
HCO_3 or citrate (mEq/L)	30	34	30	30	34	30
Glucose (g/L)	20	starch	25	20	20	25

    d. Advance diet to nonlactose formula (e.g., LactoFree, ProSobee, Isomil) for infants who are not breast-feeding; advance to BRATS (*B*ananas, *R*ice, *A*pplesauce, *T*oast, *S*altines) diet for older children × 24 hours. Continue to normalize diet as tolerated.

    e. Treat for underlying cause of diarrhea.

        (1) Treatment for bacterial and parasitic infections includes the use of the appropriate antimicrobial.

        (2) Pseudomembranous colitis resulting from *C. difficile* is treated by discontinuing the offending antimicrobial, restoring fluid and electrolyte balance, and metronidazole 15 to 35 mg/kg/d ÷ tid × 7 to 10 days or vancomycin 40 mg/kg/d ÷ q6h (maximum 2 g) × 7 to 10 days.

        (3) Other antibiotic-associated diarrheas are treated by discontinuing the drug.

        (4) Hemolytic-uremic syndrome is treated with appropriate IV fluid and electrolytes, blood transfusions (if necessary), seizure control, and management of renal disease and increased intracranial pressure.

        (5) Toxic shock syndrome should be treated with IV nafcillin 100 to 150 mg/kg/d or oxacillin 150 to 200 mg/kg/d, IV fluids, vasopressors to maintain a normal BP, and ventilatory support, if necessary.

        (6) Intussusception is treated by hydrostatic reduction with contrast enema or surgery (unsuccessful hydrostatic reduction, symptoms persisting for 2 days or more, recurrent episodes, obstruction, or peritonitis).

F. ENCOPRESIS

1. Encopresis is recurrent fecal incontinence in the absence of organic disease. Approximately 1% of 7- to 8-year-olds (the peak age) are affected, with a male-to-female ratio of 3:1. Approximately half of the children have never been completely bowel trained. A single episode of fecal incontinence should not be regarded as encopresis.

a. Hypotheses regarding possible causes include premature or coercive toilet training, fear of defecation because of previous "accidents" or pain (such as from an anal fissure), mental retardation, and isolated areas of neurodevelopmental delay. Encopresis is also associated with sexual abuse involving anal penetration.

b. Organic lesions that can cause encopresis include those discussed under Section E, Point c, as well as several others such as central and peripheral nervous system disease, defects in rectal or anal musculature, chronic constipation with resultant overflow, and chronic laxative or enema use.

2. Important historical information includes the following:

a. Onset and duration of the problem.

b. Current and previous stooling patterns.

c. Age of attainment of bowel control.

d. Appearance and consistency of stools.

e. Presence of constipation.

f. Chronic enema or laxative use.

g. Pattern of growth.

h. Psychosocial, emotional, familial, and scholastic assessments; inquire about the possibility of sexual abuse.

3. The PE is usually normal. Emphasis should be placed on the neurologic examination and abdominal/rectal examinations. The anal tone should be normal but may be patulous with chronic enema use, and the rectal vault should be of normal or enlarged size with feces present.

4. The possibility of organic disease should be obvious from the history and PE; if suspected, the workup is as discussed for chronic diarrhea and chronic constipation.

a. A U/A and urine culture may demonstrate an occult urinary tract infection secondary to chronic constipation.

b. Serum chemistry studies, ESR, CBC, and radiographic studies usually are normal in children with true encopresis.

5. Treatment of encopresis includes diet manipulation, colon evacuation with enemas or laxatives, establishment of (and reward for) a normal defecation pattern, reassurance, patience, counseling and, occasionally, psychotherapy.

G. GASTROESOPHAGEAL REFLUX

1. GER is the return of stomach contents into the esophagus as a result of increased relaxation of the lower esophageal sphincter. This incompetence may result from immaturity (as in infants), esophageal disease, obstructive lung disease, or overdistension of the stomach (because of overeating). A small degree of reflux is probably universal. GER may be accompanied by effortless vomiting (infants), aspiration pneumonia (infants), apnea (infants), belching, esophagitis (all ages), and mid-epigastric pain. Pain is worse after eating, especially if the patient is supine; in contrast, the pain of an ulcer is similarly located but is relieved by eating, especially in older children and adolescents.

2. In infants with suspected GER, the following questions are helpful:

a. Is the infant vomiting (forceful projection) or "spitting up"?

b. When does this occur (e.g., how long after a meal)?

c. How is the infant fed (sitting up, laying down)? In what position is the infant placed after feeding? Does the position make a difference as to whether the infant is likely to spit up?

d. Is the infant a rapid eater? Does he or she belch?

e. How much (and what type of) formula does the infant take with each feeding? What other foods are ingested?

f.   Does the infant appear hungry?

g.   Is the infant gaining weight?

h.   What does the vomitus look like? Is it tinged with green or red?

i.   Does the infant wheeze, cough, or turn blue? When? Has the infant ever had pneumonia? When?

j.   Are there feeding difficulties? Elaborate.

k.   Does the infant have fever or diarrhea? Elaborate on the time and degree of fever and on the onset, duration, and appearance of diarrhea.

l.   Is the infant taking any medications? Which one(s)?

m.   Have any OTC preparations or home/herbal remedies been used to stop the vomiting? Which ones?

n.   In the older patient, where is the pain (if any) located? Does it radiate? What is its relation to eating and lying down? What precipitates it? What causes relief?

o.   Is the pain accompanied by fever, vomiting, diarrhea? If yes, elaborate.

p.   Has the child ever vomited blood?

q.   Does pain interfere with activities? Does it awaken the child from sleep?

3.   The PE is usually normal. Young infants, however, may have failure to thrive or (rarely) torticollis (Sandifer's syndrome).

4.   If significant vomiting, diarrhea, or failure to thrive is present, certain laboratory tests are useful to secure a diagnosis.

a.   Except for those (especially infants) who have significant reflux and may be anemic, alkalotic, and hypochloremic, patients with GER (but without failure to thrive) usually have a normal CBC and serum chemistry profile.

b.   If there are respiratory symptoms or the chest examination is abnormal, a CXR (to R/O aspiration pneumonia) is indicated.

c.   The diagnosis of mild reflux is made by the characteristic history. With moderate-to-severe reflux (especially if accompanied by failure to thrive or respiratory symptoms), the diagnosis of GER may be confirmed by pH monitoring of the lower esophagus (to correlate reflux episodes and symptoms), measurement of lower esophageal sphincter pressure, a technetium "milk scan" (to determine if there is delayed gastric emptying), or endoscopy (with or without biopsy) to look for evidence of esophagitis and other intrinsic esophageal, gastric, or duodenal pathology.

d.   For any patient with moderate-to-severe GI symptoms or weight loss, a barium swallow should be performed to confirm normal anatomy and normal gastric emptying.

Note: Many normal infants show some reflux on barium swallow, and some infants with pathologic GER have a normal swallow because of the intermittent nature of the reflux.

5.   Treatment of the infant with GER includes small, frequent feedings in the upright position; formula thickened with cereal (1 tbsp/1 oz); and maintenance of a prone head-up position after feeding.

a. If these measures fail, a trial of a prokinetic drug, such as metoclopramide (0.1 mg/kg/dose qid before meals) or bethanechol (0.1 to 0.2 mg/kg/dose qid), may be efficacious in relieving symptoms. Because of serious adverse cardiac side effects, the prokinetic agent cisapride is no longer marketed in the U.S. It is only available through a limited access program from the manufacturer.

b. If esophagitis is present, an H_2 blocker is indicated. The use of antacids is limited by concern regarding the side effects in infants and young children. Famotidine (1 mg/kg/d divided bid) or ranitidine (2 to 5 mg/kg/d divided bid or tid) may be useful.

c. Although proton pump inhibitors such as omeprazole are used widely in adults, they should be used very cautiously in children because they suppress acid more completely than H_2 blockers, stimulate gastric hypersecretion, and may disturb the gastrointestinal milieu. Use only with the input of a pediatric gastroenterologist.

d. If medical management fails, fundoplication may be necessary.

e. Treatment of the older child with GER includes small, frequent meals; maintenance of an upright position after meals; eating slowly; and no meals after 7 PM. A prokinetic drug (see earlier) should be considered if antireflux measures do not work. An H_2 blocker (famotidine 1 mg/kg/d divided bid or ranitidine 1 to 2 mg/kg/dose q 8 to 12h bid or tid [maximum dose 6 mg/kg/d]) may be necessary for *recalcitrant* cases.

H. FOREIGN-BODY INGESTION

1. The most common foreign bodies ingested by children are metal objects (especially coins), buttons, small parts of toys, hair, tablets, and button batteries.

2. Foreign bodies that lodge in the esophagus may cause dysphagia, drooling, midsternal pain or fullness, gagging, choking, coughing, or respiratory embarrassment.

a. Diagnosis is by posteroanterior and lateral x-ray studies of the chest and neck, or by a hand-held metal detector.

b. The foreign body is usually located in the upper esophagus (C4 level) at the level of the thoracic inlet.

c. Removal may be accomplished in two ways: (1) during endoscopy in the OR (preferable approach), or (2) using a No. 8 to 14 Foley catheter. With the second method, a deflated catheter is passed into the sedated child's nose and into the esophagus; the balloon is inflated, and the foreign body is removed by traction on the catheter (this approach is still controversial). The child should be taken to the OR if there is any concern about the safety of removing the foreign body in the office or ED. Because of their potential to leach chemicals, button

8

GASTROINTESTINAL DISORDERS

batteries lodged in the esophagus must be removed as soon as possible.
3. Foreign bodies that pass into the stomach generally pass out of the body in 2 to 10 days. To localize the object's position, an x-ray study should be obtained when the child is first seen. If the object does not pass in 10 days or if GI symptoms occur, the child should return for reevaluation (and possibly treatment). Emetics and cathartics should not be used.

I. JAUNDICE

1. Jaundice is clinically obvious yellowing of the skin, mucous membranes, and sclera as a result of an excess of bilirubin in the blood. Tears, saliva, secretions, and CSF may also be icteric. Jaundice is apparent when the bilirubin reaches 6 to 7 mg/dL in neonates and 2 mg/dL in older children and adolescents.
2. Important historical information to be elicited includes the following:
a. Duration of symptoms? Worsening? Improvement?
b. Associated GI or constitutional symptoms?
c. Weight loss?
d. Stool color change (e.g., clay color)?
e. Darkening of urine?
f. Pruritus?
g. Exposure to the following:
    (1) IV drug use?
    (2) Sexual activity, especially anal sex?
    (3) Persons with known hepatitis or jaundice?
    (4) Any medications associated with chemical hepatitis?
    (5) Blood or blood products?
3. A thorough PE is mandatory, with emphasis on the following:
a. Skin color
b. Scleral color
c. Liver size (palpation and percussion)
d. Abdominal (especially RUQ) tenderness
e. Abnormal abdominal vascular pattern or distension
4. Laboratory workup includes the following:
a. CBC with differential, smear, and reticulocyte count (R/O hemolysis)
b. Bilirubin (direct and indirect); LFTs
c. SMA-7, SMA-12, amylase
d. PT/PTT
e. Hepatitis serology panel (A, B, C)
f. U/A; stool examination (acholic stools)
g. Radiographic or imaging studies if a surgical cause seems likely
5. Differential diagnosis (increased indirect bilirubin)
a. Hemolysis (e.g., ABO, Rh incompatibility, sickle cell disease, α-thalassemia, drug reaction)

b. Physiologic (neonate)
c. Hypothyroidism (neonate)
d. Hereditary/constitutional hepatic dysfunction
e. Massive internal hemorrhage
f. Pyloric stenosis, duodenal atresia, annular pancreas
6. Differential diagnosis (increased direct and indirect bilirubin)
a. Infections
   (1) Hepatitis A, B, C
   (2) Epstein-Barr virus
   (3) Cytomegalovirus
   (4) Congenital rubella
   (5) Herpes virus
   (6) Syphilis
   (7) Sepsis (bacterial)
   (8) Toxoplasmosis (congenital)
   (9) Amebiasis
   (10) Leptospirosis
b. Inborn errors of metabolism
   (1) Wilson's disease
   (2) Galactosemia
   (3) Hereditary fructose intolerance
   (4) Hereditary tyrosinemia
c. Cirrhosis
d. Chemicals, including cleaning fluids, heavy metals, certain drugs
e. Congenital/Genetic
   (1) Biliary atresia
   (2) Hypoplasia or atresia of hepatic ducts
   (3) Cystic fibrosis
   (4) α_1-antitrypsin deficiency
   (5) Inspissated bile syndrome
   (6) Dubin-Johnson syndrome
f. Cholelithiasis
g. Neoplasms
   (1) Benign
   (2) Primary malignant
   (3) Metastasis
h. Pancreatic disease
7. Treatment
a. Treatment depends on the cause of the jaundice.
b. Infectious viral hepatitis is treated by symptomatic and supportive measures; persistent viral hepatitis may respond to interferon-α.
c. Bacterial infections require appropriate antibiotics.
d. Hemolysis and internal hemorrhage require blood transfusions and control of any bleeding.
e. Surgical disorders and oncologic disease are treated in consultation with those specialists, respectively.

8

GASTROINTESTINAL DISORDERS

f.   Pancreatitis is treated supportively unless complications develop. Such patients are generally given nothing by mouth and are given IV fluids with careful monitoring of vital signs, I&O, WBC, amylase, glucose, LFTs, BUN, Ca, albumin, and oxygen saturation. Pain relief is necessary.

J. PARASITES

1. Pinworms
   a. Manifestations
      (1) Intense pruritus ani, especially at night; vulvovaginitis; urinary tract infection; irritability
      (2) No eosinophilia
   b. Diagnosis
      (1) Worms may be seen in the rectal area or stool; eggs are seen in anal skinfolds and the vaginal introitus.
      (2) Scotch tape test; press tape to perianal area (best in evening before going to bed). Mount tape over a drop of toluene on a glass slide and look for ova with a microscope.
   c. Treatment
      (1) It is often best to also treat other children at home. If recurrent, treat the entire family; make sure the mother is not pregnant.
      (2) Launder bedclothes and undergarments; make sure children sleep in underwear to avoid contact of fingers with anus.
      (3) Medication
         (a) Mebendazole (Vermox); same dosage for all ages; 100 mg × 1; not much experience in children less than 2 years of age; contraindicated in pregnant women.
         (b) Pyrantel pamoate (Antiminth) 11 mg/kg to maximum of 1 g; given in a single dose.
         (c) Consider retreatment in 2 weeks. The chance for reinfestation is very high.
2. *Giardia* infection (see Section E)

K. PEPTIC ULCER DISEASE

1. PUD is the ulceration of the gastric or duodenal mucosa and results from an imbalance between the protective mechanisms of the mucosa and the effects of acid, pepsin, injury, and infection.
2. Most primary ulcers in children under 6 years of age are gastric and equally affect boys and girls. Most ulcers found in boys more than 10 years of age are duodenal. A primary duodenal ulcer is a chronic condition; at least two thirds of patients have recurrent disease after the completion of therapy.
3. Ulcers may occur because of the use of certain drugs (e.g., steroids and antiinflammatory agents), alcohol use, the stress of critical illness (e.g., Curling's ulcer associated with burns, Cushing's ulcer associated with trauma), a secondary manifestation of certain illnesses, and

infection. Any condition that interferes with the protective mechanism of the mucosa or increases acid production contributes to the genesis and persistence of an ulcer.

4. *H. pylori* is a spirochete-like organism, specific to the gastric mucosa, which elaborates an enzyme (urease) that is capable of degrading gastric mucin. Epidemics have been related to contaminated water, travel, and raw milk. It seems to be a seasonal disease, peaking in June and November, and has been recognized as the most common cause of recurrent PUD in adults. In children, infection with *H. pylori* manifests primarily as antral gastritis. There are invasive (gastric mucosa biopsy for culture, histology, rapid urease test) and noninvasive (ELISA, latex agglutination, urea breath test) tests that can be used to document *H. pylori* infection. Workup should be carried out in conjunction with a pediatric gastroenterologist.

5. Psychological factors play a role in some patients. They have been described as bright overachievers, and they sometimes have anger or hostility (overt or covert). Peptic complaints are also common during times of divorce, an impending move, or child abuse.

6. Symptoms vary with age. In infants and young children, the symptoms are often feeding difficulties, vomiting, unexplained crying, or upper/lower GI bleeding. The pain may be periumbilical or poorly localized, may not be more prevalent at certain times of the day, and may not be affected by the types of foods or beverages ingested. On the other hand, older children and adolescents have adult-like symptoms, such as epigastric (or RUQ) pain approximately 1 hour after meals. When pain is related to esophagitis, it is relieved by eating or by antacids and is exacerbated by the ingestion of soda, juices, tomatoes, any acidic food or beverage, alcohol, and spices.

7. The PE often reveals epigastric tenderness to palpation. There may be evidence of blood in the vomitus or stools. Therefore every child with suspected ulcer disease should have a stool test for occult blood. A baseline CBC is useful to assess the degree and chronicity of bleeding.

8. If any significant or recurrent GI bleeding is noted, consultation with a pediatric gastroenterologist is advisable.

9. Treatment of uncomplicated PUD.

a. Antacids are no longer the mainstay of therapy because they are weak buffers of hydrochloric acid and cause diarrhea (magnesium) or acid-rebound (calcium). They may also interfere with the absorption (or excretion) of other medications.

b. H_2 blockers inhibit gastric secretion. Famotidine is used at a dosage of 0.5 mg/kg/d at bedtime or divided twice daily (maximum 40 mg/day). Ranitidine is used at a dosage of 1 to 2 mg/kg/dose bid or tid (maximum dose 6 mg/kg/d).

c. The use of anticholinergics is limited to severe ulcer disease in combination with H_2 antagonists.

d. The therapy of *H. pylori* in childhood includes antibiotics (amoxicillin or clarithromycin [Biaxin] plus metronidazole) and bismuth given for 3 to 6 weeks.

e. Treatment must continue for several weeks to months; exacerbations and recurrences are common. Psychotherapy may be in order for patients with marked psychological symptoms.

L. VOMITING

1. The history should differentiate between real vomiting and "spitting up."

a. Important questions about vomiting relate to its frequency, severity, appearance (blood- or bile-tinged), amount, time of occurrence, projectile nature, and duration after meals.

b. What has the child taken by mouth (foods, medicines, poison)?

c. How has the parent treated the vomiting?

d. Are there associated symptoms (e.g., fever, headache, earache, sore throat, cough, asthma, abdominal pain, diarrhea, rash, lethargy, seizures)?

e. If the patient is a young infant (1 to 3 months of age) with projectile vomiting, suspect pyloric stenosis or other gastric outlet processes (malrotation, annular pancreas).

f. Is there any possibility of an ingestion (e.g., ipecac)?

2. The PE should include an assessment of the patient's vital signs, weight, and hydration. Specific areas to highlight in the examination include the following:

a. HEENT: Fundi (papilledema), ears (otitis media), throat (pharyngitis, cervical adenopathy), fontanelle (bulging vs. sunken)

b. Respiratory tract: Coughing/wheezing

c. Abdomen: Pain, distension, bowel sounds, hepatosplenomegaly, palpable "olive"

d. Genitourinary: R/O infection, pregnancy, toxic shock syndrome

e. Skin: Rash

f. Neurologic: Lethargy, paresthesias, seizures, focal signs

3. Laboratory studies depend on the suspected cause.

a. Blood: CBC, electrolytes, glucose, BUN, creatinine, ammonia, medication or toxicology levels

b. Urine: With or without metabolic screen, urine specific gravity, glucosuria, ketonuria, microscopic, with or without culture

4. Causes include infection (viral, rotavirus, Norwalk virus, bacterial enterotoxins), metabolic (diabetic ketoacidosis, inborn error of metabolism), increased ICP (meningitis, Reye's syndrome, tumor), GI obstruction (pyloric stenosis), ingestions.

5. Treatment: Outpatient therapy should be tried if the cause appears to be a self-limited infectious process (e.g., viral, enterotoxin) and if the

patient is not significantly dehydrated and can retain sufficient liquids to maintain hydration.

a. Discontinue solid foods and milk for 12 to 18 hours.

b. Infants: Oral glucose-electrolyte solution, with frequent, small feedings × 12 to 24 hours. Advance to regular diet as tolerated over 24 to 48 hours.

c. Older children: Oral glucose-electrolyte solution (especially the flavored ones), Cola, Kool-Aid, Hawaiian Punch, popsicles; frequent, small feedings × 12 to 24 hours. Advance to BRATS diet as quickly as tolerated; finally, advance to a regular diet.

M. BIBLIOGRAPHY

8

Abdominal Pain

Ashcroft K: Acute abdominal pain, *Pediatr in Rev* 21:363, 2000.

Boyle JT: Recurrent abdominal pain, *Pediatr in Rev* 18:310, 1997.

Dern M, Stein M: He keeps getting stomachaches, Doctor. What's wrong? *Contemp Pediatr* 16:43, 1999.

Oberlander T, Rappaport L: Recurrent abdominal pain during childhood, *Pediatr Rev* 14:313, 1993.

Gastrointestinal Bleeding

Rodgers B: Upper gastrointestinal hemorrhage, *Pediatr in Rev* 20:171, 1999.

Squires R: Gastrointestinal bleeding, *Pediatr in Rev* 20:95, 1999.

Constipation

Abi-Hanna A, Lake A: Constipation and encopresis in childhood, *Pediatr in Rev* 19:23, 1998.

Felt B, Wise C, Olsom A et al: Guideline for the management of pediatric idiopathic constipation and soiling, *Arch Pediatr Adolesc Med* 153:380, 1999.

Guerrero R, Cavender C: Constipation—physical and psychological sequelae, *Pediatr Ann* 28:312, 1999.

Parker P: To do or not to do? That is the question. *Pediatr Ann* 28:283, 1999.

Diarrhea

AAP: Practice parameter—the management of acute gastroenteritis in young children, *Pediatrics* 97:424, 1996.

Burkhart D: Management of acute gastroenteritis in children, *Am Fam Physician* 60:2555, 1999.

Eliason BC, Lewan R: Gastroenteritis in children—principles of diagnosis and treatment, *Am Fam Physician* 58:1769, 1998.

Judd R: Chronic nonspecific diarrhea, *Pediatr in Rev* 17:379, 1996.

Liacouras C, Baldassano R: Is it toddler's diarrhea? *Contemp Pediatr* 15:131, 1998.

Liebelt E: Clinical and laboratory evaluation and management of children with vomiting, diarrhea, and dehydration, *Curr Op in Pediatr* 10:461, 1998.

Limbos MA, Lieberman J: Management of acute diarrhea in children, *Contemp Pediatr* 12:68, 1995.

Vanderhoof J: Chronic diarrhea, *Pediatr in Rev* 19:418, 1998.

Encopresis

Abi-Hanna A, Lake A: Constipation and encopresis in childhood, *Pediatr in Rev* 19:23, 1998.

Buttross S: Encopresis in the child with a behavioral disorder, *Pediatr Ann* 28:317, 1999.

Nolan T, Oberklaid F: New concepts in the management of encopresis, *Pediatr Rev* 14:447, 1993.

Gastroesophageal Reflux

Faubion W: Gastroesophageal reflux in infants and children, *Mayp Cl Proceed* 73:166, 1998.

Levy J: Gastroesophageal reflux and other causes of abdominal pain, *Pediatr Ann* 30:42, 2001.

Mason D: Gastroesophageal reflux in children, *Nurs Cl NA* 35:15, 2000.

Orenstein S: Gastroesophageal reflux, *Pediatr in Rev* 20:24, 1999.

Orenstein S, Izadnia F, Khan S: Gastroesophageal reflux disease in children, *Gastro Cl NA* 28:947, 1999.

GASTROINTESTINAL DISORDERS

Foreign-Body Ingestion

McGahren E: Esophageal foreign bodies, *Pediatr in Rev* 20:129, 1999.

Muniz A, Joffe M: Foreign bodies, ingested and inhaled, *Contemp Pediatr* 14:78, 1997.

Jaundice

Krugman S: Viral hepatitis A, B, C, D & E: infection, *Pediatr Rev* 13:203, 1992.

Krugman S: Viral hepatitis A, B, C, D & E: prevention, *Pediatr Rev* 13:245, 1992.

Peptic Ulcer Disease

Jones N, Sherman P: *Helicobacter pylori* infection in children, *Curr Op in Pediatr* 10:19, 1998.

Mezoff A, Balistreri W: Peptic ulcer disease in children, *Pediatr in Rev* 16:257, 1995.

Vomiting

Murray K: Vomiting, *Pediatr in Rev* 19:337, 1998.

Murray K, Christie D: Vomiting in infancy—when should you worry? *Contemp Pediatr* 17:81, 2000.

GENITOURINARY DISORDERS

A. DYSURIA, HESITANCY, URGENCY, DRIBBLING

1. Dysuria (painful urination), hesitancy (inability to start stream), urgency (heightened pressure to void), and dribbling (passing a few drops of urine after voiding is completed) may be signs of a UTI, genital infection, perineal irritation (trauma, tight clothing, harsh soaps, bubble baths, shampooing in the bath, masturbation), sexual abuse, or emotional disorder.
2. Carry out a pertinent history, PE, and laboratory workup (see Section B).
3. Treatment is directed toward the underlying disorder.

B. FREQUENCY

1. *Frequency* denotes a pattern of increased urination compared with an individual's normal pattern. There may be more frequent voiding episodes, more urine produced with each episode, or both.
2. Important historical information includes the following:
a. Age of attainment of bladder control
b. Normal voiding pattern
c. Duration of new pattern
d. Amount and types of fluids ingested each day
e. Ingestion of medications or caffeine-containing products
f. Possibility of trauma or abuse
g. Presence of other GU symptoms (dysuria, hesitancy, urgency, enuresis, change in urine color or odor)
3. The PE should be complete. Pay particular attention to the perineum (e.g., redness and swelling of urethral meatus and penile discharge; redness, bruises, swelling, or excoriations of the urethral meatus, labia, or clitoral area; vaginal discharge or odor). The perianal area should be examined for excoriations and signs of trauma.
4. Urine should be microscopically examined for blood cells and bacteria. The pH and specific gravity of the urine should be assessed; the presence of glucose, protein, ketones, blood, and bilirubin should be determined by dipstick. A culture and Gram's stain are indicated if there is penile or vaginal discharge.
5. Causes of frequency
a. UTI (see Section O).
b. Diabetes mellitus: Dipstick positive for glucose (with or without ketones) necessitates a serum glucose determination (see Chapter 6).
c. Diabetes insipidus: Failure to raise urine specific gravity above 1.010, even with 6 to 12 hours of fluid deprivation, necessitates a serum osmolality determination.
d. Vaginitis/urethritis/labial adhesions (see Section P).
e. Excessive fluid intake.
f. Diuretic, caffeine, or theophylline intake.

g. Irritation of urethra/vagina, especially trauma, tight clothing, harsh soaps, bubble baths or shampooing in the bath, masturbation.

h. Emotional problems.

i. Sexual abuse.

6. Treatment of frequency is accomplished by correcting the underlying condition.

C. ENURESIS

1. Enuresis is involuntary urination that occurs after a child has reached the age when bladder control is usually attained (4 years of age).

a. Children who have never attained bladder control have primary enuresis; those who have had such control but subsequently lose it have secondary enuresis.

b. Before 5 years of age, primary enuresis is more common; secondary enuresis is more common after 5 years of age.

c. Enuresis may be nocturnal, diurnal, or both. Diurnal enuresis in a child older than 5 years of age usually is associated with an organic disorder.

2. Important historical information includes the following:

a. Age of attainment of bladder control

b. Type of enuresis (nocturnal, diurnal); if nocturnal, the time in the night during which urination occurs

c. Frequency of accidents

d. How the child is treated after an accident

e. Possible precipitating events (e.g., too busy playing to go to the bathroom)

f. Presence of other GU symptoms (dysuria, obvious hematuria, frequency, urgency, hesitancy, dribbling, itching)

g. Presence of constipation

h. Amount and types of fluids ingested in an average day

i. Presence of psychological problems or a change in the child's familial, social, or scholastic milieu

j. Age of successful toilet training of siblings and parents

k. Concomitant presence of encopresis

3. A complete PE, including a neurologic assessment, should be performed; it is usually normal.

a. The BP should be measured (initial screen for renal pathology).

b. Give particular attention to the perineum to determine the presence of erythema, edema, signs of trauma, anatomic anomalies, or the presence of urethral/vaginal discharge. Give particular attention to the sacral area for dimpling or cutaneous anomalies that might indicate a spinal abnormality.

c. The child's abdomen should be palpated for organomegaly (bladder and kidneys), stool, and masses.

d. A rectal examination should be performed; especially note sphincter tone.

4. U/A and urine culture should be performed for all children with enuresis. Radiographic evaluation and/or ultrasound of the GU tract is necessary for children with diurnal enuresis, recalcitrant enuresis, constant dribbling, or external GU anatomic anomalies.

5. Some causes of enuresis are as follows:

a. UTI (see Section O)

b. Ectopic ureter

c. Other GU organic lesions

d. Miscellaneous GU problems (e.g., vaginal reflux of urine, labial fusion, postvoid dribble syndrome, giggle incontinence, stress incontinence, unstable bladder detrussor muscle)

e. Small bladder capacity (maturational delay in size)

f. Ingestion of increased amounts of fluids

g. Intake of caffeine, theophylline, chocolate, diuretics

h. Inattention (too busy to void)

i. Psychological problems (e.g., fear, anger, resentment, especially in conjunction with a new sibling or a change in the child's social, familial, or scholastic milieu)

j. Diabetes mellitus, diabetes insipidus

k. Post-ictal states

l. Child abuse, especially sexual abuse

m. Perineal irritation (e.g., masturbation, trauma, infection, chemical irritation)

6. Treatment of primary enuresis includes the following:

a. Reassurance (spontaneous cure rate of 10% per year after 5 years of age).

b. Bladder stretching exercises are recommended by some authorities. The family establishes the child's baseline I&O; the child is then encouraged to force fluids and hold urine for as long as possible each day; 3 to 6 months is required.

c. A reward system for a certain number of dry nights (goal should be attainable and dynamic).

d. Discouraging fluid intake after dinner.

e. Encouraging voiding before bedtime.

f. An enuresis alarm (alarm awakens sleeping child at the initiation of urination so that ultimately he or she awakens when his or her bladder is full but he or she has not yet voided).

g. Counseling, hypnotherapy, or psychotherapy (if indicated).

h. The use of imipramine had been widely advocated; it depresses both bladder contractions and REM sleep. However, recent studies have questioned the association of enuresis with a particular stage of sleep. Concerns regarding the myocardial effects of imipramine and its potential for overdosage have discouraged its use.

i. The use of intranasal DDAVP has been used in the treatment of nocturnal enuresis; it comes in both tablet form and nasal spray. The initial spray dose is 20 mcg (one spray each nostril) hs with a gradual increase to 40 mcg (2 sprays each nostril) hs if needed. The initial tablet dose is 0.2 mg (one tablet) with *gradual* increases to a maximum of 0.6 mg hs (3 tablets). Complete remission is seen in 25% of patients using nasal spray and 35% of patients taking the tablets. Side effects are few; nasal irritation is associated with use of the nasal spray, and there is a slight risk of water intoxication, especially if excessive fluids are consumed.

j. Oxybutynin has been found to be useful for children who have polysymptomatic enuresis. The dosage is 5 mg hs (5 to 12 years of age) and 10 mg hs (over 12 years of age). Its efficacy is increased with an enuresis alarm.

k. Children with secondary enuresis should have the precipitating disorder addressed and managed.

D. GLOMERULONEPHRITIS (ACUTE)

1. AGN refers to a disorder characterized by smoke-colored, tea-colored, or grossly bloody urine with proteinuria, RBC casts, hyaline casts, and granular casts.

2. Many etiologies are implicated in the genesis of AGN; the best described is poststreptococcal AGN. In this entity, immune complexes are deposited along the glomerular basement membrane and activate the complement system, which leads to a release of more inflammatory agents and recruitment of inflammatory cells to the area.

3. Clinically, a child can have brown, smoky, or red urine 1 to 3 weeks after a sore throat. Urine output may be decreased, and edema (especially periorbital) may be present. The child may (rarely) have florid CHF or acute hypertensive encephalopathy. Regardless of the etiology, any of the nephritides can appear in this manner.

4. On PE, the child may be entirely asymptomatic or severely ill depending on the amount of renal involvement at the time of presentation.

5. Laboratory tests include the following:

a. Urine for culture and for U/A; U/A shows hematuria and 2+ proteinuria or greater. Microscopic examination of the urine reveals RBC casts and leukocyturia.

b. Chemistries may be normal or markedly abnormal (decreased Na, increased K, increased BUN, increased creatinine). Total proteins may be normal or decreased (especially albumin).

c. CBC is usually normal but may show anemia depending on the amount and duration of blood loss. The ESR is elevated during the acute phase.

d. Streptococcus serologic tests (ASO, antihyaluronidase, antideoxyribonuclease), as well as ANA, C4 and C3 (decreased), should be obtained. A TC and a culture of any area of pyoderma should be obtained.

e. If the patient is hypertensive, a CXR should be obtained to assess the presence/degree of CHF.

6. Therapy

a. Admit any child with AGN who has oliguria or hypertension. If oliguria and edema are present, fluids are restricted to 300 to 400 ml/m^2 and Na intake is limited to 1 to 2 mEq/kg/d. If severe edema does not respond to furosemide, metolazone (Zaroxolyn) 0.07 to 0.14 mg/kg/d might be useful.

b. If the patient is in CHF, administer O_2, place the head up, and give 0.5 to 1.0 mg/kg furosemide IV.

Note: The daily dosage of furosemide varies between 1 and 5 mg/kg/d, depending on the degree of renal impairment.

c. If the patient is hypertensive, give a diuretic; in addition, amlodipine 0.1 to 0.3 mg/kg/dose (maximum dose 0.6 mg/kg/d) qd or bid may be required.

d. If the patient is severely hypoalbuminemic, a long-acting calcium channel blocker might be necessary.

e. If a child is only mildly affected, he or she may be discharged home. The parent should place the child on a low-sodium diet, weigh him or her each day, and measure the urine output. The parent should also be aware of signs of increasing BP and fluid retention. Follow-up is mandatory in 2 to 3 days, sooner if there are problems. Consultation with a pediatric nephrologist is advisable.

E. HEMATURIA

1. The presence of microscopic hematuria may be noted by dipstick in asymptomatic children during health assessment visits. Remember, a dipstick is very sensitive and may be positive in the presence of only 2 to 5 RBCs/HPF. When macroscopic hematuria is present, it is usually the reason for the child's visit.

2. Causes of macroscopic hematuria

a. Trauma, masturbation

b. Tumors

c. Sickle cell trait

d. Renal stones

e. Hypercalciuria without stones

f. Hyperuricosuria

g. GU disorders

h. Thin basement membrane (benign recurrent hematuria)

i. Alport's syndrome (hereditary nephritis with nerve deafness)

j. Glomerulonephritis (smoke-colored urine, hypertension, oliguria, edema)

k. Hemorrhagic cystitis

l. UTI

m. Hematospermia (in adolescent males)

n. IgA nephropathy (Berger's disease)

3. Microscopic (or variable) hematuria may be present in the conditions listed previously and also in the following:

a. Connective tissue disease-induced nephritis

9

GENITOURINARY DISORDERS

b. HUS
c. HSP
d. Leukemia
e. Certain malignancies
f. Thrombocytopenia or clotting disorders
g. Renal vein thrombosis
h. Subacute bacterial endocarditis
i. Hemangiomas of the GU tract
j. Polycystic renal disease
k. Urinary tract anomalies
l. Renal tuberculosis
m. Hydronephrosis
n. Mumps
o. Rubeola
p. Varicella
q. Malaria
r. Schistosomiasis
s. Exercise, running, boxing, wrestling
t. Drugs or toxins (e.g., aspirin, anticoagulants, amitriptyline [Elavil], lead, methicillin, phenol, sulfa drugs, and turpentine)

4. History should elicit the following:
a. Onset and duration of the hematuria
b. Urine color (or color change) and intensity
c. Any other GU symptoms; previous GU disease, surgery, or instrumentation
d. History of edema, rash, joint symptoms
e. History of trauma, chronic medical conditions, medication use or ingestions
f. Antecedent sore throat and date of its occurrence (AGN)
g. Colicky pain, back pain (stones)
h. Allergies
i. Diet history, including ingestion of red/orange/purple substances
j. Easy bleeding or bruising (hematologic disorders); history of sickle cell disease
k. Bloody diarrhea (HUS, HSP)
l. Dyspnea, fatigue, or change in a known murmur (SBE); other history of heart disease
m. Other illnesses present concomitantly (e.g., mumps, varicella, rubeola)
n. Travel history (malaria, schistosomiasis)
o. Exertion
p. History of connective tissue disease
q. Deafness in patient or other family members (Alport's syndrome)
r. Other family members with hematuria (familial hematuria) or other renal disease, connective tissue disease, or sickle cell disease

5. A complete PE must be performed. It may be normal or markedly abnormal depending on the cause of the bleeding. The child's vital signs should be assessed and stabilized if unstable. The presence or absence of the following should be noted:

a. HEENT: Periorbital edema, malformed ears, pharyngeal erythema/exudate
b. Chest: Rales or rubs, precordial activity, cardiac murmurs or gallop
c. Abdomen: Masses, ascites, bruits, trauma
d. Back: Flank tenderness
e. GU: Meatal stenosis, discharge, trauma
f. Extremities: Edema, arthritis
g. Skin: Rash, petechiae, purpura

6. Laboratory tests are dictated by the clinical findings
a. Macroscopic hematuria should be evaluated with a CBC, differential, platelet count, and clotting studies. Obtain serum BUN and creatinine, electrolytes, and sickle cell preparation (if the child is African-American and his or her sickle cell status is unknown).
b. If AGN is suspected, an ESR, ANA, IgA, serum complement (C3) level, ASO titer, and TC should be obtained.
c. If SBE is suspected, a cardiac ECHO and multiple blood cultures should be obtained.
d. When stones are suspected, an ultrasound or a flat plate of the abdomen should be obtained.
e. If trauma has occurred, an ultrasound or IVP may localize the lesion.

7. Treatment is directed toward the underlying condition.
a. Some conditions require no specific therapy but only reassurance (sickle trait, benign hematuria, Alport's syndrome).
b. Other conditions have recurrent hematuria as part of their constellation (e.g., connective tissue diseases). Patients should be alerted with instructions regarding which symptoms require attention.
c. Surgical problems and significant trauma should be addressed.
d. Infections should be treated with the appropriate antimicrobials.
e. Malignancies and tumors are treated surgically or with chemotherapy.
f. Hematologic disorders are treated with replacement therapy, when appropriate (e.g., fresh-frozen plasma, whole blood).
g. HUS and HSP are discussed elsewhere (see Sections F and G, respectively).
h. AGN is discussed in Section D.
i. Hypercalciuria may be treated with sodium citrate/citric acid (Bicitra) or a chlorothiazide diuretic.
j. Hyperuricosuria is treated with allopurinol.

F. HEMOLYTIC-UREMIC SYNDROME

1. HUS is characterized by microangiopathic hemolytic anemia (in association with glomerular endothelial injury), thrombocytopenia, and azotemia.

2. HUS occurs worldwide and in all races; it seems to be more common during the summer and fall.

3. HUS is associated with a number of infectious agents, including cytotoxic *Escherichia coli* strains (especially *E. coli* 0157:H7), *Shigella dysenteriae,* and *Streptococcus pneumoniae.*

4. Important historical information includes diarrhea (watery or bloody) 3 to 12 days before the onset of HUS symptoms with or without vomiting or abdominal pain. Inquire about consumption of ground beef. Symptoms of HUS include irritability, restlessness, pallor, oliguria/anuria, edema, and signs of fluid overload (increased BP, pulmonary congestion, and edema).

5. The PE should be complete, with careful attention to the nervous system (irritability, lethargy, ataxia, hemiparesis, focal signs, seizures, coma), the abdomen (hyperactive bowel sounds, ascites, enlarged liver), the extremities (edema), the chest (rales, rubs, cardiac gallop, new or worsening murmur), and the skin (petechiae, purpura, oozing from orifices or venipuncture sites).

6. Laboratory evaluation includes a CBC (increased WBC with shift to the left, decreased Hct), peripheral smear (evidence of fragmented RBCs), platelet count (commonly less than 40,000), fibrin degradation products (increased), PT/PTT (usually normal), electrolytes (increased K, decreased Na), BUN and creatinine (increased), uric acid (increased), P (increased), triglycerides (increased), bilirubin (sometimes increased), LFTs (increased), and an acidotic pH.

7. Differential diagnosis
a. Other renal diseases
   (1) AGN
   (2) SLE with nephropathy
   (3) Overwhelming sepsis
   (4) Vasculitis
b. Other causes of microangiopathic hemolytic anemia
   (1) Acute liver failure
   (2) Nephrotic syndrome with intravascular thrombosis
   (3) Malignant hypertension
   (4) SBE
   (5) Valvular heart disease
   (6) Coarctation of the aorta
   (7) DIC
   (8) Sepsis (especially with meningococcus or herpes)

8. Therapy
a. Renal manifestations
   (1) Follow weights carefully.
   (2) Restrict fluids to insensible losses plus measured losses.
   (3) Monitor electrolytes frequently; correct as needed.
   (4) Consider dialysis if there is severe fluid overload, severe hyperkalemia, severe acidosis, hyponatremia, or oliguria/anuria.

    (5) Control hypertension by maintaining normovolemia, avoiding overtransfusion, and using antihypertensive agents (see hypertension section in Chapter 22).

    (6) Dialysis may be necessary in cases of progressive uremia, volume overload/electrolyte imbalances/metabolic acidosis that are unresponsive to medical management.

b. Hematologic abnormalities

    (1) Maintain Hgb over 6 to 8 g/dL with infusions of washed RBCs.

    (2) Avoid platelet transfusion unless symptomatic bleeding.

    (3) Avoid plasma transfusion in pneumococcal-neuraminidase HUS.

c. Maintain caloric intake parenterally or enterally.

G. HENOCH-SCHÖENLEIN PURPURA

1. HSP is also referred to as anaphylactoid, allergic, or rheumatoid purpura; leukocytoclastic vasculitis; or allergic vasculitis.

2. The etiology of HSP is unresolved. Seventy-five percent of the cases occur in children between 2 and 11 years of age; the disease is rare in adults. The male-to-female ratio is 1.5:1 to 2.0:1. More cases occur during the spring and fall.

3. HSP is thought to be an IgA-mediated vasculitis involving the small vessels of involved organs. The renal lesions of HSP are indistinguishable from those of IgA nephropathy (Berger's disease).

4. Seventy-five percent of patients give a history of preceding upper respiratory infection.

5. The hallmarks of HSP are nonthrombocytopenic purpuric rash, abdominal pain, arthritis, and nephritis.

a. The rash may consist of urticarial wheals, erythematous maculopapules, petechiae, or purpura; there is no associated thrombocytopenia. Lesions usually occur on the lower extremities and buttocks. They may initially blanch on pressure. Purpuric lesions evolve from red to purple and become rust-colored with a brownish hue; eventually they fade. Angioedema (nonpitting) of the scalp and extremities occurs.

b. Arthralgias and arthritis occur commonly in HSP. Joint involvement (most commonly ankles and knees) tends to be periarticular; involved joints are swollen, tender, and painful on motion.

c. Most patients with HSP have colicky abdominal pain, which usually follows the skin changes in timing. Vomitus and stools may contain blood, either grossly or microscopically. The pain is a result of submucosal and intramural extravasation of fluid and blood into the intestinal wall. Intussusception (usually ileoileal) may occur and is best diagnosed by ultrasound.

d. Patients who develop renal disease do so within 3 months of the onset of rash; persistence of the rash for 2 to 3 months is associated with nephropathy. Renal disease ranges from transient microscopic hematuria to rapidly progressive glomerulonephritis. Patients may develop a nephritic syndrome (hematuria, hypertension, azotemia, oliguria) or a nephritic-nephrotic syndrome (24-hour protein excretion greater than 50 mg/kg/d and serum albumin less than 2.5 mg/dL). A syndrome with components of both nephritis and nephrosis is more predictive of renal failure and chronic renal disease than is nephritis alone, and the presence of nephrotic-range proteinuria is the most accurate predictor of long-term renal failure.

e. Patients with HSP can have thrombocytosis, increased ESR, factor VIII deficiency, vitamin K deficiency, and hypoprothrombinemia.

f. CNS involvement in HSP is rare and usually manifests as headache and mood or mental status changes. However, nearly every type of central and peripheral nervous system dysfunction has been reported anecdotally.

g. Testicular swelling or pain may result from vasculitis of the scrotal vessels.

6. Differential diagnosis

a. Abdominal symptoms: R/O acute abdomen, intussusception

b. Joint symptoms: R/O acute rheumatic fever, rheumatoid arthritis, SLE, periarteritis nodosa

c. Rash: R/O sepsis, drug reaction, hemorrhagic diathesis (e.g., immune thrombocytopenic purpura), abuse

d. Renal symptoms: R/O AGN

e. Testicular symptoms: R/O hernia, testicular torsion, orchitis

7. Laboratory tests include CBC (normal to low Hct, increased WBC with shift to the left), ESR (increased), electrolytes (normal), BUN and creatinine (increased according to degree of renal disease), serum proteins (occasionally decreased albumin), factors VIII and XIII (decreased), C3 (occasionally low), serum IgA (may be increased). Many children with HSP present with the majority of their laboratory studies in the normal range.

8. Therapy

a. No specific therapy is available.

b. Prednisone 1 to 2 mg/kg/d × 5 to 7 days is useful for abdominal colic, marked joint symptoms, and testicular swelling.

c. In the acute presentation, monitor hydration, Hct, blood in stools; D/C all unnecessary drugs.

d. For any child with HSP and a nephritic-nephrotic picture, involve a pediatric nephrologist *early* in the illness.

H. HERNIA

1. An inguinal hernia is the protrusion of abdominal structures into the scrotum or inguinal region. This protrusion is a result of the persistence of a peritoneal sac, the processus vaginalis, which normally becomes fibrotic late in gestation after testicular descent.

a. Hernias may occur in both males and females because the processus vaginalis precedes both the testis in its descent into the inguinal canal and scrotum and the round ligament in its descent into the canal and labia.

b. The male-to-female ratio of hernias is 5:1 to 6:1. In a female patient, bilateral inguinal hernias with palpable contents (gonads?) should prompt suspicion of an endocrine or intergender problem.

c. Most (85% to 90%) hernias are unilateral; the right side predominates, and the size is variable.

2. Important historical information includes duration and location of the mass, whether it changes in size (especially if it becomes larger on exertion or crying), and the events that precipitate size changes. Incarceration of the hernia is suggested by a history of vomiting, scant stooling, melena, irritability, or abdominal distension.

3. On PE, a mass may be palpated in the scrotum or labia. It may be more easily appreciated if the child is crying or straining (increased intraabdominal pressure).

a. The hernia usually does not transilluminate, and bowel sounds are usually heard on auscultation over the hernia sac.

b. Most hernias are manually reducible because the contents of the processus ordinarily slide in and out of the abdominal cavity. However, the hernia may not be reducible if the neck of the sac closes over the herniated abdominal contents (incarcerated hernia).

c. If the hernia is tender, swollen, and warm, it is strangulated. Vascular compromise may lead to bowel ischemia and perforation.

4. Treatment is surgical.

a. The hernia sac (patent processus vaginalis) is closed at the inguinal ring. Because there is a significant incidence of a contralateral hernia sac, bilateral exploration may be performed. Surgical repair should be performed as soon as possible after the hernia is discovered.

b. An incarcerated hernia may be manually reduced under sedation. If successful, a herniorrhaphy should be performed within 1 to 2 days; if unsuccessful, immediate surgery is necessary.

I. HYDROCELE

1. A hydrocele is a collection of peritoneal fluid in the scrotum. An accompanying hernia may or may not be present. If the size of the hydrocele varies over time, suspect a somewhat open tunica vaginalis (communicating hydrocele). If the size of the hydrocele is constant, the tunica vaginalis is closed.

2. Important historical information includes the duration of scrotal swelling and whether the size of the swelling varies both during rest and during times of emotional unrest (crying, fear).

3. On PE, the hydrocele feels ovoid or round, smooth, and nontender. Scrotal skin is normal. A hydrocele may be differentiated from a hernia in several ways. A hydrocele cannot be reduced; a hernia usually can. A hydrocele is translucent when transilluminated, whereas a hernia is

not. Auscultation of the scrotum reveals bowel sounds when a hernia is present but not when there is a hydrocele.

4. A hydrocele that is constant in size usually indicates that a hernia is not present; no treatment is necessary because the fluid gradually reabsorbs. If the hydrocele is accompanied by a hernia, treatment is as discussed for hernia (see Section H).

J. PENILE PROBLEMS (ACQUIRED)

1. Phimosis/paraphimosis

a. Phimosis exists when a tight foreskin precludes its ability to be retracted so that the glans can be exposed. Paraphimosis is an inability to replace the foreskin over the glans after retracting it.

b. The foreskin should never be forcibly retracted to "clean the penis" because doing so may lead to paraphimosis.

c. Paraphimosis is a medical emergency because venous and lymphatic congestion results.

d. On PE, phimosis presents as a tight foreskin incapable of any retraction; paraphimosis presents as a markedly edematous foreskin in a retracted position.

e. A child with phimosis should be referred to a urologist, especially if hygiene is a problem or if the patient has had a UTI.

f. A child with paraphimosis requires urgent care; urology consultation should be obtained when simple reduction cannot be accomplished. Steps must be taken to decompress the edema so that there is no vascular compromise to the penis. Various techniques have been suggested: applying ice or a compression dressing followed by manual pressure on the glans (similar to turning a sock inside out) to return the foreskin to its usual position (note that this procedure is performed after a local anesthetic is administered); a dorsal slit; or a "puncture" in the edematous foreskin (with subsequent manual reduction), which obviates the need for a dorsal slit.

g. Counseling must be given to parents to prevent recurrence of the problem.

2. Balanitis

a. Balanitis is an infection or inflammation of the foreskin as a result of trauma, poor hygiene, or an STD that may extend onto the glans.

b. History reveals a painful penis; PE reveals a swollen, tender, erythematous penis.

c. If there is a penile discharge, perform a Gram's stain and send a culture of the discharge. Urine should be examined microscopically and sent for culture, if appropriate.

d. Therapy includes sitz baths (warm soaks) and ampicillin 50 to 100 mg/kg/d ÷ q6h.

3. Penile trauma

a. Bruising or minor lacerations of the penis usually result from straddle injuries, falls, blunt trauma (e.g., hit with a ball or bat, toilet seat entrapment), and zipper entrapment. The possibility of abuse must always be considered.

b. The history should ascertain how the injury occurred; be careful to ascertain whether the story fits the injury. The penis can appear swollen and bruised with or without a laceration. Be sure to check for other signs of trauma, anal tears, and penile discharge. Make sure the child can void. Check urine for the presence of blood.

c. Obtain a GU consult if blood is seen at the meatus, if a large amount of blood is in the urine, or if there is significant penile laceration or swelling. A VCUG and exploration with the patient under anesthesia may be needed to verify urethral integrity.

d. If zipper entrapment is the problem, consider applying mineral oil to the foreskin and zipper, which eases the skin's release from the zipper; unfastening the zipper one tooth at a time; cutting the median bar of the zipper with a wire cutter; or cutting the cloth strips that are holding the zipper. If in doubt, call a urologist.

e. Therapy is directed toward decreasing the swelling. Sitz baths (warm soaks) are useful.

4. Strangulation

a. Strangulation of the penis may occur as a result of an encircling hair, thread, or fiber that produces venous engorgement and edema.

b. Obtain a GU consult even if the hair/thread can be cut. Sometimes it is difficult to locate the hair/thread because of the degree of edema.

c. Keep in mind the possibility of abuse.

5. Priapism

a. Priapism is prolonged, painful (because of ischemia) penile erection.

b. Common causes of priapism are trauma, sickle cell disease, and leukemic infiltration.

c. Treatment of sickle cell disease-associated priapism includes hydration and RBC transfusion or exchange transfusion.

d. Other therapies suggested are ice baths or, alternatively, warm soaks.

K. PROTEINURIA

1. When protein is present in the urine, its concentration may be estimated by a dipstick impregnated with tetrabromophenolphthalein:

a. Trace = 10 mg/100 ml

b. 1+ = 30 mg/100 ml

c. 2+ = 100 mg/100 ml

d. 3+ = 300 mg/100 ml

e. 4+ = 1000 mg/100 ml

2. Some degree of proteinuria is found in 5% to 15% of routine U/As. A falsely positive dipstick test for proteinuria may occur if the urine pH is basic.

a. Total daily protein excretion should be less than 100 $mg/m^2/d$ or less than 4 $mg/m^2/h$.

9

GENITOURINARY DISORDERS

3. Transient proteinuria

a. Transient proteinuria may result from fever, epinephrine, cold exposure, blood transfusions, burns, or exercise.

b. Orthostatic proteinuria is present in the upright position but absent in the supine position. It is diagnosed by obtaining one urine sample *before* the child gets out of bed and another *after* he or she has been up for several hours, or his or her last void before going to bed. Orthostatic proteinuria is benign; rarely is more than 1 g of protein spilled per day.

4. Other causes of proteinuria include analgesic abuse, nephritis, and nephrosis.

5. When proteinuria is discovered as an incidental finding during a health-assessment visit, the history and PE usually do not reveal its cause.

a. Questions should be asked regarding GU symptoms, edema and its location, exercise, weight gain, antecedent sore throat (especially if hematuria is also present), and family members with proteinuria.

b. The PE should determine if the kidneys can be palpated (i.e., enlargement), if there is edema, or if the perineum is abnormal in any way.

c. The urine, which is usually foamy, should be examined microscopically for evidence of infection and sent for culture as appropriate.

6. If the child has proteinuria of at least 1+, a second urine sample (on another day) should be obtained. If this sample is also positive, obtain a first morning void for urine total protein/creatinine ratio and U/A. If the U/A is normal and the protein/creatinine ratio is less than 0.2, strongly consider a diagnosis of orthostatic proteinuria.

a. If the U/A is abnormal and/or the protein/creatinine ratio is greater than 0.2, determine serum albumin, BUN, creatinine, cholesterol, and electrolytes. Also consider measurement of serum C3/C4, antinuclear antibodies, and serologies for hepatitis B and C and also HIV. A renal US might be needed.

b. Consider an ASO titer, *especially* if hematuria is present because the proteinuria may be secondary to poststreptococcal nephritis.

c. A renal biopsy may eventually be needed to secure a diagnosis.

d. Nephrotic syndrome is manifest by hypoproteinemia (serum albumin less than 3 g/dL), large proteinuria (greater than 40 $mg/m^2/h$ in a 24-hour urine examination), edema, and hyperlipidemia.

(1) There is a worldwide distribution, with males affected more commonly than females. The typical age of presentation of primary nephrotic syndrome is between 18 months and 5 to 6 years.

(2) The chief presenting sign is localized or diffuse edema. The amount of edema reflects both the lack of urine output and decreased serum albumin concentration.

(3) Laboratory tests include serum albumin and globulin (both decreased), serum cholesterol (increased), urine protein (increased), urine specific gravity (increased), U/A (check for the presence of blood), serum immunoglobulins, C3, ANA, HBsAg, Hepatitis C Ab or PCR, CBC (increased Hct), electrolytes (Na decreased), total serum Ca (decreased), BUN, and creatinine (normal or increased). Consider a renal ultrasound and a CXR.

(4) Therapy

  (a) Begin prednisone at 2 mg/kg/d or 60 mg/m^2/d (maximum 80 mg/d) ÷ q8-12h after a PPD has been placed and the need for a renal biopsy has been considered. Therapy should be for 4 to 6 weeks, followed by 40 mg/m^2 (maximum 60 mg) qod; this dose is gradually tapered and stopped after an additional 4 to 6 weeks.

  (b) Dietary sodium intake should be restricted.

  (c) Most children have a number of relapses; treat such relapses with a high-dose daily steroid until the patient is free of proteinuria for 3 days, followed by a maintenance-tapering course of alternate-day therapy for 4 to 6 weeks.

  (d) *Always* use steroid therapy in concert with a nephrologist because of the myriad side-effects associated with steroid use.

  (e) Any patient with nephrotic syndrome and fever, especially if receiving prednisone, cyclophosphamide (Cytoxan), or chlorambucil, should be considered to have a bacterial infection and be cultured and started on antibiotics to cover both gram-positive and gram-negative organisms.

(5) Admit any child who has severe dehydration, fever, refractory edema, peritonitis, or renal insufficiency. Consider admission for newly diagnosed cases.

(6) Acute and long-term management should *always* be in concert with a pediatric nephrologist, who can advise on the need for a renal biopsy, prednisone dosing (and tapering), and alkylating drugs.

L. TESTICULAR SWELLING/PAIN

1. The normal prepubertal testis is 1 × 2 cm in diameter; by adulthood, the testis measures 2.5 to 3.0 × 4.0 to 4.5 cm. Several diagnoses must be considered when there is testicular enlargement or pain.

2. Testicular torsion (torsion of the spermatic cord): This condition is an emergency because continued torsion results in gangrene of the testis. The child has sudden, unilateral testicular pain; his testis is swollen and tender, and the overlying scrotal skin is red and warm. Gently lifting the testis does not relieve the pain (Prehn's sign). The child may have fever and vomiting. A lack of urinary symptoms is the rule, and

the U/A is normal. If the diagnosis is in doubt, a technetium-99m pertechnetate scan can confirm it. However, because the risk of gangrene is high, there should be no delay in definitive treatment, which is surgery. Immediate urology consultation should be obtained. Orchiectomy is usually necessary if the torsion has been present for a prolonged period.

3. Epididymitis (inflammation of the epididymis): The child has unilateral testicular pain; the epididymis is swollen and tender, and the testis may be involved (see Point 4). Scrotal skin is red on the affected side. Unlike with testicular torsion, lifting the scrotum diminishes the pain. The child may have fever, chills, dysuria, and frequency. A microscopic urine examination may demonstrate bacteria and pyuria; *E. coli* is the common infecting agent in prepubertal boys. In postpubertal, sexually active boys (especially those with a penile discharge), a gonococcal or chlamydia infection must be considered; obtain a Gram's stain and culture of the discharge. Treatment consists of immediate antibiotic use (initially ampicillin; the final choice is based on the culture and sensitivity results of urine or urethral discharge), sitz baths tid or qid, and scrotal support. If an STD is diagnosed, sexual partners must be treated.

4. Orchitis (inflammation of the testis): The prepubertal child has fever, chills, scrotal swelling, and pain; the postpubertal boy has similar symptoms and may also have urinary symptoms and a penile discharge (usually gonorrhea). In both age groups, elevating the scrotum diminishes the pain. Urine and penile discharge should be appropriately stained, examined microscopically, and cultured. The usual cause of orchitis in a prepubertal child is mumps (with or without parotid swelling); the serum amylase level will be elevated. Treatment for self-limited (7- to 14-day) mumps orchitis consists of sitz baths and scrotal support. Treatment for orchitis resulting from gonorrhea includes sitz baths, scrotal support, and antibiotic therapy (see Chapter 20).

5. Testicular trauma: Usually results from a direct blow to the scrotum, which then is tender, bruised, and swollen. A PE may be extremely painful for the child. A urine sample should be examined for the presence of blood (urethral, renal trauma). Treatment consists of ice packs to the area (24 to 48 hours followed by sitz baths), elevation of the scrotum, or scrotal support.

6. Tumor

M. UNDESCENDED TESTIS

1. A testis may be considered "undescended" if it rides high in the scrotum or is not palpable (testicular agenesis or ectopic testis).

a. A retractile testis is normally descended but is intermittently retracted because of the action of the cremasteric muscle.

b. Undescended testes may be unilateral or bilateral. In the neonate with bilateral undescended testes, serum FSH and LH levels should be obtained to rule out anorchism.

c. An undescended testis is common in neonates, especially premature infants. If spontaneous descent is going to occur, it does so by 9 to 12 months of age.

2. A retractile testis may be brought back into the scrotum manually or may descend spontaneously when the child is relaxed, squats, or bathes in warm water. Retractile testes require no therapy.

3. The administration of human chorionic gonadotropin over several weeks may medically reposition bilaterally undescended testes. However, to preserve fertility, most children require surgery (orchiopexy with concomitant inguinal herniorrhaphy) before 2 years of age.

N. URETHRITIS

1. Urethritis is characterized by erythema of the urethra and dysuria; there may or may not be purulent discharge.

2. Etiology includes the following:

a. Purulent urethritis: *N. gonorrhoeae* (most common pathogen); also *Staphylococcus aureus,* streptococci, and enteric organisms

b. Nonpurulent urethritis: *N. gonorrhoeae, Chlamydia trachomatis, Ureaplasma urealyticum,* and *Trichomonas* and *Mycoplasma* organisms

c. Noninfectious causes: Chemicals (soaps, bubble baths, powders), trauma, physical irritation to urethra (masturbation), Reiter's syndrome (urethritis, arthritis, and conjunctivitis; cause unknown)

3. Evaluation

a. Obtain a Gram's stain. Obtain a culture for gonococci and other pathogens. *Trichomonas* and *Chlamydia* organisms require special media.

b. Obtain a wet saline preparation (look for *Trichomonas* organisms).

c. Treatment

    (1) Gonococcal: See Chapter 20, section B.

    (2) In males, nongonococcal (e.g., *Chlamydia* organisms most common): azithromycin 1 g PO × 1 or doxycycline 100 mg PO bid × 7 days; make sure partner is treated. During pregnancy, erythromycin is alternate treatment (see Chapter 20, section E).

    (3) Noninfectious: Removal of irritating factor.

O. URINARY TRACT INFECTION

1. Symptoms vary and can be nonspecific (especially in young children).

a. Symptoms include dysuria, frequency, urgency, and enuresis.

b. Nonspecific symptoms include vomiting, diarrhea, fever, lethargy, irritability, failure to thrive, and abdominal pain.

c. Dysuria and frequency also may be associated with urethritis (check for vaginal infection, history of tight underwear, bubble baths, trauma). Consider gonococci, *Chlamydia* organisms, or other STDs.

d. Some UTIs are asymptomatic; both symptomatic and asymptomatic UTIs can lead to renal compromise.

9

GENITOURINARY DISORDERS

e. Pyelonephritis is usually but not always associated with high fever, an elevated ESR, and the presence of leukocytosis.

2. The PE is often normal, but emphasis should be placed on the abdominal examination (masses, suprapubic tenderness), CVA area (tenderness), and perineum (redness, excoriations, discharge). The BP should be checked.

3. Diagnosis varies with the method of obtaining the specimen.

a. Urine culture

   (1) Clean-catch urine: Greater than 100,000 colonies/ml of single organism × 2 consecutive specimens

   (2) Catheterized urine: Greater than 100 colonies/ml of single organism × 1 specimen

   (3) Suprapubic urine: Growth of any organism

Note: The traditional standard of greater than 100,000 colonies of any organism per ml of midstream urine as diagnostic of a UTI is based on studies of adult women. This standard is probably not valid for pediatric patients; therefore strict adherence to it may result in missed diagnoses of UTIs in symptomatic patients. Make certain the patient or parent really knows how to obtain a clean-catch specimen. To obtain this type of specimen, the child's urethral meatus and surrounding area are cleaned, and the child begins to void. After the stream has started, the midstream specimen is collected.

b. U/A: Examination of the urine is valuable but is *not* sufficient to diagnose a UTI. A negative analysis does not rule out a UTI. A patient may or may not have any of the following on analysis:

   (1) Pyuria: If greater than 10 WBCs/HPF spun specimen, then positive culture rate is greater than 40%

   (2) Hematuria

   (3) Bacteriuria: greater than 1 organism/HPF on unstained, unspun urine associated with 10^5 colonies/ml (100,000 colonies/ml)

   (4) Granular casts: Associated with pyelonephritis

   (5) Also check for protein, glucose, pH, concentration

4. Causes: *E. coli* is the most common organism. Other common pathogens include enterococci and *Enterobacter, Klebsiella,* and *Proteus* organisms. *S. aureus* and *Pseudomonas* organisms are more likely to be recovered after antimicrobial therapy or instrumentation.

5. Treatment

a. Admit febrile children who are less than 1 year old, those who are vomiting, toxic, or likely to be noncompliant for at least 24 hours.

b. Parenteral therapy includes (but is not limited to) ceftriaxone 75 mg/kg qd or cefotaxime 150 mg/kg/d divided q8h, ceftazidime 150 mg/kg/d divided q8h, cefazolin 50 mg/kg/d divided q8h, or gentamicin 7.5 mg/kg/d divided q8h.

c. Oral antibiotics include (but are not limited to) sulfisoxazole (Gantrisin) 120 to 150 mg/kg/d ÷ qid (maximum 6 g/d) × 14 days *or* amoxicillin

(Augmentin) 50 mg/kg/d ÷ tid *or* TMP/SMZ 6 to 12 mg TMP, 30 to 60 mg SMZ per day ÷ bid *or* cefixime 8 mg/kg/d ÷ q12-24h *or* cefpodoxime 10 mg/kg/d ÷ q12h *or* cefprozil 30 mg/kg/d ÷ q12h *or* cephalexin 50 to 100 mg/kg/d ÷ q6-8h *or* loracarbef 15 to 30 mg/kg/d ÷ q12h *or* nitrofurantoin 5 to 7 mg/kg/d ÷ q6h.

d. If upper tract disease is suspected, use IV ampicillin 100 mg/kg/d ÷ qid or tid *and* (1) gentamicin 7.5 mg/kg/d ÷ tid *or* (2) cefotaxime 150 mg/kg/d ÷ q8h. IV therapy should be continued until fever has resolved and repeat cultures are negative. At that point, the patient can be treated with oral antibiotics to complete a 4- to 6-week course.

e. To avoid problems with equivocal urine culture results, do not start treatment until at least two clean-catch urine samples or one suprapubic or catheter specimen has been obtained.

f. Sepsis is often associated with a UTI in infants less than 8 weeks of age (some authorities would be more conservative and state 6 months of age). Work up appropriately. Treatment involves IV ampicillin (100 mg/kg/d) and gentamicin (5 to 7.5 mg/kg/d) *or* IV cefotaxime (150 mg/kg/d) for 5 days; then complete a 10- to 15-day course of therapy with oral ampicillin or a cephalosporin. The infant should receive prophylactic antibiotic coverage (one-third to half of the treatment dosage) hs until a VCUG and ultrasound or cortical scintigraphy are performed. Do not use sulfonamides or nitrofurantoins during the first 8 weeks of life.

g. Eliminate the use of bubble bath and treat constipation, if present; both are risk factors.

6. Suggested follow-up

a. Return in 48 hours for a repeat U/A and culture to document sterile urine and clinical improvement and to help identify resistant organisms.

b. Return 1 to 3 weeks after antibiotics have been discontinued for U/A and culture.

c. Obtain subsequent follow-up cultures every 1 to 3 months until patient has remained free of infection for 1 year, then yearly.

7. Recurrences

a. Recurrence in 25% of males and 30% to 80% of females within the first year; the recurrence is often asymptomatic.

b. If necessary, consider prophylaxis with TMP/SMZ (2 mg TMP/10 mg SMZ per kg hs *or* 5 mg TMP/25 mg SMZ twice a week) or nitrofurantoin (1 to 2 mg/kg qd) until imaging studies are completed; some would argue that the length of prophylaxis should be for 6 months to 1 year or longer (depending on the results of the studies).

c. Avoid urologic procedures such as cystoscopy and urethral dilation.

8. Further evaluation

a. The official recommendation of the American Academy of Pediatrics is that a radiographic workup should be performed on all children (boys and girls) younger than 2 years of age after one documented UTI.

9

GENITOURINARY DISORDERS

b. Children less than 4 years of age and boys of any age are more likely to have structural problems (e.g., vesicoureteral reflux or ureteral obstruction). Renal scarring (usually secondary to reflux or obstruction) is most likely to occur in preschool-age children.

c. The AAP has developed practice parameters for the ideal workup for a child with a first UTI.

   (1) Renal ultrasound promptly (if no or poor response to antibiotics in first 48 hours of therapy) or at the earliest convenient time (good response to antibiotic therapy).

   (2) Cystourethrography (VCUG) or radionuclide cystography (RNC) at the earliest convenient time, especially if poor or no response to therapy.

   (3) If needed, to detect renal scarring, obtain cortical scintigraphy with technetium-99m dimercaptosuccinic acid (DMSA) or ^{99m}Tc-glucoheptonate because of greater sensitivity compared with ultrasound or VCUG. This is a real issue because renal scarring can occur in the absence of reflux. Cortical scintigraphy is also recommended for an infant with a UTI.

   (4) The following types of children are likely to benefit from scintigraphy:

      (a) Children with marked reflux for whom surgery is contemplated

      (b) Children 6 to 12 years of age with moderate reflux who have been treated with antibiotic prophylaxis for several years

      (c) Children with a history of multiple UTIs or previous pyelonephritis

      (d) Children with breakthrough UTIs while on prophylaxis

      (e) Children with suspected pyelonephritis

   (5) Cortical scintigraphy is expensive but entails less radiation than a VCUG.

d. Radionuclide cystography is used to follow patients with reflux and children whose first UTI is diagnosed at 6 years of age or older. Some authorities would also advocate its use in siblings of children with reflux and in children whose parents had reflux.

P. VAGINAL PROBLEMS

1. Vulvovaginitis and vaginitis: May occur at any age

a. Symptoms include itching, discharge, dysuria (if urethritis is also present), and erythema/edema of vulva and vagina.

b. Etiology may be noninfectious or infectious.

   (1) Noninfectious

      (a) Trauma, foreign body (malodorous, often bloody discharge), labial adhesions, chemical irritant or allergen (OTC douches, powders, bubble bath), masturbation, tumor.

      (b) Nylon panties prevent evaporation of normal moisture, and therefore their use may promote vaginitis.

(2) Infectious
  (a) Nonspecific: Bacterial overgrowth of enteric organisms secondary to poor perineal hygiene; *Gardnerella vaginalis*
  (b) Specific: *N. gonorrhoeae, Monilia* or *Trichomonas* organisms, β-hemolytic streptococcus, *Chlamydia* organisms, pinworms, herpes simplex virus

c. Evaluation
  (1) Examine external genitalia for scratches, tears, redness, ulcers, discharge, or swelling. Vaginoscopy may be performed in a prepubertal female using a veterinary otoscope speculum. A gynecology consult may be needed.
  (2) A culture is indicated if clinical symptoms are present with or without discharge or ulcerations. In young girls, may need to obtain a culture using a medicine dropper filled with nonbacteriostatic saline solution; inject saline solution and aspirate for vaginal culture. Evaluate the vaginal specimen by a wet saline mount (*Trichomonas* organisms), KOH preparation (*Monilia* organisms), and Gram's stain (intracellular gram-negative diplococci). Perform both a gonococcal and a routine culture.
  (3) Foreign bodies are characteristically associated with foul-smelling discharge. Foreign bodies may be palpable by digital rectal examination in a prepubertal girl; however, toilet paper is the most common foreign body and usually is not palpable. A vaginal flush can be performed using normal saline solution introduced into the vagina via an infant feeding tube that is connected to a 30-ml syringe. Do not exert excess force to the plunger of the syringe; by doing so there is the possibility of retrograde flow up the cervix. Examination under sedation might be necessary.

d. Agent-specific treatment
  (1) Nonspecific vaginitis
    (a) Remove the irritating factor (e.g., foreign body, douche, bubble bath).
    (b) Parents should instruct the child on the proper wiping technique (front to back, not back to front).
    (c) Prescribe warm sitz baths tid.
    (d) Instruct the patient to wear loose-fitting white cotton panties.
    (e) Reassure parents about the normalcy of masturbation. If the patient is old enough to understand, she might also be counseled.
    (f) Reassess cases that are resistant to such therapies. Make sure that adequate cultures have been performed and that abuse, foreign bodies, anatomic defects, and other such conditions have been ruled out. If reassessment still does not elicit a cause, a 10-day course of oral antibiotics (e.g., amoxicillin) may be helpful.

9

GENITOURINARY DISORDERS

(2) *Monilia* organisms

    (a) Intense pruritus, thick curdy discharge, dysuria.

    (b) Predisposing factors: Oral contraceptives, antibiotics, diabetes; very common in postpubertal females.

    (c) Diagnosis is made with a KOH preparation. Darkly stained hyphae sometimes can be seen on Gram's stain. KOH may miss 50% of culture-positive specimens.

    (d) Treatment (in addition to nonspecific therapy above)

        (i) Miconazole (Monistat) cream intravaginally qhs × 1 to 2 weeks; minipad to keep cream from coming out during the day

        (ii) Clotrimazole 100-mg intravaginal tablet, 1 hs × 1 to 2 weeks

        (iii) Fluconazole 150 mg PO × 1 (pubertal patient)

(3) *Trichomonas* organisms

    (a) Greenish yellow discharge, foul odor, pruritus, dyspareunia

    (b) Diagnosis by saline wet mount

    (c) Treatment (in addition to nonspecific therapy above)

        (i) Metronidazole (Flagyl) if not pregnant, 2 g PO in a single dose (preferred) or 500 mg bid × 7 to 10 days

        (ii) Clotrimazole 100 mg intravaginally hs × 7 days if pregnant; partner should be treated to prevent reinfection

(4) *G. vaginalis* (formerly *Haemophilus vaginalis*)

    (a) Gray frothy discharge, fishy odor; pruritus not prominent.

    (b) Diagnosis is made by the presence of "clue cells" (epithelial cells covered with bacteria) and the absence of *Trichomonas* and *Monilia* organisms.

    (c) Treatment (in addition to nonspecific therapy above)

        (i) Metronidazole 500 mg bid × 7 days (This therapy is effective, but uncertainty about carcinogenicity exists.), *or*

        (ii) Clindamycin 2% cream, 1 full applicator intravaginally hs × 7 days, *or*

        (iii) Metronidazole 0.75% gel, 1 full applicator intravaginally bid × 5 days.

        (iv) It is often a good idea to treat concomitantly with nystatin cream to avoid superinfection with *Monilia* organisms.

        (v) Treat the sexual partner if antibiotics are used.

(5) Group A β-hemolytic streptococcus: Oral penicillin in same dosage as for streptococcus pharyngitis (i.e., 250 to 500 mg PO bid × 10 days)

(6) Gonococcal infection and herpes simplex virus: See Chapter 20

(7) Pinworm infestation: See Chapter 8

2. Vaginal bleeding

a. Vaginal bleeding may result from trauma (straddle injury, inanimate object penetration, sexual abuse), menstruation, spotting during early pregnancy, abortion, ingestion or improper use of birth control pills, maternal estrogen effect (neonates who may also have breast enlargement), vaginal infections, foreign bodies, and tumors.

b. Obtain a history of the duration and amount of vaginal bleeding, precipitating events, whether bleeding waxes and wanes, history of trauma, abuse, foreign body, ingestion of birth control pills, other GU symptoms.

c. Examine the perineum carefully.

   (1) Look for contusions and lacerations of the labia, vagina, and urethra.

   (2) Check hymenal integrity (virginal prepubertal hymen less than 1 cm). To visualize the hymen, separate the labia and gently pull posteriorly at a 45-degree angle *or* place traction on the labia by gently grasping the labia and pulling toward the examiner.

   (3) Is bleeding brisk, or is it slow and sporadic?

   (4) Are there any masses present?

   (5) If the patient is sexually active or has had previous pelvic examinations, perform a pelvic examination to determine if blood is coming from the cervical os (if os is open), if the cervix is eroded, or if a foreign body is present. Perform a bimanual and rectal examination to check for masses and foreign bodies.

   (6) If the child is prepubertal, she will require sedation for an adequate inspection of the vagina and cervix. Vaginoscopy may be performed using a veterinary otoscope speculum. A rectal examination should be performed to check for masses and foreign bodies.

d. If vaginal bleeding is profuse, Hct should be checked.

   (1) Clotting studies may be indicated if there are petechiae, purpura, or other bleeding sites.

   (2) If there is evidence of an infection, appropriate cultures and a Gram's stain of the discharge or exudate should be obtained.

   (3) If the girl is sexually active, a urine or serum pregnancy test should be obtained.

e. Treatment is directed toward the underlying condition.

   (1) The trauma victim may require surgical repair under sedation or anesthesia.

   (2) Foreign bodies should be removed and the vagina flushed with normal saline.

   (3) Vaginal/cervical infections should be appropriately treated (see Chapter 20).

   (4) The proper strength of oral contraceptive should be chosen, and its proper administration should be encouraged and monitored closely.

   (5) Mothers of neonates with vaginal bleeding should be reassured. Such bleeding should cease by 10 days of age.

9

GENITOURINARY DISORDERS

3. Labial adhesions
a. Labial adhesions are epithelial agglutinations that cover the hymen and sometimes the urethral meatus. They are caused by superficial inflammation of the labia minora and usually occur in prepubertal girls. Adhesions may be complete or partial. Girls with adhesions should be observed while voiding to ensure an adequate stream.
b. Adhesions disappear by puberty when estrogen levels rise.
c. If the girl has dysuria, a UTI, or chronically poor hygiene, an estrogen cream may be applied bid for 7 to 10 days to simulate the estrogen effect that occurs at puberty. Estrogen cream should not be used for more than 14 days; doing so may promote signs of precocious puberty. After separation, petroleum jelly (Vaseline) should be applied to the area tid × 4 weeks to prevent readherence.
d. Adhesions should never be cut or manually broken because they will recur.

Q. BIBLIOGRAPHY

Enuresis
Robson W: Diurnal enuresis, *Pediatr in Rev* 18:407, 1997.
Schmitt B: Nocturnal enuresis, *Pediatr in Rev* 18:183, 1997.

Glomerulonephritis
Fleisher G, Ludwig S: *Textbook of pediatric emergency medicine,* ed 3, Baltimore, 1993, Williams & Wilkins.

Hematuria
Fitzwater D, Wyatt R: Hematuria, *Pediatr in Rev* 15:102, 1994.
Roy S: Hematuria, *Pediatr in Rev* 19:209, 1998.

Hemolytic-Uremic Syndrome
Schulman S, Kaplan B: Hemolytic-uremic syndrome—prevention, recognition, management, *Contemp Pediatr* 12:61, 1995.
Stewart C, Tina L: Hemolytic-uremic syndrome, *Pediatric in Rev* 14:218, 1993.
Varade W: Hemolytic uremic syndrome—reducing the risks, *Contemp Pediatr* 17:54, 2000.

Henoch-Schöenlein Purpura
Saulsbury F: Henoch-Schöenlein purpura in children, *Medicine* 78:395, 1999.
Tizard EJ: Henoch-Schöenlein purpura, *Arch Dis Child* 80:380, 1999.

Hernia/Hydrocele
Ziegler M: Diagnosis of inguinal hernia and hydrocele, *Pediatr Rev* 15:286, 1994.

Penile Problems
Kanegaye J, Schonfeld N: Penile zipper entrapment: a simple and less threatening approach using mineral oil, *Pediatr Emerg Care* 9:90, 1993.

Proteinuria
Chesney R: The idiopathic nephrotic syndrome, *Curr Op in Pediatr* 11:158, 1999.
Crux C, Spitzer A: When you find protein or blood in the urine, *Contemp Pediatr* 15:89, 1998.
Ettinger R: The evaluation of the child with proteinuria, *Pediatr Ann* 23:486, 1994.
Hogg R, Portman R, Milliner D et al: Evaluation and management of proteinuria and nephrotic syndrome in children, *Pediatrics* 105:1242, 2000.
Hogg R, Portman R, Milliner D et al: Recognizing and treating the nephrotic syndrome, *Contemp Pediatr* 17:84, 2000.
Orth S, Ritz E: The nephrotic syndrome, *NEJM* 338:1202, 1998.

Testicular Swelling/Pain
Adelman W, Joffe A: The adolescent with a painful scrotum, *Contemp Pediatr* 17:111, 2000.
Kadish H, Bolte R: A retrospective review of pediatric patients with epididymitis, testicular torsion, and torsion of the testicular appendages, *Pediatrics* 102:73, 1998.
Kaplan G: Scrotal swelling in children, *Pediatr in Rev* 21:311, 2000.
Palmer L: Testicular torsion, *Pediatr in Rev* 15:455, 1994.
Tennebaum S, Kim S: Acute epididymitis and orchitis in children, *Pediatr in Rev* 17:424, 1996.

Undescended Testis
Berkowitz G et al: Prevalence and natural history of cryptorchidism, *Pediatrics* 92:44, 1993.
Ferrer F, McKenna P: Current approaches to the undescended testicle, *Contemp Pediatr* 17:106, 2000.
Rabinowitz R, Hulbert W: Cryptorchidism, *Pediatr Rev* 15:272, 1994.

Urinary Tract Infection
AAP: Practice parameter—the diagnosis, treatment, and evaluation of the initial urinary tract infection in febrile infants and young children, *Pediatrics* 103:843, 1999.
Benador D et al: Cortical scintigraphy in the evaluation of renal parenchymal changes in children with pyelonephritis, *J Pediatr* 124:17, 1994.
Bollgren I: Antibacterial prophylaxis in children with urinary tract infections, *Acta Paediatr Suppl* 431:48, 1999.
Conway J, Cohn R: Evolving role of nuclear medicine for the diagnosis and management of UTI, *J Pediatr* 124:87, 1994.
Hellerstein S: Evolving concepts in the evaluation of the child with UTI, *J Pediatr* 124:589, 1994.
Hoberman A et al: Pyuria and bacteriuria in urine specimens obtained by catheter from young children with fever, *J Pediatr* 124:513, 1994.
Jacobson SH, Hansson S, Jakobsson B: Vesico-ureteric reflux—occurrence and long-term risks, *Acta Paediatr Suppl* 431:22, 1999.
Johnson C: New advances in childhood urinary tract infections, *Pediatr in Rev* 20:335, 1999.
Roberts K, Akintemi O: The epidemiology and clinical presentation of urinary tract infections in children younger than 2 years of age, *Pediatr Ann* 28:644, 1999.
Rosenfeld D et al: Current recommendations for children with UTI, *Clin Pediatr* 34:261, 1995.
Schlager T: The pathogenesis of urinary tract infections, *Pediatr Ann* 28:639, 1999.
Steele R: The epidemiology and clinical presentation of urinary tract infections in children 2 years of age through adolescence, *Pediatr Ann* 28:653, 1999.
Todd J: Management of urinary tract infections, *Pediatr Rev* 16:190, 1995.

Vaginitis
Nyirjesy P: Vaginitis in the adolescent patient, *PCNA* 46:733, 1999.
Vandeven A, Emans S: Vulvovaginitis in the child and adolescent, *Pediatr Rev* 14:141, 1993.

Vaginal Bleeding
Altchek A: Finding the cause of genital bleeding in prepubertal girls, *Contemp Pediatr* 13:80, 1996.

Labial Adhesions
Wiener D: Labial adhesions, *Pediatr in Rev* 15:87, 1994.

GENITOURINARY DISORDERS

9

HEMATOLOGY

A. ANEMIA

1. Anemia is only a sign of a disease or blood loss; the cause must be determined (increased destruction, decreased production, or blood loss).
2. Normal values and indices, are shown in Table 10-1; in blacks, Hgb may run 0.5 g% lower.
3. Nadir: "Physiologic anemia" of a term infant at 8 to 12 weeks of age. Hct should not be less than 30%; after this nadir, Hct should be greater than 32% and MCV greater than 77 fL.
4. History
a. Any known blood loss (e.g., stool, urine, nosebleeds), perinatal problems
b. Source of dietary iron (breastmilk, formula, meats, cereals, vitamins with iron)
c. History of excess whole milk intake (greater than 32 oz/d)
d. History of pica (R/O lead poisoning)
e. History of prior anemia
f. Family history: Ethnic/racial background, hemoglobinopathy/ gallstones/anemia/splenectomy/jaundice
g. Any medications that may depress bone marrow or cause hemolysis
h. History of malaise, fatigue, palpitations
i. History of neonatal jaundice
j. History of prematurity or small for gestational age (decreased iron stores with accelerated growth)
5. PE: Look for pallor, tachycardia, other signs of high output cardiac failure, petechiae, purpura, icterus, lymphadenopathy, hepatosplenomegaly, positive stool test for blood, hematuria, maxillary prominence, blue sclerae, cheilosis, spooning of nails, glossitis.
6. Hematology laboratory: CBC with indices, reticulocyte count, peripheral blood smear (most important). Perform a more extensive workup (e.g., lead level/hemoglobin-electrophoresis, G-6-PD, Coombs' test, haptoglobin) as indicated in selected patients (see Table 10-2).
7. Iron deficiency anemia.
a. The highest incidence is in toddlers and adolescent girls.
   (1) Risk factors for toddlers include: preterm birth; small for gestational age; maternal iron deficiency during pregnancy; early introduction of whole cow's milk or failure to add dietary source of iron after 6 months to breast-fed infants; GI blood loss; recurrent/chronic infections.
   (2) Adolescents are at risk because of: increased demands (increase in lean body mass, expansion of total blood volume); menstrual blood loss in females; inadequate iron intake. Girls who are dieting or who are on a vegetarian diet are at particular risk.

10

TABLE 10-1

CUT-OFF VALUES FOR LABORATORY TESTS OF IRON STATUS,
AND HAEMOGLOBIN REFERENCE VALUES FOR NON-BLACK CHILDREN
WHO HAD FEWER THAN TWO ABNORMAL TESTS IN NHANES
SURVEY IN U.S.A.

	Age (Years)				
	1-2	3-5	6-11	12-15 M	12-15 F
Cut-off values					
Transferrin saturation (%)	9	13	14	14	14
Serum ferritin (mcg/l)	10	10	12	12	12
Erythrocyte protoporphyrin (mcg/dl RBC)	70	70	70	70	70
MCV (fl)	77	79	80	82	85
Reference haemoglobin values (g/dl)					
Mean	12·0	12·3	13·0	14·1	13·3
(SD)	(0·65)	(0·7)	(0·75)	(1·05)	(0·9)
Mean −2 SD	10·7	10·9	11·5	12·0	11·5

Dallman PR, Looker AC, Johnson CL, Carroll M: (1996) Influence of age on laboratory criteria for the diagnosis of iron deficiency in infants and children. *Iron Nutrition in Health and Disease* (ed. by L. Hallberg and N.G. Asp), pp. 65-74. John Libbey, London.

b. There can be a spectrum of iron deficiency.
   (1) *Iron depletion:* Erythropoiesis is normal but iron stores are reduced; serum ferritin less than 12 mcg/L.
   (2) *Iron-deficient erythropoiesis:* Abnormal RBC biochemistry (increased FEP, increased transferrin receptor); microcytosis (MCV less than 70 plus age in years); anisocytosis (RDW greater than 15%); transport iron reduced (transferrin saturation less than 10%).
   (3) *Iron-deficiency anemia:* Above plus Hgb less than 11 g/dL.
c. Think of blood loss; the incidence of nutritionally based iron deficiency anemia has decreased dramatically.
d. Smear: Hypochromic (low MCH/MCHC), microcytic (low MCV) RBCs; elevated RDW; low reticulocyte count for the degree of anemia; low serum ferritin; moderately elevated FEP.
e. Treatment of iron deficiency anemia
   (1) Correct the basic problem (e.g., dietary, bleeding sources, and similar problems).
   (2) Elemental iron (3 to 6 mg/kg/d ÷ qd or tid with meals (e.g., Fer-in-Sol drops = 25 mg Fe/ml × 2 to 3 months adequately repletes iron stores in toddlers). Check *The Harriet Lane Handbook,* ed. 15 for other preparations.
   (3) Check 5 to 7 days after initiation of iron therapy; should see elevated reticulocyte count and RDW. By 4 weeks, Hct should be

TABLE 10-2

HEMATOLOGIC PARAMETERS IN COMMON CAUSES OF ANEMIA

	Mean Corpuscular Volume	RBC Distribution Width	Anemia	Morphologic Abnormalities	Free Erythrocyte Protoporphyrin (mcg/100 ml)	Hgb A$_2$
Iron deficiency	↓	>13.5	+	1+	30-200	Normal or decreased
Lead poisoning*	↓†	>13.5†	±	1-2+	>200	Normal
α-Thalassemia trait‡	↓	<11.5	±	2+	<90	Normal or decreased
β-Thalassemia trait§	↓	<11.5	±	2+	<90	Elevated

*Pb poisoning; peak age 6 months to 4 years of age.

†Usually a result of concomitant iron deficiency.

‡α-Thalassemia trait predominant in Asians, blacks, and Mediterraneans.

§β-Thalassemia trait mainly in blacks and Mediterraneans.

10

HEMATOLOGY

normal. Smear has two populations of RBCs (normal and iron deficient). The maximum rate of increase in Hgb is usually 1 to 2 g/wk.

f. Failure to correct presumed iron deficiency anemia

    (1) Poor compliance: Did patient get iron? Teeth staining, dark stools indicate that iron was given. Ask parents to bring medication with them, or inquire how much iron is left in the bottle.

    (2) Improper administration: Iron may not be well absorbed if administered with milk or other products high in P content.

    (3) Malabsorption: Malabsorption of iron may be present in as many as 20% of patients with iron deficiency anemia who do not respond to iron.

    (4) Ongoing blood losses; check stool for blood.

    (5) Incorrect diagnosis.

        (a) Lead poisoning, thalassemia, and chronic infection are also associated with hypochromic anemia.

        (b) Check blood lead level.

        (c) Check parents' indices, smears, hemoglobin electrophoresis and family history for evidence of thalassemia. Consider direct DNA testing.

    (6) Inability to use iron: In the presence of concomitant lead poisoning or certain chronic disease states, especially those associated with inflammation, iron may be absorbed but not incorporated into Hgb.

g. Effects of iron deficiency anemia

    (1) Anorexia, fatigue, irritability.

    (2) Increased susceptibility to infection.

    (3) If present early in life, may lead to impaired growth and developmental delay.

B. HEMOPHILIA

1. General

a. Clinically, hemophilia A and B are indistinguishable; hemophilia A is much more common (1:10,000 births) than hemophilia B (1:50,000 births). The diagnosis is based on factor VIII and factor IX assays; in neonates a diagnosis of factor VIII or factor IX deficiency can be made on a cord blood assay. In 20% to 30% of patients, the family history is negative.

b. In neonates with hemophilia, there may be intracranial bleeding secondary to traumatic delivery or bleeding at the circumcision site; otherwise, bleeding complications (other than bruising) are uncommon during the first year until children become more mobile. With a positive family history, circumcision should be avoided until laboratory evaluation has excluded hemophilia in the child.

c. The highest incidence of bleeding episodes occurs from age 4 years through adolescence. Manifestations include easy bruising, palpable bruising, oral bleeding, bleeding into joints and muscles, intracranial hemorrhage, and prolonged bleeding after a laceration. Clinical severity correlates with the patient's level of factor VIII or IX: less than 1% = severe; 1% to 5% = moderate; greater than 5% = mild. Patients who have mild hemophilia bleed only after surgery, dental procedures, or severe trauma.

Note: **A child with an underlying bleeding disorder may initially be suspected to be a victim of nonaccidental trauma. In addition, a coagulation disorder may occur coincident with physical abuse. Every child with unexplained or implausible bruising should receive a coagulation screen consisting of a CBC, platelet count, prothrombin time, and partial thromboplastin time.**

10

HEMATOLOGY

d. Bleeding into joints is the hallmark of severe hemophilia. Episodes usually begin around 1 to 2 years of age coincident with ambulation and increased activity. Recurrent episodes of bleeding lead to synovitis, synovial hypertrophy, bone hypertrophy, and cartilage damage eventually resulting in a stiff, painful joint with contractures. The most frequently involved joints are the knee, elbow and ankle. In addition to treatment of acute episodes with factor replacement, patients may benefit from physiotherapy and synovectomy. Prophylaxis can be very effective in preventing hemarthrosis (see treatment section).

e. Bruises are seldom large enough to require factor replacement, but intramuscular bleeding should be treated with factor replacement; such treatment may be needed over several days. Bleeding can lead to a compression neuropathy, e.g., femoral nerve compression secondary to an ileopsoas bleed, and permanent muscle atrophy. Extensive soft-tissue bleeding into the forearm or leg may result in a "compartment syndrome." Treatment includes, ice, elevation, and factor replacement. A fasciotomy may be required to preserve function.

f. Most episodes of intracranial bleeding occur in the first decade, usually secondary to head trauma. Manifestations include headache, vomiting, irritability, hemiparesis, papilledema, cranial nerve abnormalities, behavioral changes, and seizures. Every child with hemophilia who also exhibits neurologic symptoms, including headache and vomiting, should be suspected to have an intracranial bleed and treated accordingly. Even before diagnostic studies (e.g., CT scan) are initiated, the patient should be given an initial bolus of factor to achieve 100% replacement. If an intracranial hemorrhage is present, a continuous infusion or bolus therapy is initiated to keep levels greater than 80% in the first week and then greater than 50% for an additional week. Prophylaxis (bolus dose qod) should be considered following a CNS bleed.

Note: **On occasion, an intraspinal bleed can lead to an epidural hematoma and spinal cord compression.**

g. Spontaneous hematuria usually stops without specific treatment, but GU bleeding secondary to trauma should be treated with clotting factor.

h. Tongue and mouth lacerations require clotting-factor replacement, an antifibrinolytic agent, soft diet, and, occasionally, sedation, NPO status, and IV fluids.

2. Treatment

a. Recommended dosages of factor VIII and IX concentrates for various clinical situations are shown in Tables 10-3 and 10-4. Recombinant human factor VIII products (Recombinate, Kogenate) are now available. They are as effective as plasma-derived preparations and should reduce the possibility of viral contaminants. The development of antibodies appears to be similar to that seen with plasma-derived preparations.

b. Because of the risks of DIC and thromboembolism, the repetitive use of large doses of factor IX concentrate should be avoided. The incidence of such complications is much lower with newer, highly purified products.

c. DDAVP is the treatment of choice for patients with mild-to-moderate hemophilia A or type I von Willebrand's disease. An IV dose of 0.3 mcg/kg diluted in 50 ml normal saline results in a twofold to fivefold (the average is threefold) increase in factor VIII activity. Need to monitor for hyponatremia, water intoxication, and vasospasm. Tachyphylaxis develops after 4 doses. Testing is required to ensure an adequate response for each patient before it can be prescribed routinely. A potent intranasal DDAVP preparation is also being used.

d. Patients are best managed in collaboration with a regional hemophilia center. With proper training and support, most patients can carry out much of their infusion therapy at home.

3. Prophylaxis

a. With venipuncture, apply pressure to the site for at least 5 minutes. Never use the femoral or jugular vein.

b. Immunizations should be given SQ with a 25-gauge needle or intramuscularly after factor replacement; apply pressure for 5 minutes.

c. A clotting factor infusion sufficient to raise the level to 30% of normal should be given 30 to 45 minutes before an LP.

d. For surgical procedures, give an initial bolus of clotting factor to 100% intraoperatively followed by a continuous infusion to greater than 50% levels. Maintain levels greater than 50% for 5 to 7 days and then greater than 30% for an additional 5 to 7 days. Check for "inhibitors" preoperatively.

e. For dental procedures give an antifibrinolytic agent (α-aminocaproic acid or tranexamic acid) before and for about 7 to 10 days after the procedure. A dose of factor VIII or IX is generally given before the procedure. Mandibular anesthetic blocks should be avoided.

f. For patients with severe hemophilia, primary prophylaxis can be highly effective in preventing hemarthrosis and joint complications and improving quality of life. It involves the infusion of factor (preferably a recombinant product) beginning at 1 to 2 years of age and continued indefinitely. Patients with hemophilia A are given 25 units/kg of factor

TABLE 10-3

HEMOPHILIA A: RECOMMENDED DOSAGES OF FACTOR VIII*

Type of Bleeding	Initial Dose (Factor VIII, U/kg)	Repeated Doses (Factor VIII, U/kg)	Other Treatment
Acute hemarthrosis			
Early	10	Seldom necessary	Ice packs, non–weight-bearing sling or lightweight splint; consider joint aspiration for first-time hemarthrosis or severe hemarthrosis unresponsive to factor replacement
Late	20	20 q12h	
Intramuscular hemorrhage†	20-30	20 q12h (often several days of treatment)	Non–weight-bearing support; complete bed rest for iliopsoas hemorrhage
Life-threatening situations‡	50	25-30 q8-12h or (preferably) as a continuous infusion (3-4 U/kg/h)	
Intracranial hemorrhage			
Major surgery			
Major trauma			
Tongue or neck bleeding with potential airway obstruction			
Painless spontaneous gross hematuria	None		Increased fluids by mouth; corticosteroids and factor VIII sometimes used
Severe abdominal pain‡	20-40	20-45 q12h	An antifibrinolytic agent (tranexamic acid or ε-aminocaproic acid), sedation; nothing by mouth in small child; local application of oral adhesive gauze may be beneficial for gum bleeding
Tongue and mouth lacerations‡	20	20 q12h	
Tooth extraction (permanent teeth)†	20	20 q12h (often not necessary in cases of uncomplicated extractions)	Antifibrinolytic agent beginning 1 d preoperatively; continue 7-10 d

From Lusher JM, Warrier I: *Pediatr Rev* 12:277, 1991.

*Refers to viral-attenuated factor VIII.

†In individuals who have mild hemophilia A, DDAVP (desmopressin) is the treatment of choice rather than factor VIII concentrates.

‡These situations should be treated in a comprehensive hemophilia center. If first seen in another hospital, the hemophilia center should be contacted and the patient transferred after emergency treatment is given at the local hospital.

10

HEMATOLOGY

TABLE 10-4

HEMOPHILIA B: RECOMMENDED DOSAGE SCHEDULE*

Type of Bleeding	Initial Dose (Factor IX, U/kg; and Source of Factor IX†)	Repeat Dose (Factor IX, U/kg; and Source of Factor IX†)	Other Treatment
Acute hemarthrosis‡			Seldom necessary
In association with mild hemophilia B	10-15 (FIXCC)	None	Ice packs; non–weight-bearing support, sling; rarely, joint aspiration
Early, in association with severe hemophilia B	20 (FIXCC)	None	
Late (pain, swelling, limitation of motion) in association with severe hemophilia B	30 (FIXCC)	20-25 (FIXCC) q12h	
Intramuscular hemorrhage‡			Non–weight-bearing support; complete bed rest for iliopsoas hemorrhage
In association with mild hemophilia B	15 (FIXCC)	10-15 (FIXCC) q12h	
In association with severe hemophilia B	30-40 (FIXCC)	30 (FIXCC) q12h	
Life-threatening situations§	50 (FIXCC)	20-25 (FIXCC) q12h or as a continuous infusion	AT-III concentrate as source of AT-III; add heparin to reconstituted prothrombin complex concentrate
Intracranial hemorrhage			
Major trauma			
Tongue or neck bleeding with potential airway obstruction			
Painless spontaneous gross hematuria	None		Increased fluids by mouth; corticosteroids and factor IX are used by some

Severe abdominal pain‡			
In mild hemophilia B	15 (FIXCC)	10 (FIXCC) q12h	
In association with severe hemophilia B	40 (FIXCC)	20 (FIXCC) q12h	
Tongue and mouth lacerations	30	30 (FIXCC) q12h	An antifibrinolytic agent (tranexamic acid or ε-aminocaproic acid), sedation; nothing by mouth in small children
Tooth extraction (permanent teeth)	30	30 (FIXCC) q12h (often not necessary in cases of uncomplicated extractions)	Antifibrinolytic agent beginning 1 d preoperatively; continue 7-10 d

Modified from Lusher JM, Warrier I: *Pediatr Rev* 12:278, 1991.

*FFP = fresh-frozen plasma; FIXCC = Factor IX complex concentrate; AT-III = antithrombin III. If FIXCC is not available in an emergency situation, FFP can be used (not virus inactivated). One unit of FIXCC is equivalent to 1 ml FFP.

†FIXCC refers to heat-treated or otherwise virus-attenuated FIXCC. As soon as a nonthrombogenic factor IX concentrate (coagulant FIX) is licensed and available, it will become the preferred product for most of the above situations.

‡In infants and children younger than 4 years of age, some physicians still prefer to use FFP rather than FIXCC, even in those with moderate or severe hemophilia B. However, FFP cannot be virus attenuated.

§These situations should be treated in a comprehensive hemophilia center. If first seen in another hospital, the hemophilia center should be contacted and the patient transferred after emergency treatment is given at the local hospital.

10

HEMATOLOGY

VIII 3 times weekly and patients with hemophilia B are given 50 units/kg of factor IX twice weekly. The goal is to maintain plasma trough levels greater than 1% to 3%. Using lower dosages at more frequent intervals, based on individual pharmacokinetic profiles, can be a cost-effective strategy. An added benefit of prophylaxis is the prevention of other potentially serious bleeding episodes. There is no evidence that prophylaxis results in a higher incidence of high-titer inhibitor. Therapy can be simplified by the use of a totally implantable central venous access device, but there is a risk of line failure due to thrombus formation and line sepsis.

4. Complications
a. High-titer "inhibitor" antibodies develop in 10% to 15% of patients with hemophilia A and in 1% of those with hemophilia B. Such cases can be treated with factor IX complex concentrates (standard or activated), porcine factor VIII (Hyate: C), a human recombinant factor VIIa preparation, or immune tolerance regimens.
b. Ninety percent of patients who received plasma-derived products between 1979 and 1984 have become HIV seropositive. AIDS progression in these patients is somewhat delayed compared with other risk groups. Current products are safe with respect to HIV and hepatitis, but there is a risk of parvovirus transmission. Patients who are HBsAg seronegative should be immunized with hepatitis B vaccine. Hepatitis A immunization is also recommended.
5. Carrier detection and prenatal diagnosis: In families with a history of hemophilia, carrier testing and accurate prenatal diagnosis can be carried out using DNA analysis.

C. SICKLE CELL DISEASE

The incidence of sickle cell disease is 1 in 360 African Americans; the course is very variable. In most cases, diagnosis is made as a result of neonatal screening. Because of the persistence of fetal Hgb, clinical manifestations are usually minimal before 4 months of age.

1. Clinical manifestations
a. Anemia: Patients are usually not very symptomatic at their chronic Hgb level; however, there may be an acute drop in Hgb secondary to the following:
   (1) Aplastic crisis: Usually secondary to viral infections, especially parvovirus B19 which accounts for more than 95% of cases with severe aplastic crisis. Treatment consists of blood transfusion.
   (2) Sequestration syndrome: Results from trapping sickled RBCs within an acutely enlarged spleen; peak age 6 months to 3 years
      (a) Manifestations: Precipitous fall in Hct, reticulocytosis, thrombocytopenia, with or without leukopenia, pallor, splenomegaly, hypovolemia, abdominal pain, tachycardia.

> (b) Treatment: Transfusion of packed RBCs; because of 50% recurrence rate within 2 years, elective splenectomy may be indicated after 1 or 2 episodes.

b. Infection: Because of functional asplenia, patients (especially those younger than 3 years of age) are at a significantly increased risk of overwhelming infection (sepsis, meningitis, pneumonia, osteomyelitis) with encapsulated organisms (*Haemophilus influenzae, Streptococcus pneumoniae*) and *Salmonella* organisms. It may be difficult to distinguish between a bacterial infection, self-limited viral disorder, and vaso-occlusive crisis in a patient who has fever without an obvious source.

Note: Functional asplenia occurs in most children with Hgb SS by 2 years of age and in most children with Hgb SC by 5 to 6 years of age.

> (1) Workup: CBC, blood culture, CXR; consider LP.
> (2) Management: The treatment of a child with sickle cell disease who is younger than 4 years of age and has a temperature higher than 38.6° C should include the following at a minimum:
>> (a) Evaluation by a primary care provider who is knowledgeable in the care of children with sickle cell disease.
>> (b) IV or IM administration of an antibiotic (cefotaxime or ceftriaxone) effective against *S. pneumoniae* and *H. influenzae*. In areas with a high prevalence of penicillin-resistant pneumococci, or for patients who appear acutely ill, clindamycin should be considered. If meningitis is suspected, vancomycin should be added.
>> (c) Observation for at least 4 hours after parenteral administration of an antibiotic.
>> (d) Reevaluation 24 hours after antibiotic administration.
>> (e) Continuation of antibiotic for at least 2 days.
>> (f) Hospital admission if there is no reliable source of primary care follow-up or the patient appears acutely ill.

Note: The treatment strategy previously described is recommended whether or not the child has a focal source for the fever.

>> (g) Other indications for hospitalization include the following:
>>> (i) Temperature higher than 39.4° C
>>> (ii) Patient younger than 12 months of age
>>> (iii) Toxic appearance
>>> (iv) Shock
>>> (v) Dehydration
>>> (vi) Positive CXR findings
>>> (vii) Respiratory distress
>>> (viii) Neurologic abnormalities (e.g., meningeal signs: stiff neck, altered mental status, focal signs)
>>> (ix) Rapidly enlarging spleen
>>> (x) Falling Hgb (drop of at least 2 g)

10

HEMATOLOGY

        (xi)   WBC count less than 5000 or greater than 40,000

        (xii) Severe abdominal pain

        (xiii) A significantly swollen extremity

        (xiv) Previous sepsis

        (xv) Concurrent pain crisis

Note: Outpatient management of febrile episodes should be reserved only for carefully selected patients.

c. Vaso-occlusive painful crisis: Results from areas of ischemic infarction. It may be precipitated by infection, dehydration, or cold exposure; however, in most cases no trigger is identified.

    (1) This clinical manifestation is the most common cause of hospitalization in patients with sickle cell disease, although most patients have no more than 1 episode per year requiring hospitalization. Episodes tend to recur frequently in a small subset of patients. Most episodes last 3 to 14 days.

    (2) Lower back and extremities are the most common site.

        (a) Clinical features: Pain, with or without erythema, with or without localized soft-tissue swelling, with or without localized tenderness of one or more bones or joints, with or without fever. The possibility of osteomyelitis or septic arthritis needs to be considered, although infarction is much more common than infection. Clues to infection include temperature higher than 39° C, marked elevation of ESR, WBC greater than 30,000, and systemic toxicity. A bone scan performed early can be helpful in suggesting the correct diagnosis.

Note: Young infants may have painful swelling of the hands and feet, called dactylitis.

        (b) Treatment: Hydration and analgesia

            (i)   Opioids are the cornerstone of treating moderate to severe pain. Morphine or hydromorphone should be given by a PCA device with a continuous basal infusion and boluses titrated to effect. The use of opioids should never be avoided because of fear of addiction (no evidence of increased risk in opioid-treated SCD patients). Patients who have been on IV opioids for 1 to 2 weeks need to be slowly weaned to oral drugs.

            (ii) Cognitive therapies such as distraction, biofeedback, hypnotherapy, and psychotherapy should be part of the management of acute and chronic pain.

            (iii) Codeine, NSAIDs (including ketorolac) can be useful for episodes of mild to moderate pain. Meperidine (Demerol) should be avoided because of the risk of dysphoria and seizures.

            (iv) Pain assessment using self-report instruments should be used as part of all treatment strategies.

(3) Abdominal crisis: Patient may have ileus and rebound tenderness, which mimics an acute abdomen (e.g., appendicitis). The pain may be familiar to the patient and readily recognized as "crisis pain." Because painful crises are much more common than an acute surgical abdomen, a period of careful observation of clinical response to hydration and analgesia is warranted in most cases.

(4) Acute chest syndrome
   (a) Represents the leading cause of death in patients with sickle cell disease.
   (b) Clinical: Chest pain, fever, respiratory distress, hypoxemia, rales, decreased breath sounds, egophony, infiltrates; pleural effusion; difficult to distinguish infarction vs. infection and may involve both processes.
   (c) Treatment: Antibiotics, IV hydration, oxygen; transfusion with packed RBCs, or *exchange transfusion* is indicated for severe hypoxemia.
   (d) Recurrent episodes may lead to pulmonary fibrosis and restrictive lung disease.

Note: Chronic transfusion therapy can be complicated by alloimmunization and iron overload (hemosiderosis); patients typically require chelation therapy with desferrioxamine after 1 to 2 years of transfusion therapy. Iron overload may be prevented by use of erythrocytopheresis rather than standard transfusion.

(5) Stroke
   (a) Most devastating form of vaso-occlusive crisis. In young children, its usual cause is cerebral infarct. The most common presentation is hemiplegia or hemiparesis. Patients may also exhibit severe headache, convulsions, coma, aphasia, or visual disturbances. Peak incidence occurs at 7 years of age. Incidence of symptomatic stroke is approximately 10%. Another 10% to 20% of patients will have "silent" or asymptomatic strokes.

Note: Any child with SCD who presents with a neurologic deficit or symptom should be suspected to have had a CVA.

   (b) Diagnosis is based on clinical presentation and CT and MRI findings.
   (c) Treatment consists of monitoring intracranial pressure, seizure control, and exchange transfusion.
   (d) Recurrence risk is 60% to 90% within 3 years. This can be reduced to 10% by maintaining Hgb S less than 30% with a chronic transfusion program. The duration of therapy is unknown, although most centers treat until at least 18 years of age.
   (e) Transcranial Doppler ultrasound can be used as a screen to identify patients with abnormally increased blood velocity secondary to narrow cerebral vessels, indicating an increased

10

HEMATOLOGY

risk for stroke. Such patients may benefit from a prophylactic chronic transfusion program.

(f) Some 10% to 20% of patients will have MRI evidence of a "silent" cerebral infarct; at least one third may become clinically symptomatic, including subtle cognitive deficits.

(6) Miscellaneous: Gallstones, cholecystitis, priapism, avascular hip necrosis, hepatomegaly, retinopathy, papillary necrosis, chronic renal failure, stunted growth, chronic leg ulcers, progressive CNS ischemia with neuropsychologic deficits.

2. General management

a. Comprehensive care in conjunction with a pediatric hematologist or sickle cell program.

(1) Immunization against *H. influenzae* type B, hepatitis B, influenza virus.

(2) The heptavalent conjugate pneumococcal vaccine series should be started at 2 months of age; patients should also receive the 23-valent polysaccharide vaccine at 2 years of age to expand serotype coverage.

(3) Family education, counseling, and anticipatory guidance.

(4) Consider folic acid supplementation: 0.1 mg/d from birth to 6 months of age; 0.25 mg/d from 6 to 12 months of age; 0.5 mg/d from 1 to 2 years of age; 1 mg/d after 2 years of age.

b. Penicillin prophylaxis starts at 2 months of age and continues until the second dose of 23-valent pneumococcal vaccine at 4 to 6 years of age. Prophylaxis probably can be stopped safely in children who have not had a prior severe pneumococcal infection or splenectomy and are receiving comprehensive care. However, the optimal timing of discontinuation has not been established. Parents must be counseled to seek immediate medical attention for all febrile events.

(1) Less than 2 years of age, 125 mg bid PO.

(2) More than 2 years of age, 250 mg bid PO.

(3) If compliance is poor, consider IM penicillin G benzathine q21d.

c. Operative procedures should be carried out by a surgeon who is experienced in treating patients with sickle cell disease and in conjunction with an experienced anesthesiologist and hematologist. Preoperatively, patients should be transfused to a Hgb level of 10 g/dL and/or Hgb S less than 40%.

d. New therapies.

(1) Allogenic bone marrow transplantation from an HLA-matched sibling has an 80% success rate but its use is limited by lack of HLA-matched donors.

(2) Hydroxyurea, which increases fetal Hgb production, has been shown to reduce the frequency of painful crises, but is not yet widely used in children.

D. THROMBOCYTOPENIA

1. Definition
a. Platelet count less than 150,000/mm^3. Need to confirm that low count is not spurious secondary to platelet clumping.
b. Mild-to-moderate thrombocytopenia (50,000 to 150,000/mm^3) is rarely associated with bleeding in the absence of trauma. Bleeding with trauma can occur when the count falls to 20,000 to 30,000/mm^3, but severe bleeding usually does not occur until the count is less than 10,000/mm^3.
c. Clinical manifestations include petechiae, ecchymoses, and mucosal bleeding (gums, GI, epistaxis, menorrhagia). Hematomas are rare: bleeding from superficial cuts may be persistent and profuse.

2. Etiology
a. Decreased production
   (1) Acquired bone marrow hypoplasia: Idiopathic, drug-induced, toxins, viral infection, measles vaccine
   (2) Congenital bone marrow hypoplasia: Fanconi's syndrome, TAR syndrome, Wiskott-Aldrich syndrome, amegakaryocytic thrombocytopenia
   (3) Malignancy
   (4) Drug-induced: Valproic acid, propylthiouracil, phenytoin, TMP/SMZ, penicillin, cephalothin, rifampin, acetaminophen
b. Increased destruction
   (1) Immune-mediated: Infection (TORCH), lupus erythematosus, posttransfusion, drug-induced, HIV infection, immune (idiopathic) thrombocytopenic purpura
   (2) Vascular abnormalities: Catheters, prosthetic heart valves, giant cavernous hemangioma (Kasabach-Merritt syndrome), congenital heart disease, hypersplenism (sequestration), portal hypertension, venous malformations
   (3) Vasculitis with endothelial injury, hemolytic-uremic syndrome, thrombotic thrombocytopenic purpura, DIC

Note: Thrombocytopenia due to platelet destruction is usually isolated, whereas thrombocytopenia due to decreased production is usually associated with anemia and neutropenia.

3. Neonatal thrombocytopenia
a. Alloimmune (isoimmune)
   (1) Platelet equivalent of Rh disease. Confirmed by platelet antigen typing of parents and detection of maternal antibody against the father's platelets. The mother's platelet count is normal.
   (2) Represents the most common cause of severe thrombocytopenia at birth. Affected neonates usually present with purpura; 10% to 20% have intracranial bleeding with half of such episodes occurring antenatally. The newborn is at especially high risk if a previous sibling has had an antenatal bleed.

10

HEMATOLOGY

        (3) The firstborn can be affected, but severity tends to increase in subsequent pregnancies.

        (4) Treatment options include IVIG and transfusion of washed, irradiated maternal platelets for the neonate and, in subsequent pregnancies, IVIG and high-dose prednisone for the mother. Rarely, there may be a role for weekly fetal platelet transfusions.

        (5) The thrombocytopenia is usually transient, resolving in 3 to 4 weeks or less.

   b. Autoimmune

        (1) Secondary to maternal SLE or chronic ITP and transplacental passage of platelet autoantibody. The mother's platelet count is generally low.

        (2) Only 10% to 15% will have platelet counts less than 50,000/mm^3 and risk of serious bleeding is very rare.

        (3) If severe, treatment options include IVIG and steroids.

   c. Other causes include TAR syndrome, trisomies 13 and 18, Wiskott-Aldrich syndrome, viral infection (TORCH), bacterial sepsis, cavernous hemangioma, cyanotic heart disease, and renal vein thrombosis.

4. Acute immune (idiopathic) thrombocytopenic purpura (ITP)

   a. This is by far the most common cause of thrombocytopenia in a previously well child. ITP usually occurs in an otherwise well child between 2 and 6 years of age who presents with petechiae, purpura, easy bruising and/or mucosal bleeding. The PE is otherwise normal. Intracranial and GI bleeding is uncommon.

   b. Often triggered by infection: Viral upper respiratory infection, varicella, Epstein-Barr virus, HIV, cat scratch, measles, mumps, CMV, viral hepatitis, rubella. Look for recent medication use, immunizations, HIV risk factors, family history, or symptoms of autoimmune disease.

   c. Platelet count is usually less than 20,000/mm^3; always confirm by examination of peripheral smear. Hgb concentration, WBC, and differential counts are characteristically normal. There is a slight risk (0.1% to 0.5%) of CNS bleeding when the count is less than 10,000/mm^3 and there is evidence of oral/mucosal bleeding.

   d. A bone marrow examination is not generally indicated but is mandatory with other abnormalities of CBC or smear (nucleated RBCs, blasts), lymphadenopathy, hepatosplenomegaly or failure to respond to IVIG or anti-D. The presence of at least a few large platelets on a smear is reassuring.

   e. Platelet autoantibodies can be detected in 75% of patients, but titer is of no prognostic significance and testing is not diagnostically useful.

Note: Leukemia does not present as isolated thrombocytopenia. Rarely, aplastic anemia can present this way.

   f. Course

        (1) The majority of children with ITP recover spontaneously without recurrence. The time until the return of normal platelet counts ranges from a few days to 6 months (average 3 weeks).

(2) In some patients, resolution of the initial process is followed by recurrent episodes of thrombocytopenia. Chronic ITP (more than 6 months) develops in approximately 10% to 20% of children with acute ITP, and it is more common in older children and in girls.

(3) The initial clinical and laboratory features may not distinguish between acute and chronic ITP or predict which acute patient will develop chronic ITP. However, older age, female gender, and a family history of autoimmune disease are associated with increased risk to develop chronic ITP.

Note: **In adolescents, especially girls, thrombocytopenia may present as part of an autoimmune process.**

g. Treatment

(1) Patients should be followed with serial platelet counts, close observation, and restriction of activity. In ITP, the degree of bleeding is less than what is seen with other forms of thrombocytopenia. Indications for treatment are somewhat controversial but may include: platelet count less than 20,000/mm^3 with mucosal bleeding, and platelet count less than 10,000/mm^3 with minor bleeding.

(2) Treatment options include:

(a) Single infusion of IVIG at a dose of 0.8 g/kg (rate should not exceed 4 ml/kg/h). Has the advantage of rapid platelet response but is costly and associated with side effects (headache, nausea, vomiting, myalgia, and, rarely, aseptic meningitis) in 30% to 50% of patients. Incidence may be reduced by treating with steroids, acetaminophen, and diphenhydramine during and for 48 hours after the infusion.

(b) A single IV infusion of anti-D immune globulin at a dose of 50 mcg/kg. Only indicated in patients who are Rh (o) D positive. It has the advantage of rapid platelet response, ease of administration, and fewer side effects but may be associated with a drop in hemoglobin (average 1 gm/dL) secondary to hemolysis.

(c) High-dose oral prednisone, 4 mg/kg/day × 4 to 7 days. Not often used because of slow platelet response compared to IVIG or anti-D.

(3) Platelet transfusions, along with IVIG and IV methylprednisolone, are only indicated in patients with life-threatening bleeding.

(4) Treatment of acute ITP *does not* decrease the likelihood of chronic ITP.

5. Chronic immune thrombocytopenic purpura

a. Some 10% to 20% of children with acute ITP will go on to develop chronic ITP (platelet count less than 50,000/mm^3 for more than 6 months. Higher incidence with female gender, older than 10 years of

10

HEMATOLOGY

age, higher platelet count at diagnosis of acute ITP, and family history of autoimmune disease.

b. Most children with chronic ITP have only moderate thrombocytopenia, do not have serious bleeding (ICH is rare), and do not need treatment. Spontaneous recovery may occur over a period of years.

c. For those with ongoing bleeding episodes, treatment options include IVIG, anti-D, and steriods. Use of long-term, high-dose prednisone is limited by frequent occurrence of unacceptable side effects. Other treatment options include azathioprine, cyclosporine A, cyclophosphamide, vincristine, dapsone, and alpha interferon. Chemotherapy is typically not initiated until after splenectomy.

d. Splenectomy is associated with a 60% to 85% response rate but, because of the risk of post-splenectomy infection, should be reserved for older children who have ongoing bleeding problems unresponsive to medical management.

e. Patients with chronic ITP should avoid medications that interfere with clotting. They can participate in noncontact sports if platelet counts are greater than 30,000/mm^3 and in contact sports if counts are consistently greater than 100,000/mm^3.

E. NEUTROPENIA

1. Definition

a. Newborns have elevated absolute neutrophil counts (ANCs) in the range 8×10^9/L. The lower limit of normal for patients from 2 weeks to 1 year of age is 1.0×10^9/L. Beyond 1 year of age, neutropenia is defined as an ANC less than 1.5×10^9/L, or less than 800 for African American patients.

b. ANCs are normally lower in persons of African descent and some ethnic groups in the Middle East without any associated clinical manifestations.

2. Manifestations

a. The risk for infection is inversely proportional to the ANC.

Severity	ANC	Manifestation
Mild	1000-1500	usually none
Moderate	500-1000	superficial infections, stomatitis, gingivitis, cellulitis
Severe	<500	perirectal abscess, pneumonia, sepsis

b. The occurrence of bacterial infection in patients with chronic neutropenia is significantly lower than in patients with neutropenia secondary to HIV infection or chemotherapy.

c. *Staphylococcus aureus* is the most common pathogen followed by gram-negative enteric bacilli.

3. Etiology

a. Primary bone marrow disorder

    (1) Fanconi's aplastic anemia

   (2)   Shwachman-Diamond syndrome
   (3)   Cyclic neutropenia
   (4)   Cartilage-hair hypoplasia
   (5)   Kostmann's syndrome (severe congenital neutropenia)
b. Impaired neutrophil production secondary to metabolic or systemic disease
   (1)   Familial (associated with amino-acidopathy)
   (2)   Marrow replacement (leukemia, lymphoma, solid tumor); rare cause of isolated neutropenia
   (3)   Deficiency of vitamin B_{12}/folic acid, copper, protein
   (4)   Infection
c. Infection
   (1)   Most common cause of neutropenia in childhood
   (2)   May be viral, bacterial, rickettsial, fungal, protozoal
   (3)   Often develops during first 24 to 48 hours of viral infection (Epstein-Barr virus, CMV, influenza); persists 3 to 6 days
d. Alloimmune
   (1)   May follow leukocyte transfusion or fetomaternal sensitization
   (2)   Occasionally associated with infections, especially cutaneous
   (3)   Median recovery period of 7 weeks
e. Autoimmune
f. Drug-induced
   (1)   Direct marrow suppression (TMP/SMZ, anti-retroviral drugs, beta lactams)
   (2)   Suppression by drug metabolites
   (3)   Immune neutrophil destruction
4. Evaluation
a. History
   (1)   Type, location, severity, frequency of infection
   (2)   Recent illnesses, drug or toxin exposure, family history
b. PE
   (1)   Careful attention to skin, dental, and perineal areas
   (2)   Hepatosplenomegaly, lymph nodes, congenital defects
c. Laboratory studies
   (1)   Neutrophil counts, recent and past
   (2)   Other hematologic values; bone marrow aspirate
   (3)   Serum immunoglobulins
   (4)   Special testing (e.g., anti-neutrophil antibodies) as indicated by H&P
5. Specific conditions
a. Autoimmune neutropenia (aka chronic idiopathic neutropenia, congenital neutropenia). May also include chronic, benign neutropenia.
   (1)   Most common cause of neutropenia in patients under 4 years of age: peak occurrence is 3 to 30 months. Usually not inherited. It has an autoimmune basis as anti-neutrophil antibodies are often present.

      (2) Increased incidence of infection, especially in individuals with ANCs less than 400. Infection rate tends to decrease with increasing age.

      (3) Noncyclic neutropenia may be the only hematologic abnormality, or there may be associated monocytosis, eosinophilia, and reactive thrombocytosis.

      (4) Treatment

         (a) Proper dental hygiene; all routine immunizations.

         (b) Early and comprehensive evaluation of febrile episodes; broad-spectrum antibiotic coverage, as indicated; rhG-CSF for infections and surgery.

      (5) In most cases there is spontaneous remission several months to several years after diagnosis: mean duration is approximately 20 months.

b. Congenital agranulocytosis (Kostmann Syndrome)

      (1) Frequent, life-threatening infections beginning in the first year of life. Most cases are autosomal recessive. In some cases there is a mutation in the G-CSF receptor or neutrophil elastase gene. Patients are at increased risk to develop leukemia, and this may relate to treatment with rhG-CSF.

      (2) Often severe neutropenia (ANC less than 100). Associated monocytosis and eosinophilia may be present. Bone marrow shows myeloid hyperplasia with maturation arrest at promyelocyte/myelocyte stage.

      (3) Treatment consists of aggressive treatment of infections and daily injections of (rhG-CSF). Bone marrow transplantation is an option for patients with an HLA-identical donor.

Note: Patients treated with rhG-CSF are at risk to develop severe reduction in bone mineral content.

c. Cyclic neutropenia

      (1) Repetitive superficial infections in association with marked variation in the number of circulating neutrophils. The usual cycle is 21 days but may vary from 14 to 36 days. Each cycle usually persists for 3 to 10 days. Genetic basis (autosomal dominant with variable expression) in 25% of cases.

      (2) Diagnosis based on demonstrating at least two oscillation cycles. During neutropenia, the bone marrow shows hypoplasia or maturation arrest at the myelocyte stage.

      (3) The condition is lifelong, but clinical improvement may occur as the patient ages. Usually benign, but overwhelming infection may develop in up to 10% of cases.

      (4) Treatment consists of appropriate antibiotic coverage and long-term subcutaneous administration of rhG-CSF (3 to 5 mcg/kg/d) on alternate days.

d. Shwachman-Diamond syndrome

(1) Exocrine pancreatic insufficiency, neutropenia, skeletal anomalies. Probably autosomal recessive. There is variable (sometimes cyclic) neutropenia with ANCs of 200 to 400.

(2) Treatment includes pancreatic enzyme supplements, appropriate antibiotic coverage, and daily injection of rhG-CSF.

(3) Infections usually decrease with age. However, patients are at risk to develop leukemia and aplastic anemia.

F. BIBLIOGRAPHY

Anemia

Booth IW, Aukett MA: Iron deficiency anaemia in infancy and early childhood, *Arch Dis Child* 76:549, 1997.

Dallman PR, Simes MA: Percentile curves for hemoglobin and red cell volume in infancy and childhood, *J Pediatr* 94:26, 1979.

Oski FA: Iron deficiency: facts and fallacies, *Pediatr Clin North Am* 32:493, 1985.

Stockman JA III: Office hematology: how valid are the results, *Contemp Pediatr* 3:21, 1986.

Wharton BA: Iron deficiency in children: detection and prevention, *Br J Haematol* 106:270, 1999.

Hemophilia

Bell B et al: Hemophilia: an updated review, *Pediatr Rev* 16:290, 1995.

Blanchette VS, Al-Musa A, Stain A-M, et al: Central venous access devices in children with hemophilia: an update, *Blood Coag Fibrinolysis* 8(Suppl 1):S11, 1997.

Harley JR: Disorders of coagulation misdiagnosed as nonaccidental bruising, *Ped Emerg Care* 13:347, 1997.

Ljung RC: Can haemophilic arthropathy be prevented? *Br J Haematol* 101:215, 1998.

Lusher JM: Prophylaxis in children with hemophilia: is it the optimal treatment? *Thrombosis and Hemostasis* 78:726, 1997.

Schwartz RS et al: Human recombinant DNA-derived antihemophilic factor (factor VIII) in the treatment of hemophilia A, *N Engl J Med* 323:1800, 1990.

Neutropenia

Bernina JC: Diagnosis and management of chronic neutropenia during childhood, *Pediatr Clin North Am* 43:773, 1996.

Haddy TB, Rana SR, Castro O: Benign ethnic neutropenia: what is a normal absolute neutrophil count? *J Lab Clin Med* 133:15, 1999.

Vlachos A, Lipton JM: Bone marrow failure in children, *Curr Opin Pediatr* 8:33, 1996.

Sickle Cell Disease

American Academy of Pediatrics: Health supervision for children with sickle cell disease and their families, *Pediatrics* 98:467, 1996.

Evans JPM: Practical management of sickle cell disease, *Arch Dis Child* 64:1748, 1989.

Hoppe C, Styles L, Vichinsky E: The natural history of sickle cell disease, *Curr Opin Pediatr* 10:49, 1998.

Moran CJ, Siegel MJ, DeBaun MR: Sickle cell disease: imaging of cerebrovascular complications, *Radiology* 206:311, 1998.

Pai VB, Nahata MC: Duration of penicillin prophylaxis in sickle cell anemia: issues and controversies, *Pharmacotherapy* 20:110, 2000.

Pearson HA: Sickle cell diseases: diagnosis and management in infancy and childhood, *Pediatr Rev* 9:121, 1987.

Powars DR: Management of cerebral vasculopathy in children with sickle cell anaemia, *Br J Haematol* 108:666, 2000.

Steele RW et al: Colonization with antibiotic-resistant *Streptococcus pneumoniae* in children with sickle cell disease, *J Pediatr* 128:531, 1996.

Vichinsky EP: Comprehensive care in sickle cell disease: its impact on morbidity and mortality, *Semin Hematol* 28:220, 1991.

10

HEMATOLOGY

Yaster M, Kost-Byerly S, Maxwell LG: The management of pain in sickle cell disease, *Pediatr Clin North Am* 47:699, 2000.

Thrombocytopenia

Blanchette VS et al: Randomized trial of intravenous immunoglobulin G, intravenous anti-D and oral prednisone in childhood acute immune thrombocytopenia purpura, *Lancet* 344:703, 1994.

Bolton-Maggs PHB: Idiopathic thrombocytopenic purpura, *Arch Dis Child* 83:220, 2000.

Borgna-Pignatti C, Rugolotto S, Nobili B et al: A trial of high-dose dexamethasone therapy for chronic idiopathic thrombocytopenic purpura in childhood, *J Pediatr* 130:16, 1997.

Bussel JB: Thrombocytopenia in newborns, infants, and children, *Pediatr Ann* 19:181, 1990.

Chu Y-W, Korb J, Sakamoto KM: Idiopathic thrombocytopenic purpura, *Pediatr Rev* 21:95, 2000.

Halperin DS, Doyle JJ: Is bone marrow examination justified in idiopathic thrombocytopenic purpura? *Am J Dis Child* 142:508, 1988.

Imbach P, Kuhne T: Immune thrombocytopenic purpura ITP, *Vox Sanguinis* 74(suppl 2):309, 1998.

Murphy S, Nepo A, Sills R: Thrombocytopenia, *Pediatr Rev* 20:64, 1999.

Skupski DW, Bussel JB: Alloimmune thrombocytopenia, *Clin Obs Gynecol* 42:335, 1999.

Tarantino MD: Treatment options for chronic immune (idiopathic) thrombocytopenia purpura in children, *Semin Hematol* 37(suppl 1):35, 2000.

IMMUNIZATIONS

A. RECOMMENDED CHILDHOOD IMMUNIZATION

Recommended childhood immunization schedule, United States, 2002 (Table 11-1).

1. Recommended vaccine doses should never be reduced or divided in an effort to reduce adverse events.
2. A mild acute illness with low-grade fever, mild diarrheal illness in an otherwise well child, pregnancy of mother or other household contact, current antimicrobial therapy, or recent exposure to an infectious disease are not contraindications to vaccination.
3. Permanent contraindications to vaccination.
a. Severe allergy to a vaccine component or an anaphylactic reaction to a previous dose of the vaccine.
b. Pertussis vaccine encephalopathy.
4. Temporary contraindications to vaccination.
a. Severe acute illness
b. Immunosuppression
c. Pregnancy (applies to live virus vaccines)
d. Recent receipt of blood, blood products or immune globulin (OPV not affected)

B. IMMUNIZATION OF PRETERM INFANTS

1. Prematurely born infants, including those of low birth weight, should be immunized at the usual chronologic age in most cases.
2. If a mother is HBsAg-negative, HBV vaccination of her prematurely born infant can be started at hospital discharge (if infant's weight is greater than 2 kg) or at the 2-month visit. If a mother is HBsAg-positive, HBV vaccination should begin soon after birth, along with a dose of HBIG at a different site.
3. Vaccination of small, sick, hospitalized premature infants may be associated with a 5% to 30% incidence of new or worsening episodes of apnea in the 2 to 3 days following vaccination.

C. IMMUNIZATION OF CHILDREN WITH LAPSED SCHEDULES
(See Table 11-2.)

D. IMMUNIZATION OF CHILDREN WITH IMMUNE DEFICIENCY

1. HIV-infected or HIV-exposed children should receive DTaP, HBV, *haemophilus influenzae* B conjugate vaccine, influenza vaccine, inactivated polio vaccine, and pneumoccocal conjugate vaccine according to regular ACIP and AAP guidelines.
2. Infants born to mothers infected with HIV and whose infection status is uncertain should be considered potentially HIV-infected until transmitted maternal HIV antibody is no longer detectable, at which

TABLE 11-1

RECOMMENDED CHILDHOOD IMMUNIZATION SCHEDULE UNITED STATES, 2002

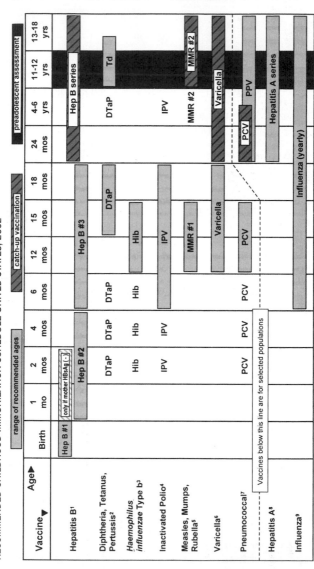

Vaccine ▼ Age ▶	Birth	1 mo	2 mos	4 mos	6 mos	12 mos	15 mos	18 mos	24 mos	4-6 yrs	11-12 yrs	13-18 yrs
Hepatitis B[1]	Hep B #1	Hep B #2 (only if mother HBsAg (-))	Hep B #2		Hep B #3						Hep B series	
Diphtheria, Tetanus, Pertussis[2]			DTaP	DTaP	DTaP		DTaP	DTaP		DTaP	Td	
Haemophilus influenzae Type b[3]			Hib	Hib	Hib	Hib	Hib					
Inactivated Polio[4]			IPV	IPV		IPV				IPV		
Measles, Mumps, Rubella[5]						MMR #1				MMR #2		MMR #2
Varicella[6]						Varicella				Varicella		
Pneumococcal[7]			PCV	PCV	PCV	PCV	PCV		PCV	PCV		
Hepatitis A[8]										Hepatitis A series		
Influenza[9]									Influenza (yearly)			

Vaccines below this line are for selected populations

Approved by the Advisory Committee on Immunization Practices (www.cdc.gov/nip/acip), the American Academy of Pediatrics (www.aap.org), and the American Academy of Family Physicians (www.aafp.org).

This schedule indicates the recommended ages for routine administration of currently licensed childhood vaccines, as of December 1, 2001, for children through age 18 years. Any dose not given at the recommended age should be given at any subsequent visit when indicated and feasible. ▨ Indicates age groups that warrant special effort to administer those vaccines not previously given. Additional vaccines may be licensed and recommended during the year. Licensed combination vaccines may be used whenever any components of the combination are indicated and the vaccine's other components are not contraindicated. Providers should consult the manufacturers' package inserts for detailed recommendations.

[1] **Hepatitis B vaccine (Hep B).** All infants should receive the first dose of hepatitis B vaccine soon after birth and before hospital discharge; the first dose may also be given by age 2 months if the infant's mother is HBsAg-negative. Only monovalent hepatitis B vaccine can be used for the birth dose. Monovalent or combination vaccine containing Hep B may be used to complete the series; four doses of vaccine may be administered if combination vaccine is used. The second dose should be given at least 4 weeks after the first dose, except for Hib-containing vaccine which cannot be administered before age 6 weeks. The third dose should be given at least 16 weeks after the first dose and at least 8 weeks after the second dose. The last dose in the vaccination series (third or fourth dose) should not be administered before age 6 months.

Infants born to HBsAg-positive mothers should receive hepatitis B vaccine and 0.5 mL hepatitis B immune globulin (HBIG) within 12 hours of birth at separate sites. The second dose is recommended at age 1-2 months and the vaccination series should be completed (third or fourth dose) at age 6 months.

Infants born to mothers whose HBsAg status is unknown should receive the first dose of the hepatitis B vaccine series within 12 hours of birth. Maternal blood should be drawn at the time of delivery to determine the mother's HBsAg status; if the HBsAg test is positive, the infant should receive HBIG as soon as possible (no later than age 1 week).

[2] **Diphtheria and tetanus toxoids and acellular pertussis vaccine (DTaP).** The fourth dose of DTaP may be administered as early as age 12 months, provided 6 months have elapsed since the third dose and the child is unlikely to return at age 15-18 months. **Tetanus and diphtheria toxoids (Td)** is recommended at age 11-12 years if at least 5 years have elapsed since the last dose of tetanus and diphtheria toxoid-containing vaccine. Subsequent routine Td boosters are recommended every 10 years.

[3] **Haemophilus influenza type b (Hib) conjugate vaccine.** Three Hib conjugate vaccines are licensed for infant use. If PRP-OMP (PedvaxHib® or ComVax® [Merck]) is administered at ages 2 and 4 months, a dose at age 6 months is not required. DTaP/Hib combination products should not be used for primary immunization in infants at ages 2, 4 or 6 months, but can be used as boosters following any Hib vaccine.

[4] **Inactivated polio vaccine (IPV).** An all-IPV schedule is recommended for routine childhood polio vaccination in the United States. All children should receive four doses of IPV at ages 2 months, 4 months, 6-18 months, and 4-6 years.

[5] **Measles, mumps, and rubella vaccine (MMR).** The second dose of MMR is recommended routinely at age 4-6 years but may be administered during any visit, provided at least 4 weeks have elapsed since the first dose and that both doses are administered beginning at or after age 12 months. Those who have not previously received the second dose should complete the schedule by the 11-12 year old visit.

[6] **Varicella vaccine.** Varicella vaccine is recommended at any visit at or after age 12 months for susceptible children, i.e., those who lack a reliable history of chickenpox. Susceptible persons age ≥13 years should receive two doses, given at least 4 weeks apart.

[7] **Pneumococcal vaccine.** The heptavalent **pneumococcal conjugate vaccine (PCV)** is recommended for all children age 2-23 months. It is also recommended for certain children age 24-59 months. **Pneumococcal polysaccharide vaccine (PPV)** is recommended in addition to PCV for certain high-risk groups. See *MMWR* 2000;49(RR-9);1-35.

[8] **Hepatitis A vaccine.** Hepatitis A vaccine is recommended for use in selected states and regions, and for certain high-risk groups; consult your local public health authority. See *MMWR* 1999;48(RR-12);1-37.

[9] **Influenza vaccine.** Influenza vaccine is recommended annually for children age ≥6 months with certain risk factors (including but not limited to asthma, cardiac disease, sickle cell disease, HIV, diabetes; see *MMWR* 2001;50(RR-4);1-44), and can be administered to all others wishing to obtain immunity. Children aged ≤12 years should receive vaccine in a dosage appropriate for their age (0.25 mL if age 6-35 months or 0.5 mL if aged ≥3 years). Children aged ≥8 years who are receiving influenza vaccine for the first time should receive two doses separated by at least 4 weeks.

For additional information about vaccines, vaccine supply, and contraindications for immunization, please visit the National Immunization Program Website at www.cdc.gov/nip or call the National Immunization Hotline at 800-232-2522 (English) or 800-232-0233 (Spanish).

11

IMMUNIZATIONS

TABLE 11-2
RECOMMENDED ACCELERATED IMMUNIZATION SCHEDULE FOR INFANTS AND CHILDREN YOUNGER THAN 7 YEARS WHO START THE SERIES LATE OR WHO ARE MORE THAN 1 MONTH BEHIND IN THE IMMUNIZATION SCHEDULE

Timing/Age	Vaccine(s)	Comment
First visit (≥4 months of age)	DTaP, IPV, Hib,* hepatitis B, MMR, varicella, pneumococcal conjugate†	Must be ≥12 months of age to receive MMR and varicella. If ≥5 years of age, Hib is not normally indicated.
Second visit (1 month‡ after first visit)	DTaP, IPV, Hib,* hepatitis B, pneumococcal conjugate†	
Third visit (1 month after second visit)	DTaP, IPV, Hib,* pneumococcal conjugate†	
Fourth visit (≥6 months after third visit)	DTaP, Hib,* hepatitis B, pneumococcal conjugate†	Preferably at or before school entry. DTaP is not necessary if the fourth dose was given on or after the fourth birthday. If the third poliovirus vaccine dose is given after the third birthday, the fourth dose is not needed
4-6 years	DTaP, IPV, MMR	
11-12 years	Varicella, MMR, and/or hepatitis B (if not already received). Td if >5 years since last dose	Repeat Td every 10 years throughout life.

Source: Centers for Disease Control and Prevention. General recommendations on immunization. Atlanta, Ga: 1994, with modifications.

*The recommended schedule for Hib vaccination varies by vaccine manufacturer and age of the child when vaccination series is started. If the series is begun at an age younger than 7 months, 4 doses are needed (only 3 doses are needed if all doses are PRP-OMP [PedvaxHib, Merck]). The last dose must be ≥2 months after the preceding dose and on or after the first birthday. If the series is started between ages 7 and 11 months, 3 total doses are needed with the third dose ≥2 months after the second dose and on or after the first birthday. If the series is started at age 12 to 14 months, 2 doses are needed ≥2 months apart. If the series is started at age ≥15 months, 1 dose of any conjugate Hib vaccine is recommended.

†The recommended schedule for pneumococcal conjugate vaccine depends on the age of the child when the vaccination series is started and on the child's health status. If the series is begun at an age younger than 7 months, 4 doses are needed. The last dose must be ≥2 months after the preceding dose and on or after the first birthday. If the series is started between ages 7 and 11 months, 3 total doses are needed. If the series is started at age 12 to 23 months, 2 doses are needed 2 months apart. If the series is started at age 24 months, or later 1 dose is recommended unless the child has a chronic illness or immunocompromising condition including human immunodeficiency virus, asplenia, and sickle cell disease, in which case 2 doses are recommended 2 months apart. These recommendations are still in the draft stage.

‡An interval of 28 or more days.

time such children can follow the same recommendations used for healthy children.

3. MMR vaccine should be given unless the child is severely immuno-compromised. The first dose should be given at 12 months of age and the second dose as soon as 30 days later.

Note: Upon exposure to wild-type measles, immune globulin prophylaxis (0.5 ml/kg, maximum 15 ml) should be administered to all HIV-infected children and adolescents and to children of unknown infection status born to HIV-infected women regardless of the degree of immunosuppression or measles immunization status.

4. Varicella vaccine (Varivax)
a. Children with impaired humoral immunity may receive varicella vaccine.
b. Varicella vaccine should not be administered routinely to children who have cellular immunodeficiency. Exceptions include:
   (1) Children who have acute lymphocytic leukemia (vaccine available through a research protocol).
   (2) HIV-infected children in CDC Class 1 with mild or no signs and symptoms; eligible children should receive 2 doses of vaccine 3 months apart.
5. Hepatitis A
a. Hepatitis A virus (HAV) vaccine is not routinely indicated in HIV-infected children unless they are more than 2 years of age and have risk factors for HAV infection.
b. Immunosuppressed children should receive immune globulin for prophylaxis of known hepatitis A exposure, regardless of vaccination status.
6. Hepatitis B
a. HBV vaccination should be followed by serologic evaluation of immunity.
b. Revaccination should be considered for children who do not develop a serum anti-HB$_s$ antibody response greater than 10 m IU/mL.
7. There are no standardized recommendations for revaccination of HIV-infected children.
8. Quadrivalent meningococcal vaccine (Menomune-A, C, Y, W-135, Aventis Pasteur) is recommended for children with anatomic asplenia, functional asplenia, or a terminal complement deficiency.
9. Temporary immunodeficiency
a. Children receiving immunosuppressive therapy should not receive live vaccines, including MMR, until the underlying condition is in remission or under control and a minimum of 3 months have passed since the cessation of immunosuppressive therapy.
b. Recommendations for the administration of live vaccines to children receiving corticosteroid therapy are shown in Table 11-3.
c. Inactivated vaccines do not pose a safety problem and may be given to children receiving immunosuppressive therapy. However, the immune

11

IMMUNIZATIONS

response is likely to be suboptimal and delaying vaccination is usually recommended.

d. The ability to generate an immune response to inactivated vaccines usually returns between 3 and 12 months after stopping chemotherapy. Children who received vaccine during immunosuppressive therapy should be revaccinated after therapy is stopped.

10. Contacts of immunocompromised children.

a. Close contacts of immunocompromised children (including those with asymptomatic HIV infection) should *not* receive oral polio vaccine.

b. MMR, varicella, and annual influenza vaccine *are* recommended for susceptible household contacts.

E. IMMUNIZATION FOR CHILDREN TRAVELING ABROAD

1. The most important step is to review and update the child's routine immunization status.

2. For travel at short notice, administration of DTaP, polio and hepatitis B vaccines can be safely accelerated according to AAP Red Book recommendations.

3. For children 6 to 12 months of age, an initial dose of MMR vaccine can be given at the time of travel, with a subsequent dose administered after 1 year of age.

TABLE 11-3

AMERICAN ACADEMY OF PEDIATRICS RECOMMENDATIONS FOR THE ADMINISTRATION OF LIVE VACCINES TO CHILDREN RECEIVING CORTICOSTEROID THERAPY

Treatment Category and Duration	Dose of Prednisone or Equivalent	Interval After Cessation of Steroids Prior to Administering Live Vaccines
Topical therapy		None*
Inhaled therapy		None*
Local injections		None*
Physiologic maintenance	Replacement doses	None
Low or moderate doses	<2 mg/kg/d or <20 mg/d if weight is >10 kg	None*
High dose, <14 days	≥2 mg/kg/d or ≥20 mg/d if weight is ≥10 kg	Discontinue steroid therapy 0-2 weeks†
High dose, ≥14 days	≥2 mg/kg/d or ≥20 mg/d if weight is ≥10 kg, daily or alternate days	Discontinue steroid therapy ≥1 month

*If prolonged treatment with topical, inhaled, or local steroids results in signs or symptoms of systemic immunosuppression, live vaccines should not be administered until steroids have been discontinued for 1 month or more.

†For short courses of high-dose steroids, some experts recommend a 2-week delay after discontinuing steroids prior to giving live vaccines. Other experts do not believe that a delay is necessary after steroids are stopped.

American Academy of Pediatrics: *Redbook Report of the Committee on Infectious Diseases,* ed 25, Elk Grove Village, IL, 2000.

4. Specific vaccine recommendations, by country, can be obtained on-line at www.cdc.gov/travel/travel.html.

F. SPECIAL CONSIDERATIONS

1. Hepatitis A virus (HAV) vaccine
a. HAVRIX (SmithKline Beecham)
   (1) Children 2 to 18 years of age—0.5 ml, repeated in 6 to 12 months
   (2) Adults more than 18 years of age—1.0 ml, repeated in 6 to 12 months
b. VAQTA (Merck)
   (1) Children 2 to 17 years of age—0.5 ml, repeated in 6 to 12 months
   (2) Adults more than 17 years of age—1.0 ml, repeated in 6 to 12 months
c. Neither vaccine is recommended for use in children younger than 2 years of age.
d. The vaccine is now *routinely recommended* for children who live in states or local areas in which the incidence of hepatitis A is 20 or more cases per 100,000 population per year.
e. The vaccine should *be considered* for children who live in areas in which the incidence of hepatitis A is 10 to 20 cases per 100,000 population per year.
f. Other indications include
   (1) Travel to developing countries
   (2) Clotting factor disorders
   (3) Chronic liver disease
g. Guidelines for immune serum globulin prophylaxis in children who have not been vaccinated are shown in Table 11-4.
2. Influenza vaccine
a. Recommended for individuals older than 6 months of age who are at increased risk of influenza-related complications.
   (1) Children having chronic pulmonary (asthma, BPD, CF), renal, and cardiac disease; cancer; and diabetes, hemoglobinopathies, and immunosuppressive disorders, including HIV.
   (2) Children and teenagers receiving long-term aspirin therapy.
b. Also recommended for children who are household contacts of persons at high risk.

11

IMMUNIZATIONS

TABLE 11-4
ISG USE IN PREVENTING HEPATITIS A VIRUS

Type of Protection Required	Duration Needed	Dose of ISG Recommended (mL/kg)
Pre-exposure	Short term (1-2 mo)	0.02
Pre-exposure	Long term (3-5 mo)	0.06
Postexposure	—	0.02

c. Annual vaccination is recommended according to the schedule shown in Table 11-5.

d. Influenza vaccine can be administered simultaneously with other scheduled vaccines.

e. The major contraindication is a history of egg allergy or allergy to other vaccine components.

3. Lyme Disease

a. A Lyme vaccine has been approved for persons 15 to 70 years of age, but because of a lack of demand, is no longer being provided by the manufacturer.

4. Meningococcal vaccine

a. A quadrivalent A, C, Y, W-135 polysaccharide vaccine (Menomune-A, C, Y, W-135, Aventis Pasteur) is available in the United States. The dose is 0.5 ml. Protective levels of antibody are usually achieved within 7 to 10 days of vaccination.

Note: A conjugate C meningococcal vaccine is in routine use in the United Kingdom and should become available in the United States.

b. Recommendations for vaccine use include the following:
   (1) Persons with anatomic asplenia, functional asplenia, or terminal complement deficiency.
   (2) Control of serogroup C meningococcal outbreaks.

c. Revaccination is indicated after 2 to 3 years for children first vaccinated at less than 4 years of age and after 3 to 5 years for older children.

d. Routine use of meningococcal vaccine in college students is controversial. College freshman living in dormitories appear to be at moderately increased risk; it is estimated that 60% of cases are vaccine preventable. Students and their families should be informed about meningococcal disease and the benefits of vaccination, and vaccine should be made available to college freshman who want to reduce their risk for meningococcal disease.

TABLE 11-5			
SCHEDULE FOR INFLUENZA VACCINE DOSAGE BY AGE			
Age	Vaccine Type	Dose (mL)	Number of Doses
6-35 mo	Split virus*	0.25	1-2†
3-8 y	Split virus	0.5	1-2†
9-12 y	Split virus	0.5	1
>12 y	Whole or split virus	0.5	1

*Split virus vaccine may be termed split, subvirion or purified surface-antigen vaccine.
Adapted from: *American Academy of Pediatrics: Redbook Report of the Committee on Infectious Diseases*, ed 25, Elk Grove Village, IL, 2000.
†Two doses administered 4 or more weeks apart are recommended for children receiving the influenza vaccine for the first time.
Vaccine should be administered in the fall, before the start of the influenza season. Vaccine should be administered intramuscularly in the deltoid area in adults and older children and in the anterolateral aspect of the thigh in infants and toddlers.

e. Routine revaccination of college students who were vaccinated as freshmen is not indicated.

f. Antimicrobial chemophylaxis

    (1) The primary means for prevention of meningococcal disease is antimicrobial chemoprophylaxis of close contacts of infected persons (Table 11-6).

    (2) Close contacts include: household members; day care center contacts, and anyone directly exposed to the patient's oral secretions.

    (3) Prophylaxis should be administered as soon as possible, ideally within 24 hours after identification of the index patient. Prophylaxis administered more than 14 days after onset of illness in the index patient is of limited or no value.

5. Pneumococcal vaccine

a. A hepatavalent pneumococcal conjugate vaccine (PCV 7, Prevnar, Wyeth-Lederle Vaccines) is licensed for use among infants 6 weeks of age or older. It is administered IM as a 0.5 ml dose and can be given at the same time as other routine childhood vaccinations in a separate syringe at a separate injection site.

b. ACIP recommendations for vaccine use are shown in Table 11-7.

c. Recommended vaccine schedules are shown in Tables 11-8 and 11-9.

11

IMMUNIZATIONS

TABLE 11-6

SCHEDULE FOR ADMINISTERING CHEMOPROPHYLAXIS FOR MENINGOCOCCAL DISEASE

Drug	Age Group	Dosage	Duration and Route of Administration
Rifampin*	Children aged <1 month	5 mg/kg every 12 hrs	2 days, orally
	Children aged ≥1 month	10 mg/kg every 12 hrs	2 days, orally
	Adults	600 mg every 12 hrs	2 days, orally
Ciprofloxacin†	Adults	500 mg	Single dose, orally
Ceftriaxone	Children aged <15 years	125 mg	Single dose, IM§
Ceftriaxone	Adults	250 mg	Single dose, IM§

*Rifampin is not recommended for pregnant women because the drug is teratogenic in laboratory animals. Because the reliability of oral contraceptives may be affected by rifampin therapy, alternative contraceptive measures should be considered while rifampin is being administered.

†Ciprofloxacin is not generally recommended for persons <18 years of age or for pregnant and lactating women because the drug causes cartilage damage in immature laboratory animals. However, ciprofloxacin can be used for chemoprophylaxis of children when no acceptable alternative therapy is available.

§Intramuscular.

CDC: Prevention and control of meningococcal disease: recommendations of the Advisory Committee on Immunization Practices, *MMWR* 49: No. RR-7, 2000.

TABLE 11-7

SUMMARY OF RECOMMENDATIONS FOR USE OF 7-VALENT PNEUMOCOCCAL CONJUGATE VACCINE (PCV7) AMONG INFANTS AND CHILDREN

CHILDREN FOR WHOM PCV7 IS RECOMMENDED

All children aged ≤23 mos

Children aged 24-59 mos with the following conditions:

- Sickle cell disease and other sickle cell hemoglobinopathies, congenital or acquired asplenia, or splenic dysfunction
- Infection with human immunodeficiency virus
- Immunocompromising conditions, including
  — Congenital immunodeficiencies: B- (humoral) or T-lymphocyte deficiency; complement deficiencies, particularly c1, c2, c3, and c4 deficiency; and phagocytic disorders, excluding chronic granulomatous disease
  — Renal failure and nephrotic syndrome
  — Disease associated with immunosuppressive therapy or radiation therapy, including malignant neoplasms, leukemias, lymphomas, and Hodgkin's disease; or solid organ transplantation
- Chronic illness, including
  — Chronic cardiac disease, particularly cyanotic congenital heart disease and cardiac failure
  — Chronic pulmonary disease, excluding asthma unless on high dose corticosteroid therapy
  — Cerebrospinal fluid leaks
  — Diabetes mellitus

CHILDREN FOR WHOM PCV7 SHOULD BE CONSIDERED

All children aged 24-59 mos, with priority given to

- Children aged 24-35 mos
- Children of Alaska Native or American Indian descent
- Children of African-American descent
- Children who attend group day care centers*

*Defined as a setting outside the home where a child regularly spends ≥4 hours per week with ≥2 unrelated children under adult supervision.

CDC: Preventing pneumococcal disease among infants and young children: recommendations of the Advisory Committee on Immunization Practices, *MMWR* 49: No. RR-9, 2000.

d. High-risk children 24 to 59 months of age who have already received the 23-valent pneumococcal polysaccharide vaccine (PPV 23) should receive 2 doses of Prevnar initiated 2 or more months after vaccination with PPV 23.

e. High-risk children who have completed the Prevnar series before age 2 years should receive 1 dose of PPV 23 at 2 years of age or older initiated 2 months or more after the last dose of Prevnar.

Note: Children under 5 years of age with functional or anatomic asplenia (including children with sickle cell disease) who have received Prevnar should continue to receive antibiotic prophylaxis through 5 years of age.

TABLE 11-8

RECOMMENDED SCHEDULE FOR USE OF 7-VALENT PNEUMOCOCCAL CONJUGATE VACCINE (PCV7) AMONG PREVIOUSLY UNVACCINATED INFANTS AND CHILDREN BY AGE AT TIME OF FIRST VACCINATION

Age at First Dose (mos)	Primary Series	Additional Dose
2-6	3 doses, 2 mos apart*	1 dose at 12-15 mos†
7-11	2 doses, 2 mos apart*	1 dose at 12-15 mos†
12-23	2 doses, 2 mos apart‡	—
24-59		
Healthy children	1 dose	—
Children with sickle cell disease, asplenia, human immunodeficiency virus infection, chronic illness, or immunocom-promising condition¶	2 doses, 2 mos apart	—

*For children vaccinated at age <1 year, minimum interval between doses is 4 weeks.
†The additional dose should be administered ≥8 weeks after the primary series has been completed.
‡Minimum interval between doses is 8 weeks.
¶Recommendations do not include children who have undergone a bone marrow transplantation.
CDC: Preventing pneumococcal disease among infants and young children: recommendations of the Advisory Committee on Immunization Practices, *MMWR* 49: No. RR-9, 2000.

TABLE 11-9

RECOMMENDATIONS FOR USE OF 7-VALENT PNEUMOCOCCAL CONJUGATE VACCINE (PCV7) AMONG CHILDREN WITH A LAPSE IN VACCINE ADMINISTRATION

Age at Examination (mos)	Previous PCV7 Vaccination History	Recommended Regimen
7-11	1 dose	1 dose of PCV7 at 7-11 mos, with a second dose ≥2 mos later, at 12-15 mos
	2 doses	Same regimen
12-23	1 dose before age 12 mos	2 doses of PCV7 ≥2 mos apart
	2 doses before age 12 mos	1 dose of PCV7 ≥2 mos after the most recent dose
24-59	Any incomplete schedule	1 dose of PCV7*

*Children with certain chronic diseases or immunosuppressing conditions should receive two doses ≥2 months apart.
CDC: Preventing pneumococcal disease among infants and young children: recommendations of the Advisors Committee on Immunization Practices, *MMWR* 49: No. RR-9, 2000.

6. Varicella vaccine
a. Recommended that all healthy children 12 months to 13 years of age receive 1 dose of live attenuated varicella vaccine (Merck). It can be given with other childhood vaccinations, but not in the same syringe. Salicylates should be withheld for 6 weeks after receipt of the vaccine.

b. Adolescents who have not had varicella should receive 2 doses of vaccine at least 4 weeks apart.

c. Post-vaccination serologic testing is not recommended.

d. Individuals with immune suppression
   (1) Children receiving high-dose corticosteroids (greater than or equal to 2 mg/kg/day or greater than or equal to 20 mg/day) for more than 1 month should not receive vaccine until the steroid has been discontinued for 3 months.
   (2) Vaccine should not be administered for 5 months after a dose of immune globulin.
   (3) Vaccine may be considered for asymptomatic or mildly symptomatic HIV-infected children in CDC class NI or AI with age-specific CD4+ T lymphocyte percentages greater than or equal to 25.

e. Approximately 6% of recipients develop a vaccine-associated rash (median 5 lesions) 10 to 21 days following vaccination and lasting an average of 2 days. Such individuals should avoid contact with immuno-compromised susceptible individuals for the duration of the rash.

f. Breakthrough cases of varicella following vaccination are significantly less severe than natural varicella (median lesions 32 to 53 versus 300 to 500).

g. Varicella vaccine appears to confer long-lasting immunity and the incidence of subsequent herpes zoster is lower than following naturally acquired varicella.

Note: If given within 3 days of exposure to varicella, the vaccine is highly effective in preventing moderate and severe disease, and it is now recommended by the AAP for this indication. Administration during the presymptomatic or prodromal stage of varicella does not increase the risk of vaccine-associated adverse events and does not result in more severe natural disease.

G. BIBLIOGRAPHY

American Academy of Pediatrics: Committee on Infectious Diseases, *Pediatrics* 109:162, 2002.

American Academy of Pediatrics: Committee on Infectious Diseases and Committee on Pediatric AIDS: Measles immunization in HIV-infected children, *Pediatrics* 103:1057, 1999.

American Academy of Pediatrics: Meningococcal disease prevention and control strategies for practice-based physicians (addendum: recommendations for college students), *Pediatrics* 106:1500, 2000.

American Academy of Pediatrics: Varicella vaccine update, *Pediatrics* 105:136, 2000.

American Academy of Pediatrics: Prevention of Lyme disease, *Pediatrics* 105:142, 2000.

American Academy of Pediatrics: *Redbook Report of the Committee on Infectious Diseases,* ed 25, Elk Grove Village, IL, 2000.

CDC: Meningococcal disease and college students: recommendations of the Advisory Committee on Immunization Practices, *MMWR* 49:13, 2000.

CDC: Preventing pneumococcal disease among infants and young children: recommendations of the Advisory Committee on Immunization Practices, *MMWR* 49: No. RR-9, 2000.

CDC: Prevention and control of meningococcal disease: recommendations of the Advisory Committee of Immunization Practices, *MMWR* 49: No. RR-7, 2000.

Chartrono SA: Varicella vaccine, *Pediatr Clin North Am* 47:373, 2000.

D'Angio CT: Immunization of the premature infant, *Pediatr Inf Dis J* 18:823, 1999.

McFarland E: Immunization for the immunocompromised child, *Pediatr Ann* 28:486, 1999.

Sood SK: Immunization for children traveling abroad, *Pediatr Clin North Am* 47:435, 2000.

Zimmerman RK: Prevention of influenza by expanded ages for routine vaccination, *J Fam Pract* 49:515, 2000.

Zimmerman RK, Burns IT: Childhood vaccination, Part 1: routine vaccines, *J Fam Pract* 49:522, 2000.

Zimmerman RK, Burns IT: Childhood vaccination, Part 2: childhood vaccination procedures, *J Fam Pract* 49:534, 2000.

11

IMMUNIZATIONS

INGESTIONS

Carl R. Baum

A. TELEPHONE TRIAGE

1. Many cases of ingestion come to attention by telephone call. Note time of call. Most parents will be frantic. *You* should remain calm.
2. Take a brief history. What was ingested and was it a sustained-release preparation? How much? (How many pills or how much liquid is missing?) The dose of ingested toxin should be calculated using a "worst case scenario." When? Where? Any vomiting? Was the event witnessed? Any treatment given? What is the child's present mental and physical status?
3. Assess urgency. Should parents come to the ED as soon as possible, or should an emergency vehicle be dispatched? If in doubt as to disposition, keep caller on hold and call local poison control center. Be sure to have parents bring ingested material with them plus the container, whether filled or empty.
4. Obtain name of caller, phone number, and address.
5. Although syrup of ipecac effectively induces emesis, clinical studies have *not* demonstrated that its use improves outcome of poisoned patients. Ipecac therefore should *not* be recommended routinely, and its use is contraindicated in cases of caustics or hydrocarbon, or if the patient is obtunded, comatose, seizing, or at risk of rapid deterioration (tricyclics) or worsening by vagal stimulation of the cardiac conduction system.
6. Although activated charcoal (AC) should not be recommended routinely, clinical studies have indicated that its use as an adsorbent is most effective if administered within one hour of ingestion of an adsorbable substance (see later discussion). Administration of AC in the home may become more common.
7. Instruct the parents to bring the child to the ED if any potentially dangerous substance has been ingested or if the child is less than 6 months of age.

B. EMERGENCY DEPARTMENT MANAGEMENT

1. Obtain a brief history as previously stated. If the nature of the ingestion is unknown, ask what medications or other toxic substances (e.g., household products, pesticides) are in and around the home.
2. PE: Note weight, vital signs, mental status, perfusion, respiratory status, cardiac status, pupils, unusual odors, and any spills on clothes.
3. Management of the highly symptomatic patient (see *The Harriet Lane Handbook*)
   a. Establish and maintain vital functions; establish and secure an airway.
   b. Insert an ETT for patients with impaired airway protection.

  c. Control hypotension, hypertension, pulmonary edema, arrhythmias, cerebral edema, renal failure, metabolic acidosis, and hypothermia as indicated.

  d. For the comatose patient, consider naloxone. Use a bedside glucometer to determine whether glucose administration is needed.

  e. For seizures, give IV lorazepam or diazepam (see Chapter 14).

 4. Laboratory

  a. Become familiar with your laboratory's toxicology capabilities. Some assays may require a time-consuming "send out" to a reference lab.

  b. Many laboratories offer urine screens for the most common drugs of abuse.

  c. Blood tests should be used selectively. Consider measurement of anion and osmolal gaps, as well as quantitation of acetaminophen, salicylates, alcohols, and glycols if clinically indicated. The management of most substances, however, does not depend on blood concentrations.

 5. GI decontamination:

  a. Syrup of ipecac (see earlier) has no role in the ED.

  b. Gastric lavage should *not* be used routinely. Clinical studies have not demonstrated with certainty that lavage improves clinical outcome, and the procedure may introduce complications.

  c. Activated charcoal (AC)

   (1) AC is indicated to prevent absorption of a wide variety of pharmaceuticals and other substances. Clinical studies have indicated that its use as an adsorbent is most effective if administered as a single dose within one hour of ingestion of an adsorbable substance. AC, however, should not be administered routinely.

   (2) For substances that undergo enterohepatic circulation (e.g., theophylline overdose), repeat doses (0.5 g/kg q2-4h) may provide effective gastrointestinal "dialysis." Experimental and clinical studies indicate that multiple-dose AC should be considered only in cases of life-threatening ingestions of carbamazepine, dapsone, phenobarbital, quinine, and theophylline.

   (3) AC is *not* effective for iron, strong acids and alkalis, and simple alcohols.

   (4) Side effects (vomiting, aspiration, constipation, and intestinal obstruction) are rare.

   (5) Contraindications include the absence of bowel sounds, intestinal obstruction, GI bleeding, and lack of adequate airway protection, in which case a cuffed endotracheal tube should be placed before AC is given.

   (6) Usually given as a slurry in water. It is best tolerated if the liquid is cold and sipped through a straw from an opaque container (e.g., covered Styrofoam cup) to hide the appearance, although many patients object to its texture. If refused, AC may be given

via a nasogastric or orogastric tube. Metoclopramide (Reglan) may also improve tolerance.
(7)   The usual dose is 1 g/kg (minimum 15 g).
d.   Cathartics (sorbitol, magnesium citrate, magnesium sulfate) may cause diarrhea, but clinical studies of their use alone or in combination with AC have not demonstrated improved clinical outcome. Multiple doses may cause severe fluid and electrolyte disturbances.
e.   Whole bowel irrigation (WBI)
(1)   WBI should not be used routinely. Volunteer studies have indicated that WBI may decrease bioavailability of ingested substances (particularly enteric-coated or sustained-release drugs), but there are no controlled clinical trials that have demonstrated improved clinical outcome.
(2)   WBI remains a theoretical possibility for iron, lead, zinc, and packets of illicit drugs.
(3)   Use an osmotically balanced polyethylene glycol electrolyte solution (such as GoLYTELY) via a nasogastric tube at a rate of 0.5 L/h in children to 2 L/h in adolescents. A clear rectal effluent is often used as the endpoint for WBI, but a variety of clinical factors may shorten or extend the therapy.

C. SPECIFIC ANTIDOTES
(See Table 12-1.)

D. SPECIFIC INGESTIONS
The toxins that may be ingested by children are too numerous to list in this section. The local Poison Control Center (PCC) can provide up-to-date information on management of poisonings. The PoisIndex database is also useful. Some of the more common ingestions are outlined as follows:
1.   Acetaminophen
a.   Toxicity
(1)   Rapid intestinal absorption; peak plasma level in 70 to 120 minutes; possibly earlier (30 minutes) with liquid preparations in children. GI symptoms such as abdominal pain, nausea, vomiting, and lethargy occur within hours. There may be a latent period of 1 to 5 days between ingestion and the onset of hepatic symptoms.
(2)   Assessment of risk
(a)   Amount ingested less than 140 mg/kg: No treatment. Hepatotoxicity is rare, but remains a possibility in cases of chronic exposure to therapeutic doses. Consult with Poison Control Center if round-the-clock acetaminophen administration has exceeded 1 to 2 days.
(b)   Amount ingested greater than 140 mg/kg: Potentially toxic dose in children. Send to ED.

12

INGESTIONS

TABLE 12-1

SPECIFIC ANTIDOTES (CONTACT LOCAL POISON CONTROL CENTER FOR GUIDANCE IN SPECIFIC CASES)

Indication	Antidote	Dose	Comments
Acetaminophen	N-acetylcysteine (Mucomyst 20%)	Loading dose 140 mg/kg PO, then 70 mg/kg q4h × 17 doses	Dilute to 5%; give with soda on ice in covered cup; consult medical toxicologist via Poison Control Center if alternate courses are considered
Anticholinergic agents (includes antihistamines)			Physostigmine has a brief duration of action and therefore is more likely to be diagnostic than therapeutic; may induce arrhythmias, including asystole
Benzodiazepines			Empiric use of flumazenil (Romazicon) is controversial; may not reverse benzodiazepine-induced respiratory depression and may precipitate convulsions, particularly if TCA co-ingested
Calcium-channel blockers	Glucagon	0.05 mg/kg bolus; if no response, 0.1 mg/kg	May cause vomiting; consider infusion of 2-10 mg/h
Carbon monoxide	Oxygen	FiO2 1.0 by non-rebreather	Consider hyperbaric oxygen, although transport to facility may present logistical difficulties
Digoxin (and other cardiac glycosides)	Digoxin-immune Fab fragments (Digibind)	Each vial (38 mg) binds 0.5 mg digoxin	Reserve for life-threatening arrhythmias and hyperkalemia refractory to usual measures; dose calculations may be required for chronic overdoses that have reached steady-state concentrations
Dystonic reaction (variety of causative agents)	Diphenhydramine (Benadryl)	1 mg/kg IV	Consider continuation of diphenhydramine 1 mg/kg PO q6h × 1-2 days following ingestion

Ethylene glycol or methanol	15 mg/kg, then 10 mg/kg × 4 doses q12h, then 15 mg/kg q12h until ethylene glycol or methanol level <20 mg/dl	Reserve for levels >20 mg/dl; dialysis may be necessary; change dosing frequency to q-4-h during dialysis (Note: traditional antidote is ethanol, but difficult to maintain adequate levels by infusion; may cause CNS depression and hypoglycemia)
Fomepizole (Antizol)		
Deferoxamine (Desferal)	Start at 15 mg/kg/h IV; max 24 h	Reserve for levels >500 mcg/dl; avoid IM route
Iron		
Methemoglobin	1-2 mg/kg IV (0.1-0.2 ml of 1% solution)	Contraindicated in G-6-PD deficiency and methemoglobin reductase deficiency
Methylene blue		Consider repeat dose of 2 mg if no response; may require infusion
Opiates	0.1 mg/kg	
Naloxone (Narcan)		
Organophosphates/ Carbamates	0.02 mg/kg (min 0.1 mg) IV	Consider addition of pralidoxime (2-PAM) for organophosphates only
Atropine sulfate		
Salicylates	1-2 mEq/kg IV bolus, then infusion of 3 ampoules (132 mEq) in D5W at 1.5-2 times maintenance to maintain urine pH at 7.5-8	Urinary alkalinization may require addition of 35-40 mEq/L of potassium (if renal failure is not present) to IV fluids
Sodium bicarbonate		
Sulfonylureas (oral hypoglycemic agents)	1-2 mcg/kg per dose q8-12h SC	Optimal dose not known (Note: traditional antidote of dextrose may paradoxically increase severity of hypoglycemia)
Octreotide		
Tricyclic antidepressants	1-2 mEq/kg IV bolus	Repeat as necessary; maintain serum pH between 7.45 and 7.55
Sodium bicarbonate		

12

INGESTIONS

b. Diagnosis
   (1) An acetaminophen level is not considered reliable before 4 hours. If the 4-hour level is greater than 300 mcg/ml, there is a 90% chance of severe toxicity. If the level is less than 150 mcg/ml, toxicity is unlikely (Fig. 12-1).
c. Management
   (1) N-acetylcysteine (NAC) is most effective if administered within 8 to 10 hours of ingestion, and therefore the decision to treat in early-presenting cases may often await the acetaminophen level. Do not delay NAC treatment if timing of the ingestion is uncertain.
   (2) The U.S. oral protocol requires 72 hours, although shorter protocols (including intravenous protocols considered investigational in this country but in routine use around the world) may be considered in consultation with the PCC or a medical toxicologist. Acetaminophen levels that fall subsequently are an expected consequence of first-order kinetics and should not be used in isolation to discontinue NAC treatment prematurely.
   (3) If coingestants require the use of AC, its administration should be separated from NAC by 1 to 2 hours. Activated charcoal is not necessary if only acetaminophen has been ingested.
   (4) The administration of NAC may be associated with vomiting; the dose may be repeated one time if vomited within 1 hour of administration. NAC can be made more palatable by putting it in juice or soda, on ice, and in a covered cup with a straw. If it is vomited, it may need to be administered by a slow drip via a tube in the duodenum; IV administration of high-dose metoclopramide (0.5 to 1 mg/kg following premedication with diphenhydramine 1 mg/kg may decrease vomiting. Ondansetron may be used in refractory cases of vomiting.
   (5) In all patients with acetaminophen levels in the toxic range, AST and PT (as markers of hepatic damage and function, respectively) should be followed daily beginning 24 hours postingestion.
   (6) Prognosis
      (a) Significant toxicity is rare in children less than 6 years of age.
      (b) Adolescents have a higher incidence of toxic plasma levels following ingestion, and are more likely to develop severe hepatotoxicity (AST greater than 1000 IU/L). The presence of severe hepatotoxicity does not predict outcome, and the mortality rate is very low. Patients who recover have no sequelae.
2. Caustics
a. Toxicity
   (1) Acids tend to cause a self-limiting coagulation necrosis.
   (2) Alkalis cause a liquefaction necrosis that penetrates more deeply than acids.

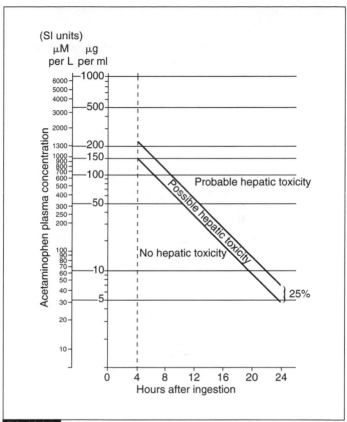

FIG. 12-1

Rumack-Matthew nomogram for acetaminophen poisoning. Semilogarithmic plot of plasma acetaminophen levels vs. time. The following are cautions for the use of this chart: (1) time coordinates refer to time after *ingestion*, (2) serum levels drawn before 4 hours may not represent peak levels, (3) the graph should be used only in relation to a single acute ingestion, and (4) *lower solid line* 25% below the standard nomogram is included to allow for possible errors in acetaminophen plasma assays and estimated time from ingestion of an overdose. (From Rumack BH, Matthew H: Acetaminophen poisoning and toxicity, *Pediatrics* 55:871, 1975.)

      (3)   Button batteries are generally tightly sealed and leakage of contents is rare; batteries larger than about 25 mm may become impacted in the esophagus.

  b. Diagnosis

      (1)   Oral pain, chest pain, abdominal pain, dysphagia, drooling, stridor, and hoarseness may indicate oral or esophageal burn or impaction.

      (2)   The absence of oral burns does not rule out esophageal burns.

      (3)   A CXR may reveal mediastinal air from perforation or an impacted button battery.

  c. Management

      (1)   If esophageal involvement is possible, keep patient NPO and arrange for endoscopic evaluation for esophageal burns and removal of impacted batteries.

      (2)   Button batteries that have passed into the stomach generally pass through the gastrointestinal tract without event; subsequent impaction is rare. Consider abdominal x-rays for batteries that do not pass within 1 week or in patients who develop abdominal symptoms. The National Button Battery Hotline (202-625-3333) may be called collect and is interested in examining recovered batteries for leakage.

3. Hydrocarbons

  a. Toxicity

      (1)   Hydrocarbons include gasoline, kerosene, lamp oil, lighter fluid, turpentine, paint thinner and remover, furniture polish, paraffin wax, and lubricating oil.

      (2)   Because of their unpleasant taste, large volumes of hydrocarbons are rarely ingested (usually less than 1 oz).

      (3)   Pulmonary injury results from aspiration, *not* GI absorption. Aspiration may occur in the absence of vomiting.

  b. Diagnosis

      (1)   Signs and symptoms of hydrocarbon ingestion include coughing, choking, hemoptysis, tachypnea, dyspnea, cyanosis, rales, rhonchi, and wheezes. Respiratory symptoms almost always begin within 4 to 6 hours of ingestion.

      (2)   Somnolence is the chief neurologic manifestation (probably related to hypoxia and acidosis).

      (3)   Fever may occur but usually does not correlate with infection.

  c. Management

      (1)   Evacuation of gastric contents is not indicated unless an aromatic (xylene, toluene) or complex hydrocarbon is ingested or heavy metals, pesticides, or other toxins contaminate the material. Activated charcoal is *not* indicated.

      (2)   All patients should be observed for at least 4 to 6 hours. A CXR should be obtained on all patients; most abnormal x-ray studies become abnormal within 4 hours. The x-ray study may show

evidence of aspiration pneumonia/pneumonitis, patchy densities, consolidation, hyperinflation, atelectasis, and pneumatoceles.

(3) All symptomatic patients should be admitted; there may be rapid deterioration over 24 to 48 hours.

(4) Treatment is primarily respiratory support. Steroids are not effective, and prophylactic antibiotics are not indicated. Even in patients with fever and leukocytosis, bacterial pneumonia is unusual.

(5) The course usually lasts 3 to 8 days. There may be fever up to 8 to 10 days. The CXR may show pneumatoceles 2 to 3 weeks after ingestion.

4. Iron

a. Toxicity

(1) Generally associated with an ingested dose of elemental iron greater than 60 mg/kg.

(2) Prenatal iron preparations (rather than multivitamins with iron) tend to be implicated in cases of serious toxicity.

b. Diagnosis

(1) History: Always assume that the maximum number of tablets missing has been ingested. Most prenatal vitamins contain 65 mg of elemental iron per tablet.

(2) A serum iron level obtained 2 to 4 hours postingestion is the best predictor of toxicity. Relationship of this level to TIBC, leukocytosis, and hyperglycemia has not been demonstrated to be a reliable indicator of iron toxicity.

    (a) When less than 350 mcg/dL: Toxicity unlikely

    (b) When 350 to 500 mcg/dL: Mild toxicity

    (c) When greater than 500 mcg/dL: Toxicity likely

(3) Consider an abdominal x-ray examination for iron tablets and fragments. Small fragments may not be visible.

(4) The use of a test dose of deferoxamine and subsequent urinary color change to a pink "vin rose" has been demonstrated to be unreliable and should *not* be used to rule iron ingestion in or out.

(5) Clinical features: four phases of iron poisoning.

    (a) 0.5 to 6 hours after ingestion: Hemorrhagic gastroenteritis (vomiting and bloody diarrhea), fever, metabolic acidosis, coagulation defects, shock, coma

Note: If signs and symptoms of toxicity do not appear within 4 to 6 hours, the process is unlikely to progress.

    (b) 6 to 24 hours: Period of relative improvement (may be the calm before the storm!)

    (c) 24 to 48 hours: Delayed profound shock, acidosis, pulmonary edema, hepatic failure, hypoglycemia, bleeding diathesis, renal shutdown, coma

    (d) 1 to 2 months: Gastric scarring, pyloric obstruction, bowel stricture, cirrhosis

12

INGESTIONS

    c. Management
        (1) If abdominal x-ray is positive, WBI (see earlier) should be considered.
        (2) Supportive care.
            (a) Correction of fluid and electrolyte abnormalities and acidosis
            (b) Maintenance of intravascular volume: Blood, colloid, pressors
            (c) Correction of clotting abnormalities
        (3) Support of ventilation.
        (4) Follow CBC, LFTs, clotting studies, electrolytes, ABGs, renal function, and serial iron levels.
        (5) Chelation therapy.
            (a) Indication: Serum iron exceeds 500 mcg/dL 2 to 4 hours after ingestion.
            (b) IV deferoxamine: 15 mg/kg/h; decrease rate if hypotension occurs. Other toxicities of the antidote include infection (the deferoxamine-iron complex facilitates the growth of siderophile organisms) and acute respiratory distress syndrome (ARDS) (possibly related to free-radical formation). Limiting chelation to less than 24 hours may prevent these complications.
            (c) IM deferoxamine cannot be titrated and is not recommended.
            (d) Hemodialysis is not effective unless iron is bound to deferoxamine and the patient has developed renal failure.

5. Salicylates
    a. Toxicity
        (1) Nausea, vomiting, abdominal pain, fever, hyperpnea, tinnitus, coma, convulsions, hyperglycemia (early), hypoglycemia (late), oliguria, bleeding diathesis. Severe poisoning is associated with seizures, coma, as well as respiratory and cardiovascular failure.
        (2) Respiratory alkalosis (early), metabolic acidosis (late).
        (3) May be confused with diabetic ketoacidosis, Reye's syndrome, encephalitis, and other ingestions.
    b. Diagnosis
        (1) Toxicologists have abandoned use of the Done nomogram. The nomogram is now considered unreliable, in part because it does not reflect the tendency of salicylate metabolism to change from first-order to zero-order (i.e., Michaelis-Menten) kinetics in acute overdose.
        (2) In an acute overdose, the clinical appearance of the patient should guide therapy. Rising salicylate levels and/or levels greater than 50 to 80 mg/dL should prompt vigilance.
    c. Management
        (1) Administer AC.
        (2) Hospitalize the patient who is symptomatic or whose peak serum level exceeds 50 mg/dL.
        (3) Replace fluid/electrolyte deficits (aim for urine output of 3 to 6

ml/kg/h). Start with 10 to 15 ml/kg/h for the first 2 hours and then adjust.

(4) Alkalinize the urine; give sodium bicarbonate 1 to 2 mEq/kg IV as a loading dose followed by an infusion of sodium bicarbonate 3 ampoules (132 mEq) in D_5W at 1.5 to 2 times maintenance to maintain urine pH at 7.5 to 8. Alkalinization may require the addition of 35 to 40 mEq/L of potassium (if renal failure is not present) to IV fluids.

(5) Follow serial salicylate levels, as well as urine pH and volume, plasma pH, LFTs, electrolytes, PT, and calcium.

(6) Administer vitamin K if PT is prolonged.

(7) Consider hemodialysis; indications include chronic overdose, renal failure, unresponsive acidosis, intractable seizures, coma, and a serum salicylate level greater than 80 to 100 mg/dL.

6. Tricyclic antidepressants
a. Toxicity
(1) The manifestations of TCAs are those of autonomic dysfunction: fever, dry mouth, tachycardia, flushing, dilated pupils, excitation along with confusion, arrhythmias, hallucinations, hypotension, ataxia, seizures, and coma.

b. Diagnosis
(1) The triad of anticholinergic signs, acute alteration of mental status, and sinus tachycardia suggests tricyclic poisoning.
(2) Prolongation of the (QRS) complex (greater than 100 msec) on an ECG has been correlated with severe overdoses: greater than 100 msec, seizures; greater than 160 msec, ventricular arrhythmias.
(3) Serum drug levels are not usually helpful in acute ingestions; treatment should be based on the clinical picture and QRS duration.

c. Management
(1) Administer AC.
(2) Sodium bicarbonate, 1 to 2 mEq/kg, administered as a bolus is probably the single most effective therapy for TCA overdose.
(3) Support BP and cardiac output; manage arrhythmias.
(4) Administer IV lorazepam (Ativan), or phenobarbital for seizures.
(5) Correct acidosis and electrolyte disturbances.
(6) Physostigmine is contraindicated, and dialysis is not indicated.
(7) A depressed level of consciousness (Glasgow Coma Scale score less than 8) predicts serious complications of TCA overdose. Significant complications almost always occur within 4 to 6 hours of ingestion. Patients who remain awake after 6 hours of observation in the ED are at low risk for serious complications.
(8) All symptomatic patients should be admitted to an intensive care unit for supportive management and cardiac monitoring.

INGESTIONS

E. HOUSEHOLD PRODUCT INGESTION

Be suspicious of household product ingestion if any of the following are true:

1. Child of 1 to 5 years of age with a previous history of ingestion
2. Nonfebrile illness; multisystem involvement without obvious explanation
3. Unusual odor, stains on clothing, burns around mouth or on oral mucosa, lip or tongue swelling, dysphagia, drooling
4. Unexplained hematemesis

Note: Caustics can cause severe burns to the esophagus or stomach in the absence of other symptoms.

F. MUNCHAUSEN SYNDROME BY PROXY
(see Chapter 4, Section J)

1. Accidental ingestion *may not be* accidental. Some children may be abused by the administration of drugs. In many cases the abuse continues while the patient is in the hospital. The abuser is often pleasant, cooperative, and appreciative.
2. Be suspicious if any of the following are true:
a. Child less than 1 or more than 5 years of age
b. More than one ingestion episode
c. Bizarre clinical manifestations. Such poisonings may have an insidious onset or an inexplicable presentation.
d. Presence of risk factors for abuse

G. ANOREXIA NERVOSA

1. Adolescents with anorexia nervosa are at a particularly high risk for intentional self-poisoning, some as a result of purging attempts.
2. Common agents include psychotherapeutic drugs, cathartics, and analgesics; multiple toxins may be involved.
3. Management may be complicated by the following:
a. Unreliable history and a delay in seeking medical attention
b. Presence of underlying electrolyte disturbances
c. Underlying GI abnormality (e.g., delayed gastric emptying)

H. BIBLIOGRAPHY

American Academy of Clinical Toxicology, European Association of Poisons Centres and Clinical Toxicologists: Position statement: ipecac syrup, *J Toxicol Clin Toxicol* 35:699, 1997.

American Academy of Clinical Toxicology, European Association of Poisons Centres and Clinical Toxicologists: Position statement: gastric lavage, *J Toxicol Clin Toxicol* 35:711, 1997.

American Academy of Clinical Toxicology, European Association of Poisons Centres and Clinical Toxicologists: Position statement: single-dose activated charcoal, *J Toxicol Clin Toxicol* 35:721, 1997.

American Academy of Clinical Toxicology, European Association of Poisons Centres and Clinical Toxicologists: Position statement: cathartics, *J Toxicol Clin Toxicol* 35:743, 1997.

American Academy of Clinical Toxicology, European Association of Poisons Centres and Clinical Toxicologists: Position statement: whole bowel irrigation, *J Toxicol Clin Toxicol* 35:753, 1997.

American Academy of Clinical Toxicology, European Association of Poisons Centres and Clinical Toxicologists: Position statement and practice guidelines on the use of multi-dose activated charcoal in the treatment of acute poisoning, *J Toxicol Clin Toxicol* 37:731, 1999.

American Academy of Pediatrics: Committee on drugs: acetaminophen toxicity in children, *Pediatrics* 108:1020, 2001.

Boehnert MT, Lovejoy FH: Value of the QRS duration versus the serum drug level in predicting seizures and ventricular arrhythmias after an acute overdose of tricyclic antidepressants, *N Engl J Med* 313:474, 1985.

Howland MA: Deferoxamine. In *Goldfrank's toxicologic emergencies,* ed 6. Goldfrank LR et al, eds. Stamford, CT, 1998, Appleton & Lange.

Kim S: Salicylates. In *Poisoning & drug overdose,* ed 3. Olson KR, ed. Stamford, CT, 1999, Appleton & Lange.

Liebelt EL: Iron. In *Clinical management of poisoning and drug overdose,* ed 3. Haddad LM, Shannon MW, Winchester JF, eds. Philadelphia, 1998, WB Saunders.

Liebelt EL: Newer antidotal therapies for pediatric poisonings, *Clin Ped Emerg Med* 1:234-243, 2000.

Meadow R: Munchausen by proxy, *Arch Dis Child* 57:92, 1982.

Mullen WH: Caustics. In *Poisoning & drug overdose,* ed 3. Olson KR, ed. Stamford, CT, 1999, Appleton & Lange.

Rumack BH, Matthew H: Acetaminophen poisoning and toxicity, *Pediatrics* 55:871, 1975.

Smilkstein MJ, Knapp GL, Kulig KW, et al: Efficacy of oral N-acetylcysteine in the treatment of acetaminophen overdose, *N Engl J Med* 319:1557, 1988.

Woolf AD, Gren JM: Acute poisonings among adolescents and young adults with anorexia nervosa, *Am J Dis Child* 144:785, 1990.

Woolf AD, Wenger T, Smith TW, et al: The use of digoxin-specific Fab fragments for severe digitalis intoxication in children, *N Engl J Med* 326:1739, 1992.

12

INGESTIONS

NEONATAL PROBLEMS

A. BLOODY STOOLS

1. The differential diagnosis includes bacterial enterocolitis, Meckel's diverticulum, intussusception, GI duplication, Hirschsprung's disease, milk protein allergy, swallowed maternal blood, polyps, rectal injury (thermometer), and anal fissure (most common cause of bloody stool in a well-looking infant).
2. Evaluation
a. Meticulous examination of the anal canal for fissures
b. Stool examination for leukocytes (methylene blue), culture (enteric pathogens, *Campylobacter*), and *Clostridium difficile* toxin
c. Meckel scan
d. Radiographic studies
e. Milk protein precipitins
f. Endoscopy/biopsy
3. Treatment depends on the specific diagnosis. For anal fissures, give a stool softener such as malt soup extract 1 to 2 tsp tid, and clean the perianal area with water following bowel movements.

B. BREAST ENGORGEMENT

1. Breast engorgement secondary to the transfer of maternal hormones is physiologic in neonates. It is usually bilateral and may be associated with breast secretions.
2. Peak enlargement (1 to 3 cm) may not be reached until 4 to 6 weeks and may persist for several months.
3. No treatment is indicated.

C. BREAST INFECTION

1. Breast infection is most common during weeks 2 and 3 and presents as *unilateral* firm swelling with tenderness and warmth. Systemic manifestations, except for low-grade fever, are rare.
2. It may be helpful to aspirate material for Gram's stain and culture; infection usually results from *Staphylococcus aureus.*
3. Admit patient for IV antistaphylococcal therapy. Incision and drainage may be needed.

D. CEPHALHEMATOMA

1. Cephalhematoma is a traumatic subperiosteal hemorrhage that usually involves a parietal bone. Predisposing factors are large head size, prolonged labor, vacuum extraction, and forceps delivery (most important).
2. Firm swelling is fixed at suture lines without discoloration of overlying skin; it may not become apparent until hours to days after birth. An underlying linear skull fracture is present in 1% to 5% of cases, but

routine skull x-ray studies are not indicated (obtain only with CNS signs and symptoms).

3. Spontaneous resolution occurs over weeks; 1% to 2% calcify. No treatment is required, but watch for jaundice and anemia (rare).

E. CLEFT LIP AND PALATE

1. Incidence is 1:1000 births. Caused by a combination of genetic and environmental factors. Can be diagnosed antenatally by ultrasound.

2. Some 50% of cases involve both the lip and palate, 25% the palate only, and 25% the lip only.

3. The degree of clefting can vary tremendously. A cleft lip may manifest as a small notch in the vermilion border to a complete separation extending into the nose. It may be unilateral (80%) or bilateral (20%). Palatal clefts can occur in association with a cleft lip or as an isolated defect, which can vary from a bifid uvula to extension through the hard and soft palates.

4. In 15% to 20% of cases (especially with isolated cleft palate or bilateral cleft lip) there are associated anomalies, and cleft lip or palate or both may be a component of more than 250 syndromes.

5. A neonate with a cleft lip or palate is at high risk for problems with sucking, feeding, and weight gain.

a. A neonate with a cleft lip should be able to breast-feed, but with a cleft palate, breast-feeding can be very difficult.

b. For bottle feeding, frequent small feedings in the sitting position using a long soft lamb's nipple with an enlarged crisscross may be helpful.

6. Refer immediately to a multidisciplinary craniofacial team for treatment and counseling. Surgical correction of a cleft lip is usually carried out during infancy, while a cleft palate is repaired at about 18 months of age.

F. CONSTIPATION

1. Constipation is defined by stool consistency (hard and dry) and not frequency. The number of stools can be variable, ranging from 8 to 10 per day to one every 3 to 4 days, even in nursing infants.

2. Causes of constipation include inadequate milk intake and switching from breast to bottle. Consider hypothyroidism, hypotonia secondary to neuromuscular disease, and Hirschsprung's disease. A rectal examination is indicated; look for anal fissures, a tight anal sphincter, and a lack of stool in the rectum (Hirschsprung's disease).

Note: Almost all cases of Hirschsprung's disease are symptomatic by 4 weeks of age.

3. If specific causes are ruled out, treat with 1 to 2 tsp malt soup extract tid, 4 to 6 oz of glucose water per day, or the occasional use of glycerine suppositories.

G. FRACTURED CLAVICLE

1. A fractured clavicle is present in 1.5% to 3.0% of vaginal deliveries, with the right clavicle involved more often than the left (2:1). Predisposing factors are large size, shoulder dystocia, and traumatic delivery. May be associated with brachial plexus injury.
2. Findings include swelling/fullness over the fracture site, crepitus, decreased arm movement, and irritability during arm movement; however, 80% have no symptoms and only minimal physical findings. It is often diagnosed when callus is detected at 3 to 6 weeks of age. Radiography is not usually indicated.
3. No specific treatment is needed; if both ends of the bone are in the same room, good healing will occur. Advise parents to avoid tension on the affected arm.

H. HYPOSPADIAS

1. Occurs in 8:1000 newborn males.
2. With hypospadias, the urethral meatus is on the ventral surface of the glans (87%), the penile shaft (10%) or, in severe cases, on the perineum (3%). May be accompanied by ventral curvature of the penis (chordee), a dorsally hooded prepuce, or torsion of the penile shaft.
3. Familial tendency; 7% of patients have a brother or father with hypospadias. Some cases may be related to maternal exposure to progestins at 8 to 14 weeks' gestation.
4. Examine carefully for other anomalies, especially genital (micropenis, cryptorchidism). Additional diagnostic studies are not indicated in infants who have mild hypospadias without other abnormalities. Patients with urinary tract symptoms, a family history of reflux, or multiple anomalies should have a complete evaluation for other GU abnormalities. Among infants who have both hypospadias and undescended testes, 25% will have mixed gondal dysgenesis. Immediate urology, endocrine, and genetic evaluation is indicated.

Note: Rarely, chordee and torsion of the penile shaft occur in the absence of a meatal abnormality. Surgical correction will be required.

5. Management
a. Circumcision withheld
b. Refer for urologic evaluation
c. Surgical repair at 6 to 12 months, usually after a short course of parenteral testosterone

I. OMPHALITIS

1. During the first week, faint erythema of the rim of the umbilical stump is common and of no consequence.
2. Omphalitis is defined by the following:
a. Foul-smelling discharge
b. Periumbilical erythema, induration, and tenderness to palpation
c. Purulent or serosanguineous drainage

3. Simple omphalitis can rapidly progress from a localized infection to necrotizing fasciitis of the abdominal wall or ascending infection via the umbilical vein to the liver and portal system. Skin that is violaceous or has a peau d'orange appearance indicates involvement of deep tissue layers.
4. Treatment
a. In the absence of periumbilical spread, use alcohol wipes and a topical antibiotic containing neomycin, polymyxin, and bacitracin.
b. With purulent discharge or periumbilical involvement, (usually associated with polymicrobial flora) use oral or parenteral antibiotics on the basis of culture and sensitivity.

Note: With serous umbilical secretion, need to rule out a vitelline duct or urachal remnant.

Note: A wet malodorous stump with minimal inflammation can be seen with group A β-*hemolytic streptococcus* infection.

J. PYLORIC STENOSIS

1. Pyloric stenosis usually appears at 3 to 6 weeks of age but has been observed from birth to 5 months of age; it is more common in first-born males. There is an increased risk in siblings and the offspring of affected children.
2. Signs and symptoms include persistent and progressive vomiting (usually projectile, occasionally bloody, *never* bilious), failure to thrive, palpation of a hypertrophic pylorus ("olive") in the epigastrium just to the right of midline, visible peristaltic waves, and hypochloremic metabolic alkalosis. A modest degree of indirect hyperbilirubinemia is a common associated finding.
3. Diagnosis is based on clinical findings, including palpation of an "olive." If an "olive" is not palpable (10% to 25% of cases), an ultrasound is the imaging procedure of choice. An upper GI study is usually unnecessary.
4. Treatment consists of hydration, correction of metabolic alkalosis, and pyloromyotomy.

K. RASHES

1. Acne: Multiple comedones, inflammatory papules, and small pustules on the cheeks and nose are present in up to 20% of newborns. Lesions occur within the first 1 to 2 months (occasionally at birth) and involute spontaneously within 1 to 3 months. It may be confused with milia. No specific treatment is needed; moisturizing creams and lotions should be avoided.
2. Acropustulosis: Recurrent crops of pruritic vesiculopustules on the hands and feet, which last 7 to 10 days and recur every few weeks to months over the first 2 to 3 years. Gram's stain reveals numerous PMNs and occasional eosinophils. The etiology is unknown, and there is no specific therapy. Antihistamines and short courses of moderate

potency topical steroids to the palms and soles may provide temporary relief.

3. Bullous disease: Several varieties of epidermolysis bullosa have their onset in the neonatal period, with bullae involving the skin and mucous membranes. Bullae often occur at sites of trauma. Any bullous lesions (blistering) in the neonatal period require immediate dermatology consultation.

4. Café-au-lait spots: Discrete tan macules that appear at birth or during childhood in 10% to 20% of normal individuals; may involve any site on the skin surface. In the neonatal period, the presence of six or more lesions larger than 1.5 cm, especially when associated with axillary freckling, is highly suggestive of classic neurofibromatosis (NF). In children with NF, café-au-lait spots may increase in size and number during first few years of life. Café-au-lait spots are also seen in McCune-Albright syndrome, epidermal nevus syndrome, Bloom syndrome, ataxia-telangiectasia, and Russell-Silver syndrome.

5. Erythema toxicum: Evanescent papules, vesicles, and pustules on an erythematous base occur on the face, forehead, chest, trunk, and extremities (*not* the palms and soles) of a high percentage of full-term neonates. They usually appear between 24 and 72 hours but may be seen at birth. A Wright's or Giemsa stain of contents reveals sheets of eosinophils. Peripheral eosinophilia is seen in 7% to 15% of cases. The condition resolves over 3 to 5 days without therapy but recurrences may be noted for several weeks.

6. Miliaria (prickly heat): Pruritic, erythematous 1-mm to 2-mm papulovesicular lesions with predilection for the face and clothed areas of the body. A Gram's stain of the contents is negative. This condition may occur during the first few weeks of life. Treatment consists of less heat, less clothing, and cool soaks.

7. Neonatal lupus syndrome: Occurs in the setting of maternal auto-immune disease, but 30% to 40% of mothers may be aysmptomatic. Lesions consist of an erythematous, oval (discoid), slightly atrophic plaque with scaling. The condition may appear from birth up to 12 weeks. It is primarily localized to the face (periorbital areas) scalp, and neck but may spread. It may be associated with hepatic dysfunction, aseptic meningitis, anemia, leukopenia, and thrombocytopenia; 15% have congenital irreversible A-V block. Serum is positive for antibodies to SSA/Ro and SSB/La antigens. Most cases are transient, with resolution of skin lesions by 6 to 8 months, but some may progress to subacute or acute SLE. Affected infants should be protected from excessive sun exposure. Topical steroids may be helpful.

8. Pustular melanosis: Appears at or shortly after birth as brownish 3-mm to 4-mm vesicles and pustules on a nonerythematous base on the neck, face, palms, and soles. Within a few days the pustules shed, leaving pigmented macules with scaling. Wright's stain reveals PMNs.

Lesions tend to recur in crops but gradually resolve by 3 to 4 months without scarring. It is seen mainly in darker-pigmented infants. The etiology is unknown, and there is no treatment.

9. Pustulosis (neonatal impetigo)

a. Pustulosis involves small vesicles to larger bullae that rupture easily and leave a red, moist, denuded base that crusts over. It occurs in periumbilical and diaper areas, appears at 7 to 10 days of age, and usually results from *Staphylococcus aureus*.

b. Obtain a Gram's stain and culture of fluid; start an oral antistaphylococcal agent (cephalexin). Lesions usually clear in 5 to 7 days. Most patients can be treated at home. It is rarely associated with systemic manifestations.

Note: It is important to report all cases of pustulosis to the nursery of origin; the condition may be a harbinger of a staphylococcus outbreak in the nursery.

L. STRIDOR

1. Stridor is a harsh sound produced by turbulent airflow through a partial obstruction. It is a description, not a disease entity, and it may be inspiratory, biphasic, or expiratory. Differential diagnosis includes the following:

a. Laryngomalacia, tracheomalacia

b. Subglottic stenosis

c. Vascular ring

d. Laryngeal ring, laryngeal cleft

e. Subglottic hemangioma

f. Vocal cord paralysis (unilateral or bilateral)

g. GER with aspiration

Note: Laryngomalacia and vocal cord paralysis are the most common causes of stridor in the neonate.

2. Evaluation

a. History: Onset and duration, aggravating and alleviating factors, quality of cry, hoarseness, cough, color change, relation to feeding and position (Table 13-1)

TABLE 13-1
SYMPTOMS ASSOCIATED WITH SITE OF AIRWAY OBSTRUCTION*

Site of Obstruction	Inspiratory Stridor	Expiratory Stridor	Feeding Problems	Abnormal Cry
Nose	++		++	+
Oropharynx	++		++	+
Supraglottic	++		++	++
Glottis/subglottic	++	++		++
Trachea		++		

*+, Mild; ++, moderate-to-severe.

b. Examination: Facial and chest configuration, retractions, nasal flaring, cyanosis. Define the portion of the respiratory cycle affected by the stridor.
   (1) Inspiratory: Above laryngeal glottis (i.e., supraglottic larynx, pharynx, or nose).
   (2) Biphasic: Glottic or subglottic lesion.
   (3) Expiratory: Intrathoracic tracheobronchial tree. Auscultate for the location of loudest stridor and abnormal or asymmetric breath sounds. Examine for neck masses, tongue abnormalities, and cutaneous hemangiomas.

c. Diagnostic studies (Table 13-2)

Note: Up to 20% of patients will have more than one airway diagnosis.

3. Treatment

a. If there is stridor with airway compromise, the first step is establishment of a stable airway with endotracheal intubation. A tracheostomy may be needed.

b. Subsequent treatment is guided by the specific cause.

M. THRUSH

1. Oral candidiasis has peak incidence during the second week of life.
2. Cheesy white plaques on an erythematous base over gingiva, tongue, palate, and buccal mucosa that cannot be removed easily.
3. Often associated with candidal diaper rash.
4. Treatment: Nystatin suspension 100,000 to 200,000 U PO qid × 7 to 10 days. Recurrent and persistent infection should raise the suspicion of immunodeficiency.

Note: In a breast-fed infant, it may help to have the mother apply nystatin (Mycostatin) cream to the areola/nipple area. If thrush is recurrent or refractory to treatment, consider a work-up for endocrinopathy or immunodeficiency (and, possibly, AIDS).

TABLE 13-2

DIAGNOSTIC TESTS FOR INFANTS WITH STRIDOR*

	Neck/Airway X-ray Films	Airway Fluoroscopy	Barium Esophagram	Fiberoptic Laryngoscopy	Operative Laryngoscopy, Bronchoscopy
Laryngomalacia	−	−	−	++	++
Tracheomalacia	−	+	−	−	++
Subglottic stenosis	+	+	−	−	++
Vascular ring	−	+	+	−	++
Laryngeal web	−	−	−	++	++
Laryngeal cleft	−	−	+	+	++
Vocal cord paralysis	−	−	−	++	++
Subglottic hemangioma	+	+	−	−	++

*−, Usually not diagnostic; +, often suggests diagnosis; ++, diagnostic procedure of choice.

13

NEONATAL PROBLEMS

N. TORTICOLLIS

1. When a head tilt is recognized in the early neonatal period, the usual cause is congenital muscular torticollis. It occurs in 0.4% of live births and affects male infants more than female infants. It may be noted at birth and is almost always obvious by 2 to 4 weeks of age.

2. Clinically, the head is tilted toward the involved side, and the face is turned toward the opposite side. A firm, nontender, discrete fusiform mass ("tumor") that is 1 to 3 cm in diameter may be palpable in the body of the sternomastoid. It may increase in size gradually over the first month but then regresses; by 4 to 6 months it is usually no longer palpable.

3. The cause is unknown; it may be secondary to an intrauterine positional deformity or an intrauterine or perinatal compartment syndrome.

4. The differential diagnosis includes congenital anomalies of the cervical vertebrae, vertebral dislocation, cystic hygroma, and a branchial cleft cyst.

5. Treatment consists of passive stretching exercises and positioning. Surgery (open bipolar tenotomy) is indicated if torticollis persists beyond 1 year of age or if there is residual craniofacial deformity or a 30% loss of range of motion.

Note: Associated musculoskeletal disorders such as talipes equinovarus, metatarsus adductus, and hip dysplasia occur in up to 20% of cases.

O. UMBILICAL GRANULOMA

1. The umbilical cord usually separates within 8 to 10 days following birth (2 to 3 days later if cesarean section) and heals within 3 to 5 days. Delayed separation and/or mild infection may result in a moist granulating area at the base of the cord with slight mucoid discharge. Treat with alcohol swabs several times a day.

2. Occasionally there may be persistence of reddish-pink, soft, granular, meaty tissue (granuloma) protruding from the base of the umbilicus. Treatment consists of a single application of silver nitrate cautery; be careful to swab only over the area of granuloma.

3. If a granuloma does not respond to silver nitrate, it may represent a remnant of the vitelline duct or urachus.

Note: Infants with delayed separation of the umbilical cord (more than 3 weeks) should be screened for complement receptor (CR3) deficiency.

P. UMBILICAL HERNIA

1. An umbilical hernia is a central fascial defect resulting from incomplete closure of the umbilical ring; it may pinpoint in diameter to greater than 5 cm and is easily reduced. Incarceration is possible but rare. It is common in black infants and premature infants and is also associated with hypotonia (e.g., Down syndrome, hypothyroidism).

2. Most close spontaneously by 2 to 3 years of age. Surgery is not indicated unless it is larger than 5 cm or is still large once the child has passed 5 years of age. Pressure or adhesive dressings with coins and metallic or plastic objects are popular but useless (and may lead to contact dermatitis).

Note: Surgical repair probably is needed if there is progressive enlargement of the skin over the umbilicus until a downward-pointing proboscis is formed.

Q. VAGINAL DISCHARGE/BLEEDING

1. During the first week of life, a thick, milky-white vaginal discharge and vaginal bleeding (a result of estrogen withdrawal) are common; only reassurance is indicated.

2. Older infants may develop labial adhesions secondary to mild irritation (see Chapter 9).

R. VOMITING

1. Vomiting involves forceful expulsion of the GI contents as compared with regurgitation, which is more passive and effortless; 80% of all infants younger than 3 months of age regurgitate feedings at least once a day. Persistent regurgitation without other signs or symptoms usually represents uncomplicated GER.

2. Etiology
a. Nonbilious vomiting
   (1) Overfeeding
   (2) Milk/formula protein sensitivity
   (3) Infection (sepsis, urinary tract infection, meningitis)
   (4) Necrotizing enterocolitis
   (5) Pyloric stenosis
   (6) Electrolyte/metabolic abnormalities
   (7) Hirschsprung's disease
   (8) Lactobezoars
b. Bilious vomiting: Congenital anomalies (malrotation, atresia, stenosis, webs, annular pancreas, persistent omphalomesenteric duct)

3. Management
a. Review of feeding history; examination for signs of infection; serum electrolytes
b. Plain abdominal x-ray examination with upright and cross-table lateral
c. Upper GI series to R/O obstructive anomalies
d. Abdominal ultrasound to R/O pyloric stenosis
e. Passage of gastric tube if obstruction is suspected
f. Prompt surgical consultation if there is bilious vomiting or hematemesis

S. BIBLIOGRAPHY

Davids JR et al: Congenital muscular torticollis: sequela of intrauterine or perinatal compartment syndrome, *J Pediatr Orthop* 13:141, 1993.

13

NEONATAL PROBLEMS

Dinkevich E, Ozuah PO: Pyloric stenosis, *Pediatr Rev* 21:249, 2000.

Fanaroff A, Martin RJ: *Neonatal-perinatal medicine,* St Louis, 1996, Mosby.

Findlay RF, Odom RB: Infantile acropustulosis, *Am J Dis Child* 137:455, 1983.

Joseph PR, Rosenfeld W: Clavicular fractures in neonates, *Am J Dis Child* 144:165, 1990.

Mancuso RF: Stridor in neonates, *Pediatr Clin North Am* 43:1339, 1996.

O'Donnell KA, Glick PL, Caty MG: Pediatric umbilical problems, *Pediatr Clin North Am* 45:791, 1998.

Tseng C-E, Buyon JP: Neonatal lupus syndromes, *Rheum Dis Clin North Am* 23:31, 1997.

Tunkel DE, Zalzal GH: Stridor in infants and children: ambulatory evaluation and operative diagnosis, *Clin Pediatr* 31:48, 1992.

Yasunaga S, Rivera R: Cephalhematoma in the newborn, *Clin Pediatr* 13:256, 1974.

Yip WC et al: Sonographic diagnosis of infantile hypertrophic pyloric stenosis: critical appraisal of reliability and diagnostic criteria, *J Clin Ultrasound* 13:329, 1985.

NEUROLOGY

A. ALTERED MENTAL STATUS

1. Altered mental status includes any change in sensorium or behavior. In the extreme, there is stupor or coma and hyperirritability; in milder cases, there is confusion, sleepiness, aggressive behavior, and decreased school or social performance.

2. Important historical information includes the following:

a. A complete description of the altered sensorium (e.g., acute vs. gradual onset, duration, waxing and waning vs. steady progression)

b. Previous mental status

c. Possible precipitating events, trauma, psychologic stressors, medication, or illicit drug use

d. Signs of illness, especially fever, headaches, visual disturbances

e. Chronic medical condition or preexisting neurologic problem

f. History of depression or a change in school or social performance

3. The PE must be thorough. Special emphasis should be placed on the neurologic examination, fundoscopic assessment, nuchal rigidity, and skin findings (e.g., herpetic lesions, bruises). Note any odor on the breath that might suggest an ingestion or a metabolic disturbance, such as diabetic ketoacidosis.

4. Causes of altered mental status

a. CNS infection (meningitis, encephalitis)

b. CNS mass (usually a gradual onset of symptoms)

c. CNS hemorrhage (may be acute or gradual and may be preceded by headache) or infarct

d. CNS trauma

e. Medication/drug overdose

f. Alcohol and illicit drug use, including secondhand exposure to "crack" cocaine

g. Hypertensive encephalopathy

h. Hypoglycemia

i. Diabetic ketoacidosis

j. Reye's syndrome

k. Depression

l. Ictal/post-ictal states

5. Laboratory tests are dictated by the history, PE, and type of mental status change.

a. For the comatose, stuporous, and hyperirritable patient, CBC, electrolytes, glucose, ammonia, BUN, LFTs, and a toxicology screen should be obtained.

b. If vital signs are stable and there are no localizing neurologic signs or evidence of increased ICP, an LP should be considered (CSF sent for glucose, protein, Gram's stain, cell count, culture/ELISA). Consider obtaining an opening pressure.

   c. A CT scan should precede the LP in a patient who is unstable or has localized neurologic signs.

   6. Treatment is directed toward the underlying cause of the altered mental status.

B. HEADACHE

1. Headache is a common presenting complaint, especially in the older pediatric age group and in febrile children.

2. Important historical information includes the following:

a. Location, day(s), and time(s) of occurrence; frequency, duration, precipitating factors, ameliorating factors, and associated symptoms (e.g., fever, neck pain, scotoma, photophobia, nausea, vomiting). Is the headache acute or chronic, progressive or nonprogressive? (See Figure 14-1.)

b. Does the patient have a chronic medical condition or take medications on a long-term basis?

c. Is there a family history of headaches? If so, who has them and what are they like?

d. Does the patient have a history of head trauma, seizures, cranial surgery, allergies, decreased vision or hearing, pain on chewing? Has the headache ever awakened him or her from sleep?

e. Is the patient stressed? Have there been changes in his or her personality, school performance, or growth?

3. The PE should be complete. Place emphasis on the skull, eyes, ears, teeth, temporomandibular joints, sinuses, and neurologic examination. Look for areas of tenderness, asymmetry, and bruits.

4. No single laboratory test is mandatory for the patient with a headache. Laboratory tests and radiographic studies are dictated by the results of the history and PE. A CT scan or MRI is not indicated unless abnormal neurologic findings are present.

5. Frontal headaches may result from viral illnesses (especially when accompanied by fever), sinus infection, sinus edema (resulting from exposure to allergens or noxious environmental stimuli such as smoke), stress, or fatigue.

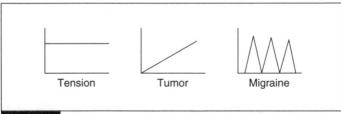

FIG. 14-1

Pain course over time.

a. The presence of pain on palpation over the sinuses and a purulent nasal discharge suggests sinusitis; an imaging study confirms the diagnosis.

b. The presence of suborbital edema/cyanosis, edematous bluish nasal turbinates, and watery ocular/nasal discharge suggests allergic disease.

6. Facial pain may result from dental disease, middle ear disease, temporomandibular joint dysfunction, or maxillary sinusitis.

7. Pain in the temples or neck pain (tightness) may result from stress (especially if the pain occurs during stressful situations) or depression.

8. Frontal and occipital headaches may be associated with intracranial disease (bleeding, tumor, abscess, pseudotumor cerebri), especially if the pain occurs upon arising in the morning, is relieved by vomiting, and is accompanied by visual field or acuity changes or alterations in mental status, mood, motor function, or sensation.

9. Generalized (or poorly localized) headaches may result from fatigue, stress, migraines, medications such as sympathomimetics, illicit drugs such as amphetamines, encephalitis (often associated with sensorium changes), meningitis (usually associated with positive Kernig's and Brudzinski's signs), severe anemia, hypertension, hyperventilation, hypoglycemia, hypoxia, hypercapnia, carbon monoxide poisoning, and trauma.

10. A severe headache may herald a subarachnoid bleed, especially if the patient is confused or unconscious.

11. Migraine headaches are "classically" paroxysmal, either bilateral or unilateral, and are preceded by an aura or accompanied by nausea and vomiting. However, not all patients have this classic presentation. Young children may have abdominal pain and vomiting. A family history of migraine is helpful.

12. Treatment of uncomplicated headaches includes analgesics and rest.

a. Headaches resulting from bacterial processes respond to antibiotic therapy of the underlying disease.

b. Headaches resulting from allergen exposure respond to the elimination of the offending agent. Antihistamines may be useful if other histamine-mediated symptoms are present.

c. Headaches resulting from stress or depression respond to the elucidation and resolution of the psychic conflict. Biofeedback techniques may be useful.

d. Headaches resulting from intracranial mass lesions or bleeding are usually treated surgically.

e. Once a migraine headache has been firmly established, it cannot be resolved easily; ice packs, remaining in a dark and quiet place, and biofeedback may be useful.

   (1) If vomiting is a problem, promethazine (Phenergan) (0.5 to 1.0 mg/kg up to 25 mg as an initial dose, followed by 0.25 to 1.0 mg/kg q4 to 6h) can be used if there are no contraindications.

14

NEUROLOGY

(2) Simple analgesics may be used, such as acetaminophen (20 mg/kg PO followed by 10 to 15 mg/kg q4h up to a maximum dose of 65 mg/kg/d); ibuprofen (1 to 12 years old: 10 mg/kg PO q4-6h; more than 12 years of age: 200 to 400 mg PO q4h up to maximum dose of 1200 mg/d); or naproxen 5 mg/kg PO q12h up to 750 mg/d.

(3) When simple analgesics do not give relief, a selective serotonin agonist such as sumatriptan (Imitrex) 6 mg subcutaneously, or dihydroergotamine (DHE) mesylate 0.5 to 1.0 mg IV over 3 minutes in those older than 10 years of age may be given. DHE can be given q8h, and is often used in combination with metoclopramide (0.1 to 0.2 mg/kg PO, maximum 10 mg). Sumatriptan is useful for adult migraine, but studies in adolescents have yielded mixed results. Its safety and efficacy in young children are unknown.

(4) Propranolol 0.5 to 4 mg/kg/d ÷ q8h for children 12 years of age or older can prevent episodes or abort a headache if taken early in its course. Start with the lower dose and increase slowly. Propranolol should be avoided in those with asthma, diabetes mellitus, and heart disease. Another useful drug in adolescents is amitriptyline; it is most useful in those with migraines, muscle contraction headaches, and headaches associated with depression. For adolescents, the dose is 10 to 50 mg/d divided tid.

(5) Other helpful modalities for all ages include regular sleep and meal schedules, elimination of any foods that seem to be associated with headaches, biofeedback, and counseling.

C. HEAD TRAUMA

1. Evaluation: The main objective is to sort out patients who have treatable complications (e.g., intracranial bleeding, depressed fractures) from those who do not; doing so can be difficult.

a. The history should include a detailed description of the type of trauma (e.g., fall, blow), loss of consciousness and duration, amnesia (especially retrograde), lethargy, vomiting, seizures, vision difficulties, and a history of other medical problems (especially a shunt). Many patients have a period of sleepiness, headaches, and vomiting a few times without sequelae. Consider the possibility of child abuse.

b. The PE should be complete and include vital signs (increased ICP causes reduced HR, increased BP, irregular respirations); look for direct signs of trauma (e.g., soft-tissue swelling, hematoma, skull depression, lacerations). Give particular attention to the following:

(1) Fundus: Retinal hemorrhage; papilledema (usually a *late* sign of increased ICP). Do not use mydriatics to dilate pupils.

(2) Tympanic membrane: Blood behind eardrum, CSF discharge.

(3) Ecchymosis behind ear (Battle's sign), or orbital (raccoon sign).

(4) Nose: CSF rhinorrhea.
(5) Neck examination: Make sure cervical spine is not injured. If in doubt, (e.g., patient cannot interact reliably, patient complains of neck pain or has neurologic symptoms), stabilize head with sandbags and obtain cervical spine x-ray studies.
(6) Skin: Check for signs of abuse.
(7) Neurologic examination: Emphasize level of consciousness (probably the most important observation) and general mental state; serial observations are mandatory.
  (a) Eyes: Unequal pupils signify compression of the third nerve by a herniating temporal lobe.
  (b) Diplopia: Sixth nerve (to lateral rectus) is particularly vulnerable to increased ICP.
  (c) Motor: Use of arms and legs normal? Ataxic gait?
  (d) Reflexes: Symmetric? Toes turn down?

c. Imaging studies
  (1) Skull x-ray studies are expensive, overused, and of limited usefulness. In general, fractures are poor predictors of intracranial injury.
    (a) Patient treatment is rarely affected by skull x-ray examination findings.
    (b) A cranial CT scan is preferred over skull x-rays. However, most patients with minor head trauma need *no* imaging studies.
  (2) Cervical spine stabilization and an imaging study are indicated if the head injury is severe. Cervical abrasions and upper spine tenderness suggest a neck injury.
d. A CT scan is indicated if intracranial bleeding is suspected (e.g., patient with persistent or progressing neurologic signs). In infants and toddlers, a subdural hemorrhage indicates abuse, whereas an epidural hemorrhage makes a diagnosis of abuse less likely.
e. An MRI is superior to a CT scan for visualizing diffuse axonal (shear) injury and subarachnoid hemorrhage. It is also useful for detecting traumatic hematomas of varying duration, brain ischemia, and edema. However, a consensus statement from the AAP noted that there is not really a difference between CT and MRI in the diagnosis of significant acute head injury/bleeding that requires neurosurgical intervention; also, CT scans are both more available and less costly than MRI scans. Hence, a CT scan is felt to be the more advantageous scanning technique for minor head injury in pediatric patients.
f. An EEG is not indicated in the initial evaluation or in uncomplicated cases.

2. Management
a. The patient may be sent home when the level of consciousness and neurologic function are back to normal.

14

NEUROLOGY

b. If the post-injury CT scan is normal, the patient may be discharged to home with specific instructions (see Point c).
c. Give the parent instructions for home care. The level of alertness should be evaluated every few hours for the first 24 hours. The parent should also look for evidence of blood or clear fluid from the nose or ear; an inability to use limbs properly; difficulty speaking, hearing, or seeing; seizures; repeated vomiting; or behavior changes. The parent should note any fever, headaches, or change in mental status or behavior during the next 2 weeks, and the child should return if such problems develop.
d. The patient is usually hospitalized if any of the following are present:
  (1) Any sign of deterioration
  (2) Clear-cut abnormal neurologic findings
  (3) The level of function does not return promptly to normal (sometimes the patient may be sent home if parents are reliable, overall examination results are reassuring, and neurology consultant and primary physician agree)
  (4) Fracture across area of middle meningeal artery or a depressed skull fracture
e. A seizure in the first 24 hours after the injury does not necessitate an automatic admission, nor does the presence of a skull fracture.
f. If there are any questions, get a neurology/neurosurgery consult, especially if the CT shows an abnormality.
g. Give parents written instructions for follow-up at home, including the information in point c.

D. ACUTE INCREASED INTRACRANIAL PRESSURE: EMERGENCY DEPARTMENT MANAGEMENT

1. Signs and symptoms include headache, nausea, vomiting, spectrum of altered mental status, and papilledema.
a. Note vital signs and any change suggestive of increased ICP (reduced HR, slow respirations, increased BP with widening pulse pressure).
b. The patient with severe increased ICP may be delirious and thrashing about or may be completely obtunded.
2. Causes include trauma, infection, metabolic (Reye's syndrome), tumor, hypoxic/ischemic damage, and shunt malfunction.
3. Priorities are to establish and maintain appropriate ventilation and perfusion and to decrease ICP.
a. Elevate head of bed to 30 degrees. Midline positioning of head and maintenance of normal body temperature should be accomplished.
b. Provide controlled intubation and hyperventilation. Hyperventilation (goal is Pco_2 of 30 to 35 mm Hg) is the most rapid means to decrease ICP. If the patient is obtunded, intubation should neither be difficult nor require premedication (e.g., muscle relaxants). If the patient is thrashing about, diazepam (Valium) 0.1 to 0.2 mg/kg by IV push or

lidocaine 1.5 mg/kg IV should be adequate to allow intubation; neither drug increases ICP.

Note: **Some consultants prefer to avoid the use of pancuronium (Pavulon) because its use interferes with the assessment of neurologic status during the first critical hours. In cases that involve significant crush or burns, succinylcholine may lead to fatal hyperkalemia. Diazepam (Valium) is a safe "relaxant" to use in the ED until the patient can be transferred to an intensive care unit.**

c. Hypertonic agent: Mannitol (0.75 to 1 g/kg IV initially over 10 to 20 minutes) has been used to help decrease cerebral edema and thereby decrease ICP (additional boluses of 0.25 to 0.5 g/kg/dose IV can be given q3-5h). Its use in initial emergency management has been debated recently; check with a neurology consultant before administering it.

d. Diuretic: Furosemide 1 to 2 mg/kg/dose IV (maximum 6 mg/kg) q6-12h has both a diuretic and independent effect on decreasing ICP (probably by decreasing CSF production).

e. Isotonic intravenous fluid (normal saline, lactated Ringer solution, colloid, or blood products) should be titrated to maintain adequate tissue perfusion, blood pressure, and central venous pressure; initial resuscitation may require one or more boluses of 10 to 20 ml/kg of isotonic fluids to restore normal vascular volume. Some acute care physicians recommend IV administration of hypertonic saline, but the most efficacious osmolarity is still a matter of debate.

f. If seizures occur, either diazepam (0.1 mg/kg/dose IV) or lorazepam (0.05 to 0.1 mg/kg/dose IV) can be used.

14

NEUROLOGY

E. CENTRAL NERVOUS SYSTEM INFECTIONS

1. CNS infections include bacterial meningitis, aseptic meningitis, encephalitis, and brain abscess.

a. Patients with these processes may have nuchal rigidity, headache, behavior changes, seizures, sensorium changes, focal neurologic signs, and fever.

b. Depending on the etiologic agent, other signs may be present (e.g., rash, vomiting, diarrhea, pneumonia).

2. Important information includes a history of immune compromise, antibiotic use, immunizations, travel, animal/insect exposure, and the duration and character of any of the signs listed under point 1. With a confused or comatose patient, drug ingestion must be considered.

3. A complete PE is mandatory, with special emphasis on the neck (nuchal rigidity), skull (trauma, tenderness, split sutures), skin (rash, especially petechiae/purpura), and the neurologic examination (e.g., focal findings, sensorium, orientation, cranial nerves). Check for lymphadenopathy (generalized or local). Optimally, the fundi should be visualized (to R/O papilledema) before an LP is performed.

4. Laboratory tests are usually crucial.

a. Spinal fluid is examined for cell count, protein, glucose (compare with a simultaneous serum glucose), and organisms (Gram's stain).

b. CIE and latex particle agglutination of CSF, blood, and urine may help to rapidly diagnose *Haemophilus influenzae, Streptococcus pneumoniae, Neisseria meningitidis,* and group B streptococcus infections. When a viral cause is suspected, the appropriate PCR study can be useful.

c. Blood and urine cultures should be obtained.

d. Serum electrolytes, BUN, creatinine, and a CBC with differential and smear may be helpful.

e. If an ingestion is suspected, a toxicology screen is indicated.

f. LP is contraindicated if there are focal findings (e.g., if a brain abscess is suspected) because herniation is possible. Instead, an emergent CT scan is indicated.

5. Causes

a. Bacterial meningitis: *H. influenzae* (now uncommon because of HIB vaccine), *S. pneumoniae, N. meningitidis,* group B streptococcus, *Listeria* organisms, *Staphylococcus aureus, Pseudomonas* organisms. The latter four occur in neonates.

b. Aseptic meningitis: Most commonly enterovirus.

c. Encephalitis: S/P measles, varicella, mumps, influenza, Epstein-Barr infection, herpes.

d. Abscess: *S. aureus,* group A streptococcus, *H. influenzae* (uncommon), anaerobes, gram-negative enteric bacteria, fungi.

6. Treatment

a. Bacterial meningitis beyond the neonatal period: Cefotaxime 75 mg/kg/dose q6-8h or ceftriaxone 80 to 100 mg/kg/dose q12h × 1 day and then q24h. If a penicillin-sensitive *S. pneumoniae* or *N. meningitidis* is the etiologic organism, ampicillin 50 to 75 mg/kg/dose q6h is used. Initial therapy with one of the aforementioned cephalosporins or ampicillin must also include vancomycin 60 mg/kg/d ÷ q6h; the dosage should be adjusted depending on serum concentrations. Vancomycin should be discontinued if the bacterial isolate demonstrates sensitivity to either penicillin or the cephalosporin.

(1) Follow vital signs and neurologic status carefully; fluid restrict (NPO × 24 hours, then oral and IV total fluids at 60% to 75% maintenance) to prevent SIADH.

(2) In infants and toddlers, follow head circumference; may need CT scan to R/O subdural fluid accumulation if focal neurologic signs, focal seizures, or increasing head circumference occur.

(3) For seizures: Phenobarbital (loading dosage 15 to 20 mg/kg no faster than 30 mg/min; maintenance dosage 3 to 5 mg/kg/d ÷ q12h) or phenytoin (Dilantin) (loading dosage 15 to 20 mg/kg in normal saline no faster than 50 mg/min; maintenance dosage

5 to 10 mg/kg/d ÷ qd or q12h). Fosphenytoin may also be used. See Section G regarding status epilepticus.

b.   Aseptic meningitis: If CSF cell count is confusing or contaminated with blood, may need to give cefotaxime 75 mg/kg/dose q6h or ceftriaxone 80 to 100 mg/kg/d ÷ q12h × 1 day and then qd for 3 days pending negative cultures.
  (1)   Fluid restrict to avoid SIADH, administer IV fluids and analgesics/antipyretics, and incline head of bed 30 degrees.
  (2)   For herpes encephalitis, give acyclovir 1500 mg/m^2/d divided q8h × 14 to 21 days. Treat seizures as above.

c.   Bacterial meningitis (*H. influenzae* and pneumococcal): dexamethasone 0.6 mg/kg/d ÷ bid or qid × 2 to 4 days. Because dexamethasone can decrease the CNS penetration of vancomycin, *in initial therapy,* either dexamethsaone is omitted *or* rifampin 10 mg/kg/dose q12h is given in addition to dexamethasone, vancomycin, and the cephalosporin/penicillin.

d.   If *N. meningitidis* or *H. influenzae* is the etiologic agent, rifampin should be given to all household (and other close) contacts. For *H. influenzae,* the rifampin dose is 20 mg/kg (maximum 600 mg) qd × 4d. For *N. meningitides,* the rifampin dose is 10 mg/kg/dose (maximum 600 mg) q12h × 2 days for all individuals older than 1 month of age, and 5 mg/kg/dose q12h × 2 days for infants younger than 1 month of age.

F. RETT SYNDROME

1.   Characterized by the following:
a.   Female gender
b.   Normal prenatal/perinatal period and normal development in the first 6 to 18 months of life
c.   Normal head circumference at birth with deceleration of head growth between 6 months and 4 years of age
d.   Early behavioral, social, and psychomotor regression with evolving communication dysfunction and dementia
e.   Loss of purposeful hand skills between 1 and 4 years of age
f.   Hand wringing/clapping/washing stereotypies between 1 and 4 years of age
g.   Gait apraxia and truncal apraxia/ataxia between 1 and 4 years of age

2.   Four stages of Rett syndrome
a.   Stage 1: Onset of slowing of development, some hypotonia
b.   Stage 2: Obvious loss of acquired skills, onset of hand stereotypies, loss of contact with environment and autistic affect, evolving dementia, loss of speech and purposeful hand use, screaming episodes, sleep disturbances
c.   Stage 3: Seizures, disappearance of autistic affect, prominent hand stereotypies and jerky apraxic movements, disappearance of screaming

14

NEUROLOGY

episodes, improvement of sleep, onset of apnea spells, loss of gross motor skills, hypertonia

d. Stage 4: Spasticity; muscle wasting; immobility; cool, mottled extremities; cachexia; constipation; profound mental retardation

3. Incidence is 0.4 to 1.0 per 10,000 girls.

4. Etiology is unknown, but a genetic cause seems likely.

5. Various CNS biochemical abnormalities have been noted; EEG is abnormal.

6. Life span per se is not shortened.

7. Referral to a pediatric neurologist is in order.

G. SEIZURES, FEBRILE SEIZURES, AND STATUS EPILEPTICUS

1. Seizures are a common problem in children; approximately 3.5% of children have at least one seizure by 15 years of age. Most have a single seizure or recurrent seizures over a limited time. Only a small percentage (0.5% to 1%) have epilepsy.

2. Causes of seizures

a. Neonatal: Hypoxic-ischemic insult, CNS bleed, infection, CNS malformation, metabolic derangement

b. Infants older than 28 days: Infection, dehydration, fever (older than 6 months of age), inborn errors of metabolism, electrolyte imbalance, birth injury, CNS trauma, malformations

c. Children: Head trauma; noncompliance with, change of, or inadequate dose of anticonvulsant medication; intercurrent infection in a known seizure patient; toxin ingestion (do not forget lead); tumor; fever (up to 6 years of age)

d. Adolescents: Causes similar to those of children, but remember illicit drug ingestion

e. In up to two thirds of cases, no obvious cause is found

3. Initial evaluation of nonfebrile seizure

a. Assess whether a real seizure occurred (or, perhaps, a choking spell, breath-holding spell, or syncope). Is the child ictal or post-ictal? Any seizure activity (lateralization, eye deviation, focal vs. generalized)?

b. Prior seizures? Medications? Fever? Other signs of illness? Aura? Circumstances preceding the seizure? Precipitating event? History of drug abuse or ingestion? Trauma (remember occult trauma such as abuse)? Presence of preexisting neurologic disease?

c. Vital signs.

d. PE (quick and pertinent): Assess neurologic (pupils, response, signs and symptoms of increased ICP, fontanelle), cardiovascular (BP, perfusion), and respiratory (cyanosis, irregular breathing, ineffective ventilation) status. Note breath odor, rash, signs of trauma, liver size, signs of infection (sepsis, meningitis). *Keep reassessing*—condition may change quickly!

e. Initial laboratory evaluation in acute situation.

(1) Dextrostix or Chemstrip
(2) Electrolytes, Ca, glucose, BUN, CBC, anticonvulsant levels (if applicable)
(3) Toxicology screen on blood and urine (and vomitus, if indicated)
(4) Sepsis workup, including LP, may be indicated
(5) Consider need for LFTs, Mg, Pb, NH_4^+
(6) CNS imaging (CT scan or MRI) may be indicated
(7) EEG will be needed at some point in the patient's care

f. Treatment
(1) After a complete assessment, decide if the patient needs an anticonvulsant drug and, if so, the drug most appropriate for the seizure type. These decisions are best made in conjunction with a pediatric neurologist.
(2) When initiating therapy, perform the following procedures:
  (a) Start with a single drug and begin with the lowest dose needed to achieve a therapeutic serum level. Increase the dose as needed to achieve a clinical response.
  (b) Switch to a second drug if the first is not effective.
  (c) If monotherapy fails, add a second drug.
(3) It is important to monitor serum drug levels at onset of therapy, again when well-controlled, and if there are side-effects reported (to evaluate for toxicities).
(4) Most children with recurrent seizures remain on an anti-convulsant medication for at least a 2-year seizure-free period.

4. Febrile seizures
a. Some 2% to 5% of all children will develop a febrile seizure. Although most are simple seizures, a minority are complex.
b. Onset: Most febrile seizures occur between 6 weeks and 6 years of age, with a peak between 1 and 3 years of age. There is a 50% recurrence rate if onset is before 1 year of age.
c. Duration: 50% less than 5 minutes, 75% less than 20 minutes, 2% to 3% more than 30 minutes.
d. Type: Typically generalized tonic-clonic, but 15% are focal. Usually only one seizure occurs during any febrile illness.
e. Most occur with a temperature greater than 39° C and at the onset of fever. A seizure that occurs after a fever has been present for more than 24 hours is more likely to be associated with a significant infection.
f. Evaluation
(1) LP is indicated if any of the following are present:
  (a) Any suspicion of meningitis
  (b) Abnormal postseizure neurologic examination
  (c) History of illness for several days before seizure
  (d) Slow recovery from febrile seizure
  (e) Strongly consider an LP if the patient is less than 12 months of age, and consider an LP if the patient is between 12 and 18 months of age

14

NEUROLOGY

(2) CBC, electrolytes, glucose, Ca, Mg, CNS imaging, and EEG are *not* indicated with simple febrile seizures.

g. Treatment
(1) No treatment is needed for simple febrile seizures.
(2) Give lorazepam for acute control of status epilepticus (dosages are given later in this section).
(3) Attempt to reduce fever with tepid water sponging and rectal acetaminophen to make child more comfortable.

h. Consider long-term prophylaxis with phenobarbital or valproic acid *only* if the patient has multiple risk factors as follows:
(1) Prior history of abnormal neurologic or neurodevelopmental examination
(2) Family history of nonfebrile seizures
(3) Seizure duration more than 15 minutes
(4) Seizure with focal component or associated with transient or persistent neurologic abnormalities
(5) More than one seizure during the same illness within a 24-hour period

Note: **There is no evidence that prophylaxis reduces the risk of subsequent nonfebrile seizures and no evidence that recurrent febrile seizures, even when complex, increase a child's risk for epilepsy or neurodevelopmental problems.**

5. Status epilepticus
a. Status epilepticus describes seizure activity that lasts 30 minutes or longer or in which there is incomplete recovery between recurrent seizures for that period of time.
b. Immediate management includes the following:
(1) Maintain airway and maximize ventilation (oral airway or intubation); provide oxygen as indicated.
(2) Suction secretions and insert NG tube to prevent aspiration.
(3) Establish IV access; if that is not feasible, establish intraosseus access.
(4) If febrile, provide tepid sponging and rectal acetaminophen to make the child more comfortable.
(5) Check Dextrostix; if hypoglycemia (less than 60 mg/dL) is present, give IV bolus of $D_{25}W$ 1 to 4 ml/kg followed by continuous glucose infusion of $D_5/0.25$ normal saline or $D_{10}/0.25$ normal saline.
(6) Also check electrolytes, BUN, creatinine, Ca, CBC, and anticonvulsant levels (if applicable).
(7) IV anticonvulsant therapy
(a) Lorazepam 0.1 mg/kg (maximum 4 mg) at a rate of 1 to 2 mg/min. One dose usually stops status in 2 to 3 minutes. The half-life is 10 to 12 hours. Lorazepam may be less likely than diazepam to cause respiratory depression and hypotension,

but both can occur, especially if the patient has been taking a barbiturate, *or*

(b) Diazepam 0.1 to 0.5 mg/kg (maximum 5 mg in infants and 10 mg in older children) at a rate of 1 mg/min by IV push; may repeat in 10 minutes. The rectal route (0.2 to 0.5 mg/kg) can be used if IV access is a problem; it can be repeated once.

    (i) Advantage: Rapidly effective.

    (ii) Disadvantage: Respiratory and cardiovascular depression, especially if the patient has been taking a barbiturate. In addition, the drug is quickly redistributed throughout the body, and seizures may recur as redistribution occurs.

    (iii) After initial therapy with lorazepam or diazepam, the patient needs to be started on a long-acting anticonvulsant such as phenytoin or phenobarbital.

(c) Phenytoin 15 to 20 mg/kg (maximum 1 g) is administered slowly IV in normal saline at 0.5 to 1.0 mg/kg/min (not to exceed 50 mg/min). As an alternative, fosphenytoin (15 to 20 mg phenytoin equivalents [PE]/kg) can be used.

    (i) Advantage: Phenytoin does not alter mental status (useful in patients with head trauma) and has a longer half-life than benzodiazepines.

    (ii) Disadvantage: Seizures do not respond as quickly as with benzodiazepines; when given parenterally, need to monitor ECG for arrhythmia.

(d) Phenobarbital 10 to 20 mg/kg (maximum 30 mg/kg or 1 to 2 g) is administered by IV no faster than 30 mg/min. If seizures continue, may give second dose of 10 mg/kg after 20 minutes. The maintenance dose is 5 mg/kg/d. The disadvantage is slow onset of action (takes up to 15 minutes to cross blood-brain barrier) compared with benzodiazepines.

6. Maintenance therapy for generalized tonic-clonic and partial seizures in children

a. Carbamazepine: Initial dosing of 3 mg/kg/d, gradually increasing to a maintenance of 20 to 40 mg/kg/d divided bid or tid.

b. Valproic Acid: Initial dosing of 10 to 15 mg/kg up to a maximum of 60 mg/kg; increase slowly to a maintenance dose of 15 to 30 mg/kg/d divided bid.

c. Phenytoin: Initial dosing of 3 to 10 mg/kg/d divided bid or tid.

H. SHUNT MALFUNCTION

1. Anything that goes wrong with a patient with shunted hydrocephalus results from a shunt problem until proven otherwise. Shunt obstruction and shunt infection (usually a result of *S. aureus* or *Staphylococcus epidermidis*) are common.

14

NEUROLOGY

2. Signs and symptoms of acute obstruction include headache, irritability, lethargy, vomiting, acute strabismus, eye movement dysfunction, bulging fontanelle, and behavior change. If present, evaluate as an emergency.
3. Shunt infection may or may not be accompanied by fever. Most shunt infections occur within 2 months of initial shunt placement.
4. Do not waste time pumping the device; doing so may result in misleading information. Perform a general/neurologic evaluation and call a neurosurgeon for probable tap of pump device. Imaging studies may or may not have diagnostic value depending on the study selected, the age of the child, and the acuity of the obstruction. In general, shunt series and head CT scan should be ordered if obstruction is suspected.

I. SYNCOPE

1. Syncope is the sudden, transient loss of consciousness (persisting for only seconds to a minute or more) as a result of cerebral hypoperfusion or anoxia.
2. Important historical information includes the following:
a. A complete description of the episode and antecedent events or patient's feelings (e.g., palpitations, dizziness, nausea, light-headedness)
b. A history of similar events and their precipitating factors
c. Presence of aura or ictal stereotypic movements during the episode (R/O seizure)
d. Cardiac symptoms (exertional dyspnea, palpitations)
e. History of cardiac, endocrine, CNS, pulmonary disease
f. Chronic medication use
g. Family history of syncopal episodes
3. The PE is usually normal. It should be complete with special emphasis on cardiac (murmurs, arrhythmias, tachyarrhythmias) and neurologic assessment, especially the patient's mental state and recollection of the event.
4. Causes of syncope
a. Vasovagal: Preceded by light-headedness, dizziness, diaphoresis, and pallor. This type of syncope may be preceded by physical discomfort, emotionally charged situations, or fright (e.g., seeing blood).
b. Hysteria: The clue is that the patient is seemingly unconcerned about the event.
c. Hyperventilation: Prolonged deep breathing intentionally or unintentionally during stress may lower P_{CO_2} enough to cause syncope. Other symptoms include chest tightness, weakness, and light-headedness.
d. Breath-holding: Usually precipitated by injury or anger. There may be cyanosis following crying or there may be pallor and collapse without antecedent crying.

e. Cardiac lesions: Aortic stenosis, pulmonic stenosis, truncus arteriosus, transposition of the great vessels, tetralogy of Fallot, pulmonary hypertension, carotid sinus syncope.
f. Cardiac arrhythmias: Paroxysmal atrial tachycardia, atrioventricular block, paroxysmal ventricular fibrillation, long QT syndrome (episodes precipitated by physical or mental exertion), mitral valve prolapse (chest pain may also be present).
g. Postural hypotension.
h. Prolonged coughing.
i. Micturition.
j. Severe anemia.
k. Antihypertensives/antihistamines.
l. Hypoglycemia.
m. Cerebellar or brainstem tumor.
5. History and PE guide the choice of laboratory tests.
a. Most individuals with a simple faint require no laboratory evaluation, except perhaps a Dextrostix or glucometer reading.
b. An ECG is in order if there is a history of recurrent faints or "seizures" or if there are cardiac symptoms. Holter monitoring may be helpful.
c. The patient's BP should be measured in the supine, sitting, and standing positions.
6. For most patients with syncope, treatment is usually reassurance.
a. Patients with hyperventilation should be taught to breathe into a paper bag (to increase P_{CO_2}) during episodes.
b. Patients with transient hypoglycemia should be encouraged not to skip meals.
c. Patients with chronic or recurrent hypoglycemia are managed as described in Hypoglycemia (see Chapter 6).
d. Individuals with postural hypotension should be instructed to go slowly from a supine to a standing position.
e. Correction of anemia, discontinuation of offending medications, and therapy for tumors should aid patients with these causes.
f. Individuals with cardiac processes should be managed together with a cardiologist, especially if there are episodes of syncope during exercise.

J. TICS AND TOURETTE'S SYNDROME

1. A tic is a sudden, involuntary, repetitive, rapid, random, nonrhythmic, purposeless, and highly stereotypic movement. The stereotypic nature differentiates it from chorea, myoclonus, athetosis, dystonia, and hemiballism. Other than the tics, affected children generally have a normal PE.
2. The etiology of tics is not well understood.
a. Dopamine may play a role because drugs that increase dopamine metabolites suppress tics, whereas drugs that decrease dopamine levels worsen symptoms.

14

NEUROLOGY

b. Psychologic factors play some role because tics tend to increase when a child is stressed and tend to be precipitated by traumatic events.

3. Tics may be transient (duration of weeks) or chronic (duration longer than 12 months).

4. Average age of onset is 7 years, and there is a male predominance.

5. Tics may occur singly or in groups. A child with a simple tic disorder has only one type of tic at any one time, but this tic may be replaced serially by other tics.

6. Tics typically wax and wane in severity. There is usually an ability to voluntarily suppress tics for minutes to hours, and they disappear during sleep.

7. Types of tics include the following:

a. Motor: Commonly involve the head, face, and neck (eye blinking, eye rolling, mouth twitching, head bobbing, facial grimacing, shoulder shrugging). Individuals may also display hopping, jumping, skipping, squatting, twisting, compulsive touching, and ritualistic acts.

b. Vocal: Coughing, sniffing, throat clearing, high-pitched cries, screams, barking, hiccuping, belching, echolalia, palilalia (repeating one's own words), coprolalia (involuntary utterance of obscenities), and animal sounds.

c. Complex: Multiple motor and vocal tics simultaneously; usually begins with a single tic.

8. Tourette's syndrome represents a subset of tic disorders that usually has its onset between 2 and 15 years of age (mean age is 7 years). The incidence is 5 per 1000, with a 3:1 male predominance.

a. Historically, the child has multiple motor tics and multiple vocal tics that have waxed and waned for more than 1 year.

b. The tics wax and wane over weeks; the child can suppress them temporarily, but the syndrome itself lasts for years or even a lifetime.

c. Familial clustering of affected individuals is common. A genetic etiology is likely (perhaps an autosomal dominant with variable expression).

d. Some investigators believe the syndrome may be precipitated or exacerbated by the use of methylphenidate (Ritalin) and other stimulants used for attentional problems commonly associated with Tourette's syndrome.

9. No laboratory abnormalities have been detected in patients with tics or Tourette's syndrome. The PE is normal except for the tics.

10. Treatment

a. Simple tics: Because of the side effects of the medications used to control tics, transient tics that are not socially objectionable should be permitted to spontaneously abate. Counseling of the patient and parents is necessary, but psychotherapy and medication are unnecessary and do not hasten resolution.

b. Complex tic disorder and Tourette's syndrome

(1) Management in consultation with a pediatric neurologist is *essential.*

14

NEUROLOGY

(2) No drug is curative or alters the long-term prognosis. Medication only suppresses symptoms so that a child is better able to function.

(3) For chronic tics and Tourette's syndrome, haloperidol (starting with 0.25 to 0.5 mg hs, with 0.5 mg incremental increases q4-5d until the desired effect is achieved) has been used with success. The usual dosage requirement is 0.75 to 2.0 mg/d in 2 to 3 divided doses. Side effects include lethargy, dysphoria, depression, and diminution of cognitive functioning. Extrapyramidal side effects (dystonia, tardive dyskinesia) have also been reported. To decrease the likelihood of the occurrence of acute dystonia, routinely administer benztropine (0.5 mg) with haloperidol at the beginning of treatment.

(4) Pimozide (starting with 0.05 mg/kg hs, with 1 mg increases q5-7d until relief of tics or side effects). The maximum dose is 0.2 mg/kg/day or 10 mg/day. Cardiotoxicity is seen with dosages greater than 0.2 mg/kg/d. Side-effects include lengthening of the QT interval, sedation, impaired motivation, dysphoria, phobia, weight gain, ocular changes, dry mouth, gynecomastia or lactation, akathisia, acute dystonic reactions, tardive dyskinesia, and decreased libido. However, these effects occur less commonly than with haloperidol.

(5) Clonidine has been statistically less efficacious than haloperidol and pimozide in reducing tics but has fewer side effects and improves other symptoms such as hyperactivity. The starting dosage is 0.025 to 0.05 mg/d hs, with increases of 0.025 to 0.05 mg q2wk. The usual daily oral dose is 0.2 to 0.3 mg/d. Clonidine transdermal patches are available. Sedation and orthostatic hypotension are the most common side effects.

c. Counseling (psychotherapy) of the patient and parents is necessary. Educational and social counseling is also important.

K. BIBLIOGRAPHY

Headache

Annequin D, Tourniaire B, Massiou H: Migraine and headache in childhood and adolescence, *PCNA* 47:617, 2000.

Farkas V: Appropriate migraine therapy for children and adolescents, *Cephalgia* 19(suppl 23):24, 1999.

Forsyth R, Farrell K: Headache in childhood, *Pediatr in Rev* 20:39, 1999.

Head Trauma

AAP: The management of minor closed head injury in children, *Pediatrics* 104:1407, 1999.

Coombs J, Davis R: A synopsis of the AAP practice parameter on the management of minor closed head injury in children, *Pediatr in Rev* 21:413, 2000.

Goldstein B, Powers K: Head trauma in children, *Pediatr Rev* 15:213, 1994.

Kaufman B, Dacey R: Acute care management of closed head injury in childhood, *Pediatr Ann* 23:18, 1994.

Increased Intracranial Pressure

Larsen G, Goldstein B: Increased intracranial pressure, *Pediatr Rev* 20:234, 1999.

Central Nervous System Infections
Phillips E, Simor A: Bacterial meningitis in children and adults, *Postgrad Med* 103:1998.
Wubbel L, McCracken G: Management of bacterial meningitis—1998, *Pediatr in Rev* 19:78, 1998.

Rett Syndrome
Kozinetz C et al: Epidemiology of Rett syndrome, *Pediatrics* 91:445, 1993.

Seizures, Febrile Seizures, and Status Epilepticus
Baumann R, Duffner P: Treatment of children with simple febrile seizures—the AAP practice parameter, *Pediatr Neurol* 23:11, 2000.
Bebin M: The acute management of seizures, *Pediatr Ann* 28:225, 1999.
Greenwood R, Tennison M: When to start and stop anticonvulsant therapy, *Arch Neurol* 56:1073, 1999.
Haafiz A, Kissoon N: Status epilepticus—current concepts, *Ped Emerg Care* 15:119, 1999.
McAbee G, Wark J: A practical approach to uncomplicated seizures in childhood, *Am Fam Physician* 62:1109, 2000.
Pellock J: Treatment of seizures and epilepsy in children and adolescents, *Neurology* 51(suppl 4):S8, 1998.
Rivera R, Laureta E: Emergency management of seizures—what fits for fits, *Contemp Pediatr* 16:49, 1999.
Russell RJ, Parks B: Anticonvulsant medications, *Pediatr Ann* 28:238, 1999.
Tasker R: Emergency treatment of acute seizures and status epilepticus, *Arch Dis Child* 79:78, 1998.

Shunt Malfunction
Key C et al: Cerebrospinal fluid shunt complications: an emergency medicine perspective, *Pediatr Emerg Care* 11:265, 1995.

Syncope
Hardy C: Syncope and chest pain: to worry or not? *Contemp Pediatr* 11:19, 1994.
Lewis D, Dhala A: Syncope in the pediatric patient, *PCNA* 46:205, 1999.
Prodinger R, Reisdorff E: Syncope in children, *Emerg Med Cl NA* 16:617, 1998.
Rodriguez-Nunez A, Fernandez-Cebrian S, Perez-Munuzuri A et al: Cerebral syncope in children, *J Pediatr* 136:542, 2000.

Tics and Tourette's Syndrome
Frantz D: Tremor in childhood, *Pediatr Ann* 22:60, 1993.
Golden G: Tic disorders in childhood, *Pediatr in Rev* 8:229, 1987.
Pranzatelli M: Miscellaneous movement disorders in childhood, *Pediatr Ann* 22:65, 1993.
Singer H: Tic disorders, *Pediatr Ann* 22:22, 1993.
Vedanarayanan VV: Paroxysmal movement disorders, *Pediatr Ann* 26:402, 1997.
Zinner S: Tourette disorder, *Pediatr in Rev* 21:321, 2000.

OPHTHALMOLOGY

A. CONJUNCTIVITIS (PINK EYE)

1. The differential diagnosis of a red eye in an infant or child includes: conjunctivitis; misdirected lashes; corneal abrasion; foreign body; hyphema; traumatic iritis; keratitis; glaucoma; and systemic disorders such as Stevens-Johnson Syndrome, juvenile rheumatoid arthritis, Kawasaki Disease, lupus erythematosus, and inflammatory bowel disease.
2. Evaluation: Conjunctivitis must be differentiated from a more serious ocular inflammation (e.g., keratitis, iritis).
a. Conjunctivitis: Diffuse redness of conjunctiva (more prominent on palpebral surface); associated with watery or purulent discharge; usually no photophobia; minimal pain; near-normal vision; normal pupillary and red reflexes. Causes are bacterial, viral, allergic, and chemical.
b. Keratitis: Acute inflammation of the cornea associated with extreme pain, tearing, and photophobia. Causes are bacteria, viruses, fungi, and ultraviolet light (e.g., sun, sunlamps).

Note: Do not miss corneal ulcers or lacerations; a clue might be an irregular corneal light reflex or corneal haze. Corneal injury may precede keratitis. The patient may have combined keratoconjunctivitis.

c. Iritis: Red eye with tearing, circumlimbal injection (not seen in conjunctivitis), photophobia, pain, and little or no discharge. The pupil may be smaller and possibly irregular; red reflex may be lost. Vision is often blurred. Refer to ophthalmologist if iritis or keratitis is suspected.
3. Diagnosis and therapy
a. Neonatal
    (1) Chemical
        (a) Secondary to silver nitrate drops or antibiotic ointment
        (b) Begins during the first 24 to 48 hours and clears in the next 24 to 48 hours; no treatment needed
    (2) Bacterial
        (a) There are a wide variety of gram-positive and gram-negative organisms, but by far the most serious is *Neisseria gonorrhoeae.*
        (b) Gonococcal conjunctivitis presents as bilateral purulent eye drainage 2 to 6 days after birth. There may be marked lid edema and chemosis. It is especially likely in settings of inadequate prenatal care and maternal substance abuse.
        (c) Diagnosis is confirmed by Gram's stain and culture.
        (d) Treatment options
            (i)   IM or IV ceftriaxone 50 mg/kg (maximum 125 mg) as a single dose. Use cautiously in infants at risk for hyperbilirubinemia.

(ii) IM or IV cefotaxime 100 mg/kg as a single dose.

(iii) IV penicillin G 100,000 U/kg/d in two divided doses × 7 days.

(iv) Buffered saline eye flushes until discharge disappears.

(v) Mother and sexual partner(s) should be referred for evaluation and treatment.

(3) *Chlamydia trachomatis* (inclusion blennorrhea)

  (a) Most common identifiable cause of neonatal conjunctivitis; incubation period 5 to 14 days

  (b) Presents as mild hyperemia with scant discharge to severe hyperemia, copious purulent discharge, pseudomembrane formation, and chemosis

  (c) Diagnosis

    (i) Giemsa stain of conjunctival scrapings showing basophilic cytoplasmic inclusions

    (ii) Direct fluorescent antibody test (e.g., MicroTrak)

    (iii) PCR assay

    (iv) Enzyme immunoassay

    (v) Culture

  (d) Treatment

    (i) PO erythromycin estolate or ethylsuccinate 50 mg/kg/d in four divided doses × 14 days.

    (ii) No need for topical therapy.

    (iii) Treatment should be offered to mother and sexual partner(s), even if they are asymptomatic.

(4) Viral: Isolated HSV infection is rare in neonates. It usually occurs in association with infection at other sites.

b. Older infants and children

  (1) Bacterial

    (a) Presents as unilateral or, more commonly, bilateral purulent exudate and crusting of lashes. There may be lid edema but pain and photophobia are rare. It is often associated with otitis media in infants and toddlers.

    (b) The most common pathogens are nontypable *Haemophilus influenzae* (beta-lactamase producers) and *Streptococcus pneumoniae* (¼ penicillin-resistant). *Staphylococcus aureus* is probably not a common pathogen except after trauma or surgery. Conjunctivitis secondary to *N. gonorrhoeae* in children may occur secondary to close contact with an infected adult and should raise suspicion of sexual abuse.

    (c) Diagnosis is based on the clinical presentation. Gram's stain showing abundant PMNs is helpful, but cultures are not routinely indicated.

    (d) Treatment

(i) Topical trimethoprim-polymixin B, ciprofloxacin 0.3%, ofloxacin 0.03%, tobramycin 0.3%. Sulfonamides are no longer an appropriate choice.

(ii) Although bacterial conjunctivitis is self-limited, topical therapy is associated with faster symptom resolution and bacterial eradication.

Note: A short (3- to 5-day) course of an oral antibiotic (e.g., amoxicillin-clavulanate) effective against beta-lactamase producing haemophilus species is effective against bacterial conjunctivitis and may prevent the subsequent development of otitis media in young children who present with conjunctivitis. Also, using an oral antibiotic is easier than administering drops to a struggling infant or toddler.

(2) Viral

(a) Often unilateral with erythema, pain, watery discharge, with or without photophobia. It may be associated with preauricular adenopathy and pharyngitis (pharyngo-conjunctival fever).

(b) Most cases are due to adenovirus. Commonly seen in fall and winter.

(c) Treatment is not usually indicated, but it is often difficult to differentiate a viral from a bacterial etiology; if in doubt, a short course of topical antibiotic is the best course of action.

Note: Epidemic keratoconjunctivitis (adenovirus type 8 and others) is extremely contagious. To minimize spread, thorough hand washing and contact precautions are imperative for family members, as well as day-care, school, and medical personnel.

(d) Primary HSV infection may involve the eyelid, conjunctiva, and cornea.

(i) HSV infection usually presents as unilateral follicular conjunctivitis with mucoid discharge, pain, preauricular adenopathy, photophobia, tearing, and blurred vision; there may be satellite vesicular lesions. Recurrent HSV infection usually presents as dendritic keratitis.

(ii) Diagnosis is suggested by finding a dendritic ulcer on fluorescein uptake examination and then confirmed by Tzanck smear and culture.

(iii) Treatment (in conjunction with ophthalmologist) (a) Trifluorothymidine 1% solution (Viroptic) applied q2h while awake × 10 to 15 days (b) Vidarabine (Vira-A) or idoxuridine 0.5% ointment for lid involvement.

Note: Topical steroids are contraindicated for conjunctivitis if there is any possibility of HSV infection. In general, ophthalmic preparations containing corticosteroids, either with or without an antibiotic, should be prescribed only by an ophthalmologist.

(3) Allergic

15

OPHTHALMOLOGY

(a) Bilateral conjunctivitis with itching, redness, periorbital edema, tearing, with or without photophobia. There is usually a seasonal pattern with other atopic manifestations; there may be a secondary bacterial infection.

(b) Treatment

(i) Decongestants: Naphazoline-Antazoline (Vasocon-A), Naphazoline-pheniramine (Naphcon-A).

(ii) Topical antiinflammatory and antihistamine ophthalmic solutions: ketorolac 0.5% (Acular); nedocromil sodium 2%; lodoxamide 0.1% (Alomide); emedastine 0.05% (Emadine); ketotifen 0.025% (Zaditor).

(iii) Systemic antihistamine.

(iv) Attempt to identify and eliminate the allergen (a topical medication may be the culprit).

Note: **Vernal conjunctivitis is a severe form of allergic conjunctivitis that may be present year-round. It exhibits redness, itching, tearing, photophobia, foreign body sensation, thick stringy mucoid discharge, "cobblestone" conjunctival papillae, and superficial punctuate keratitis. The mast-cell stabilizers lodoxamide (Alomide) 1% ophthalmic solution (1 to 2 gtt qid) or cromolyn sodium 4% provide effective prophylaxis.**

(4) Chronic conjunctivitis (persisting for more than 2 weeks)

(a) In young infants, the usual cause is nasolacrimal duct obstruction or chlamydia infection.

(b) In older children, consider allergy, blepharitis, *Chlamydia* (sexually active teenagers), chemical irritants (chlorine, mascara, antibiotic eyedrops), retained foreign body, contact lens cleansing and wetting solution, and Parinaud's oculoglandular syndrome.

(c) Corneal problems, uveitis, and glaucoma may produce a red eye and be confused with conjunctivitis.

(5) Refer a patient with conjunctivitis to an ophthalmologist when any of the following are present:

(a) History of ocular injury or recent eye surgery

(b) Loss of visual acuity or significant pain

(c) Use of contact lenses

(d) Vesicles or ulceration

(e) Chronic or recurrent episodes

B. ORBITAL CELLULITIS

1. Orbital cellulitis is an infection of the orbital contents posterior to the orbital septum. It usually (90% of occurrences) represents contiguous infection from an adjacent sinus, especially the ethmoid sinus.

2. Etiology: *S. aureus,* group A streptococcus, *S. pneumoniae, H. influenzae* type B

3. Onset is often insidious and is characterized by lid edema, chemosis, proptosis, pain on eye movement, decreased ocular mobility, and

decreased visual acuity. Marked proptosis, globe displacement, and impaired vision indicate abscess formation.

4. Treatment
a. Admit patient for IV antibiotic therapy directed at the pathogens listed previously, including resistant *S. pneumoniae.*
b. Obtain ophthalmology consult, blood culture, culture of any aspirated material (from abscess or sinus), and a CT scan of the orbit and sinuses.
c. Surgical drainage of the sinus or orbital abscess may be necessary.

C. PERIORBITAL CELLULITIS (PRESEPTAL CELLULITIS)

1. Periorbital cellulitis is the acute onset of unilateral eyelid edema, erythema, a well-demarcated purplish hue *(H. influenzae),* tenderness of the overlying skin, and fever. The eye itself is usually normal. Differential diagnosis includes insect bite and chemosis secondary to severe conjunctivitis.
2. It may result from hematogenous spread (*H. influenzae* type B, *S. pneumoniae*) or local trauma *(S. aureus).*
3. Blood culture and CIE of tears and urine may help identify the organism; obtain a CT scan of the sinuses if no source is evident.
4. Treatment.
a. Usually requires IV antibiotic therapy.
b. Oral antibiotics may be adequate in mild cases.

Note: There is a 1% to 2% incidence of bacterial meningitis in children who have orbital or periorbital cellulitis. An LP is indicated if there are signs and symptoms of meningeal irritation.

D. STYE (HORDEOLUM)

1. A stye is an acute focal infection (usually *S. aureus*) of one of the sebaceous glands along the lid margin. It causes a small, red, tender swelling that usually suppurates and drains spontaneously.
2. Treatment consists of applying warm moist compresses × 15 minutes qid and continuing until several days after clinical resolution.
3. A topical ophthalmic ointment (bacitracin, erythromycin) may be helpful.
4. Systemic antibiotics and incision and drainage are rarely indicated.

E. CHALAZION

1. A chalazion is a sterile granulomatous inflammation of a meibomian gland (one of the sebaceous glands in the eyelid tarsus). It results in a slow-growing, firm, nodular swelling that most often points on the conjunctival aspect of the lid and usually causes little discomfort.
2. If the chalazion becomes secondarily infected (inflammation, tenderness, and lid edema), apply warm, moist compresses × 15 minutes qid; continue until 1 week after clinical resolution. A topical antibiotic is indicated if there is significant blepharitis.

3. If a chalazion persists for several months, it can be injected with a steroid (triamcinolone) or surgically treated by incision and curretage.

F. CHEMICAL BURNS

1. Burns from strong acids and (especially) strong alkalis can be devastating.
2. Profuse irrigation of the eye with tap water or available neutral fluid should be instituted as soon as possible. If a family member calls with such an injury, instruct that person to irrigate the eye immediately at home (being careful to retract both lids) and then bring the patient to the ED.
3. In the ED, apply 1 to 2 gtt of a topical anesthetic, proparacaine HCl 0.5% (Ophthestic), to the eye to facilitate irrigation with an elevated bottle of normal saline and an IV tubing set. This procedure is a convenient way to provide a controlled and copious flow of irrigation fluid. Swab the upper and lower fornices to remove foreign material. Litmus paper touched to the conjunctival surface should register in the neutral pH range when irrigation is satisfactory.
4. Refer to an ophthalmologist for assessment of the extent of injury.

G. CORNEAL ABRASIONS AND FOREIGN BODIES

1. Corneal abrasions and foreign bodies are usually unilateral. Perform a fluorescein stain. Otherwise, refer to an ophthalmologist.
2. If the abrasion is large or over the central cornea, refer to an ophthalmologist.
3. A simple abrasion with no suspicion of a retained foreign body is treated with a single application of erythromycin or bacitracin ointment and often a tight eye patch × 24 to 48 hours.
4. Foreign bodies require removal by an ophthalmologist, usually followed by a local antibiotic and patching.

H. BLUNT OCULAR TRAUMA (BLACK EYE OR SHINER)

1. With blunt ocular trauma, a complete eye and retinal examination is indicated, including an eye movement test to detect injury to muscle, especially the inferior rectus.
2. Look for a blow-out fracture of the orbital floor, retinal detachment, hyphema, a dislocated lens, and traumatic iritis.
3. Refer to an ophthalmologist if there is any suspicion of these complications, and always if vision is reduced.

I. PENETRATING OCULAR TRAUMA

1. A perforation site can usually be seen with the naked eye. Another sign is distortion of the pupil.
2. Apply a metal shield over the eye, and do *not* put pressure on the eye.
3. Refer to an ophthalmologist.

Note: Do not forget to measure visual acuity during the initial evaluation of a patient with ocular trauma. Use the Snellen chart, Allen picture cards, or the "E" game. For children under 2 years of age, observe the ability to reach for a small object using only the damaged eye.

15

OPHTHALMOLOGY

J. DACRYOSTENOSIS

1. Dacryostenosis is usually due to congenital nasolacrimal duct obstruction and is characterized by excessive tearing in the involved eye and crusting of the lids on awakening. There may also be mild conjunctival infection and a purulent discharge. Symptoms usually begin in the first few days to weeks of life, and 90% of cases remit during the first 8 to 12 months.
2. Treatment involves massaging the lacrimal sac bid and applying trimethoprim-polymixin B drops, or erythromycin ointment if purulent drainage is present.
3. Probing of the nasolacrimal duct is indicated if the obstruction persists for more than 8 to 12 months.

K. DACRYOCYSTITIS

1. Dacryocystitis represents delayed canalization of the nasolacrimal duct with superimposed infection characterized by swelling, tenderness, and erythema below the medial canthus.
2. Treat with IV or PO antibiotics effective against *S. aureus, H. influenzae,* and *S. pneumoniae.*
3. Warm compresses may speed resolution.
4. Once inflammation has diminished, lacrimal drainage system probing should be performed.

L. BLEPHARITIS

1. Blepharitis represents an inflammatory condition of the eyelid margin.
2. It exhibits erythema of the lid with flaking scales along the lid margin, plugs of fibrinous exudate encircling the eyelashes, and breakage and loss of eyelashes; it may lead to chalazion formation.
3. It may be associated with seborrhea. Other causes include HSV infection and lice infestation. There may be secondary bacterial infection *(S. aureus, S. epidermidis).*
4. Treatment
   a. Lid hygiene, debridement with diluted (1:1) tearless baby shampoo, topical antibiotic.
   b. For severe pruritus, a short-term course of topical ophthalmic steroid (e.g., dexamethasone phosphate 0.05%) may be helpful.
   c. In older children with blepharitis and recurrent chalazia, oral doxycycline or tetracycline may be helpful.

M. OCULAR MEDICATIONS

1. Caution must be exercised in using topical ocular medications in children.

2. Some eye drops, such as dilating agents and antiglaucoma medications can have serious systemic side effects.

3. It is estimated that a newborn requires only half of the adult eyedrop dosage to obtain an equivalent ocular concentration; two thirds of the adult dosage is required at age 3, and 90% of the adult dosage at age 6.

4. Approximately 80% of each drop passes through the nasolacrimal system and is available for rapid systemic absorption. Systemic absorption may also occur through the conjunctiva, nasolacrimal duct, oropharynx, digestive system, and skin.

N. BIBLIOGRAPHY

Baker JD: Treatment of congenital nasolacrimal system obstruction, *J Pediatr Ophthalmol Strabismus* 22:34, 1985.

Bodor FF et al: Bacterial etiology of conjunctivitis: otitis media syndrome, *Pediatrics* 76:26, 1985.

El-Mansoury J et al: Results of late probing for congenital nasolacrimal duct obstruction, *Ophthalmology* 93:1052, 1986.

Friedlander MH et al: Diagnosis of allergic conjunctivitis, *Arch Ophthalmol* 102:1198, 1984.

Gigliotti F: Acute conjunctivitis, *Pediatr Rev* 16:203, 1995.

Gigliotti F et al: Efficacy of topical antibiotic therapy in acute conjunctivitis in children, *J Pediatr* 104:623, 1984.

Gross RD, Hoffman RO, Lindsay RN: A comparison of ciprofloxacin and tobramycin in bacterial conjunctivitis in children, *Clin Pediatr* 36:435, 1997.

Hammerschlag MR: Neonatal conjunctivitis, *Pediatr Ann* 22:346, 1993.

Hammerschlag MR et al: Enzyme immunoassay for diagnosis of neonatal chlamydia conjunctivitis, *J Pediatr* 1076:741, 1985.

Knox DL: Uveitis, *Pediatr Clin North Am* 34:1467, 1987.

Lavrich JB, Nelson LB: Disorders of the lacrimal system apparatus, *Pediatr Clin North Am* 40:767, 1993.

MacEwen CJ, Yang JD: Epiphora in the first year of life, *Eye* 5:596, 1991.

Newell FW: *Ophthalmology: principles and concepts,* ed 5, St Louis, 1982, Mosby.

Ogawa GSH, Gonnering RS: Congenital nasolacrimal duct obstruction, *J Pediatr* 119:12, 1991.

Persaud D, Moss WT, Munoz JL: Serious eye infections in children, *Pediatr Ann* 22:379, 1993.

Rettig PJ: Chlamydial infections in pediatrics: diagnostic and therapeutic considerations, *Pediatr Infect Dis J* 5:158, 1986.

Robb RM: Probing and irrigation for congenital nasolacrimal duct obstruction, *Arch Ophthalmol* 104:378, 1986.

Sandstron KI et al: Microbial causes of neonatal conjunctivitis, *J Pediatr* 105:706, 1984.

Wald ER: Conjunctivitis in infants and children, *Pediatr Infect Dis J* 16:517, 1997.

Wallace DK, Steinkuller PG: Ocular medications in children, *Clin Pediatr* 37:645, 1998.

ORTHOPEDICS

Paul D. Sponseller

A. BOWLEGS (GENU VARUM)

1. Infants are physiologically bowlegged because of their intrauterine position; however, this physiologic state corrects itself by 18 to 24 months of age. The child's knee then develops decided valgus at about 3 years of age before assuming the mild valgus of adulthood (Fig. 16-1). The degree of bowleggedness is appreciated on examination by bringing the medial malleoli together and measuring the distance between the knees. Parents of children with *physiologic* bowing are often reassured if shown the graph in Figure 16-1.

2. If correction has not begun by 24 months of age or if the degree of bowing is greater than 20 degrees, x-ray studies of the lower limbs should be obtained to rule out Blount disease or rickets (see Points 3 and 4). Physiologic bowing generally corrects by 2 to 3 years of age.

3. Blount disease (tibia vara) is the defective formation of the medial corner of the proximal tibial epiphysis, perhaps as a result of epiphyseal overload caused by early or excessive weight-bearing in a child with severe physiologic bowing. There are two variants, infantile and adolescent.

   a. The infantile variant occurs between 1 and 4 years of age.

      (1) Initially, infants with Blount disease are indistinguishable from infants with physiologic bowing.

      (2) However, after 2 to 3 years of age, x-ray studies of children with Blount disease demonstrate angulation beneath the medial proximal epiphysis (Fig. 16-2), metaphyseal irregularities, proximal tibial breaking, and proximal epiphyseal wedging.

      (3) Bracing with a valgus-producing brace may be effective if the condition is detected between 24 and 30 months of age.

      (4) If no improvement occurs, surgery is usually indicated after 3 to 4 years of age.

   b. The adolescent variant develops in obese children (more than 8 years of age) or in adolescents whose legs have been in slight varus; it is much less common and milder (less than 20-degree bowing) than the infantile variant. Previous epiphyseal injury may be present. Spontaneous regression may occur; however, progressive cases require surgery.

4. Rickets represents deficient mineralization of the growing skeleton. The most common cause worldwide is deficient dietary vitamin D. The most common cause in the United States is familial hypophosphatemia.

Note: There has been a resurgence of nutritional (vitamin D deficient) rickets in the United States among African-American breast-fed infants not receiving vitamin D supplementation and among older infants on a reduced dairy product intake (often related to a macrobiotic or vegan diet). Sunshine deprivation may be an additional risk factor.

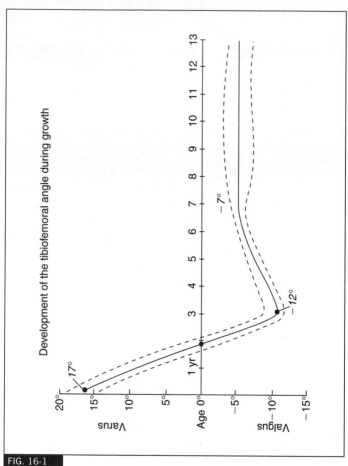

FIG. 16-1

"Bowed legs" and "knock knees." Note broad variation with age. Varus corrects to neutral at approximately 20 months of age and changes to valgus by 3 years of age, with slight valgus persisting to adulthood.

B. DEVELOPMENTAL DYSPLASIA OF THE HIP

1. DDH refers to a spectrum of disease that includes hips that are unstable, subluxed, dislocated, and/or have malformed acetabula. The incidence of true dislocation is 1:1000 to 2:1000. Two common factors in its causation are ligamentous laxity and intrauterine breech position. The left hip is involved in 60% of cases; the right hip in 20%,

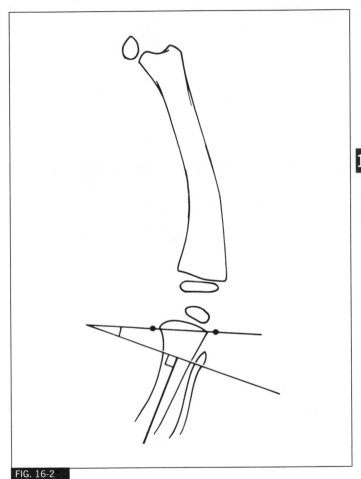

FIG. 16-2

In early Blount disease, the metaphyseal-diaphyseal angle is greater than 11 degrees.

and both hips in 20%. The male-to-female ratio is 1:6. Genetic predisposition seems likely.

2. Infants with DDH usually (but not universally) have the following:

a. A positive Barlow's sign (hip is dislocatable by flexion, adduction, and axial pressure) (Fig. 16-3) and a positive Ortolani's sign (as the flexed hip is slowly abducted, the femoral head shifts into the acetabulum,

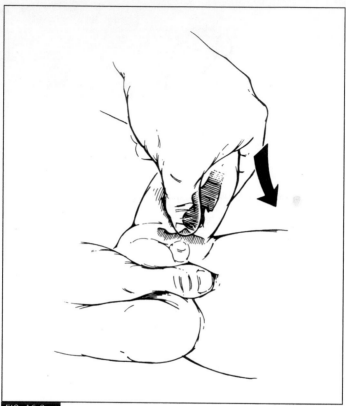

FIG. 16-3

Barlow's test. Flexion-adduction and axial pressure elicit laxity or a "clunk" in an abnormal hip in a child up to 3 to 5 months of age.

producing a "soft clunk") (Fig. 16-4). These maneuvers should be performed on one hip at a time.

b. After age 2 months when muscle contractures develop, the Barlow and Ortolani tests are less helpful. Thigh-fold asymmetry, leg-length discrepancy (which is best observed when the infant is in the supine position and the hips and knees are flexed to 90 degrees), and limitation of hip abduction on the affected side are then seen (Fig. 16-5).

3. Older children with untreated DDH have a characteristic gait. Because the abductor muscles on the affected side are shortened and weakened, the opposite side of the pelvis drops during the stance phase on the affected side (Trendelenburg gait). Children with bilateral

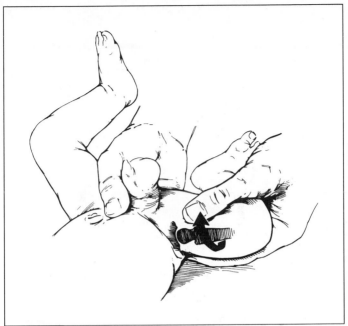

FIG. 16-4

Ortolani's test involves reduction of the dislocated hip by abduction in the flexed position. Examine only one hip at a time. This test is useful in children up to 3 to 5 months of age.

DDH have wide-set hips, a double Trendelenburg (waddling) gait, and exaggerated lumbar lordosis.

4. The diagnosis of DDH depends on a careful hip examination by an experienced practitioner. A newborn with a positive Barlow or Ortolani sign should be referred to an orthopedist (an ultrasound of the hip is not necessary).

Note: During a hip examination, high pitched clicks are commonly elicited with flexion and extension and are inconsequential. If the newborn examination is equivocal (soft click, mild asymmetry), it should be repeated in two weeks. If the results are equivocal or positive, the infant should be referred. If the results are negative, hips should continue to be examined at all routine visits through age 1 year. If the examination becomes positive or equivocal, the infant should be referred for a real-time ultrasound (through age 6 months) or plain radiographs (after 6 months when the femoral head has ossified) and orthopedic evaluation. The use of triple diapers when abnormal physical signs are detected

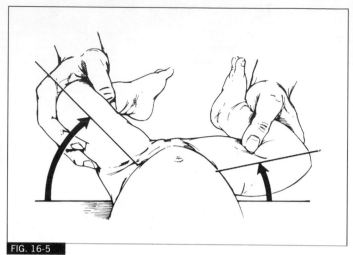

FIG. 16-5

In the older child with fixed dysplasia and in whom Barlow's and Ortolani's signs cannot be elicited, the main signs are limited abduction and apparent shortening.

during the newborn examination is not recommended. In instances of frank dislocation, such an approach may delay the initiation of appropriate treatment.

5. Treatment of DDH in the neonatal period is most reliably achieved by the use of a Pavlik harness; this device holds the hip in reduction (hyperflexion [90 to 100 degrees] with no more than 60 degrees of abduction), allows the infant to be diapered and cleaned, and permits some movement by the infant. Duration of harness use is based on clinical evaluations and follow-up ultrasound studies. The success rate is approximately 85%.

a. Extremes of flexion and abduction must be avoided because such extremes are associated with avascular necrosis and severe hip deformity.

b. Infants 6 to 18 months of age at diagnosis usually require reduction under arthrographic control, preceded in some patients by traction, and subsequent casting. Open surgery may be needed if closed reduction is not possible. Avascular necrosis may still occur.

c. Children 18 to 48 months of age at diagnosis require surgery (muscle release, open reduction, and pelvic or femoral osteotomy) to obtain a stable hip. Avascular necrosis is a more common complication.

d. Children older than 48 months of age at diagnosis require more extensive surgical intervention. The risks and benefits of surgery with potential complications must be carefully discussed.

C. IN-TOEING (FEMORAL ANTEVERSION AND INTERNAL TIBIAL TORSION)

1. In evaluating the child who is in-toeing, the following three common conditions should be considered: metatarsus adductus (see Section H), which is usually seen before 18 months of age; internal tibial torsion, 18 months to 4 years of age; and femoral anteversion, 3 to 8 years of age. These conditions can be sorted by a systematic examination (Fig. 16-6). The angle of the foot in walking should be noted. The child should be placed in the prone position, and the thigh-foot angle, shape of the foot, and hip rotation should be checked.

2. Tibial torsion measures 0 to 20 degrees at birth; with growth, derotation occurs until the adult configuration of 0 to 40 degrees (average 20 degrees) of *external* tibial torsion is reached.

a. The angle is measured as follows: The knee is flexed to 90 degrees. The medial and lateral malleoli are palpated; in a neonate, the malleoli may be parallel or the medial malleolus may lie posterior to the lateral malleolus; in the adult, the medial malleolus is anterior to the lateral one.

b. The angle may also be measured (with the child in the prone position and the knee flexed) by estimating the angle between the foot axis and the long axis of the thigh (see Figure 16-6).

3. Growth alone corrects the vast majority (99%) of cases of tibial torsion by 3 to 4 years of age.

a. Night splints (Denis Browne splints) are believed to be of no real benefit.

b. Shoe modifications are of no value.

c. Rarely (1 per 1000 cases) is surgery needed.

4. Excessive femoral anteversion occurs when the femoral neck is rotated forward or anteriorly more than usual from the femoral shaft (Fig. 16-7). When the child stands, the leg rotates internally to accommodate the femoral head into the acetabulum. The underlying cause of excessive femoral anteversion is unknown. The child with femoral anteversion may have internal rotation of the leg, flexible flat feet, genu recurvatum, and increased lumbar lordosis. On examination with the child in the prone position, internal rotation markedly exceeds external rotation (up to 90 degrees vs. 30 degrees); normally, external exceeds internal rotation.

5. Treatment consists of reassurance. By 8 years of age, 99% of all children with this condition experience resolution. Even if it persists, anteversion generally results in no functional hindrance and no increased risk for arthritis.

a. Surgery is an option for the 1% of children with severe deformity (internal hip rotation greater than or equal to 80 degrees, external rotation less than or equal to 15 degrees, severe gait deformity, and absence of compensatory external tibial torsion).

b. Braces and cables have no influence on femoral anteversion.

16

ORTHOPEDICS

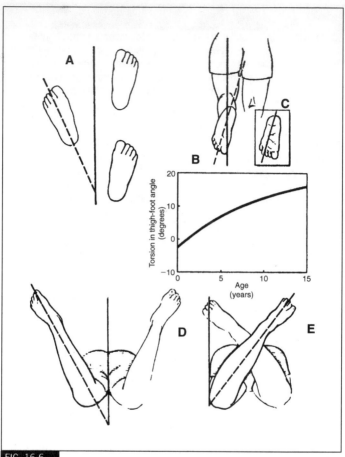

FIG. 16-6

Steps in assessing rotational abnormality. **A,** Angle of the foot during walking should be observed. **B,** Thigh-foot angle reflects tibial torsion and becomes more external with age. **C,** Bleck's line indicates the degree of forefoot adduction. Heel bisector should normally fall between the second and third toe. Here it falls lateral, indicating metatarsus adductus. **D,** Hip rotation occurs if internal rotation is significantly greater than that of external rotation. **E,** Anteversion or capsular tightness contributes to in-toeing.

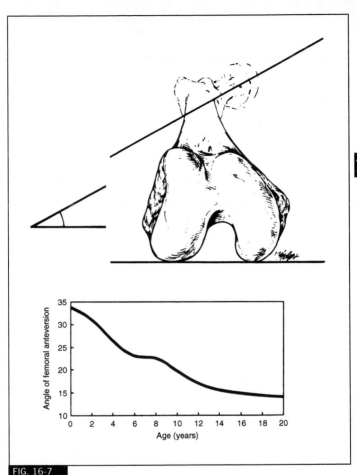

FIG. 16-7

Definition of anteversion and its normal variation.

D. JOINT PAIN AND JOINT SWELLING

1. Arthritis vs. arthralgia
a. Arthritis: Swelling of a joint or limitation of motion accompanied by heat, pain, and tenderness
b. Arthralgia: Subjective complaint of joint pain or tenderness without swelling or limitation of motion

   c. Joint swelling can occur secondary to the following:
- (1) Periarticular soft-tissue swelling (angioneurotic edema, tenosynovitis)
- (2) Thickened synovium (JRA, hemophilia)
- (3) Joint effusion (septic arthritis, Lyme disease, acute rheumatic fever, transient synovitis, JRA, trauma)
- (4) Bony enlargement (traumatic arthritis)

2. General: Joint complaints are common in children. In most cases the problem is transient and is the result of trauma or strenuous activity. The patient needs to be evaluated for evidence of tendonitis, myositis, myalgia, and muscular or ligamentous strain. Pain and loss of motion can result from changes at musculoskeletal sites other than joints. Bone, muscle, nerve, and referred pain can be confused with arthritis.

3. Evaluation

   a. History: Which joints are involved? Characteristics (large joints, small joints; monarticular, polyarticular, symmetric, migratory, duration)? Systemic manifestations (fever, rash, weight loss, stool abnormalities)? Response to antiinflammatory drugs? Family history? Recent trauma, new activities, immunizations, exposure to infections (e.g., hepatitis, rubella, gonorrhea, mononucleosis)?

   b. PE should be complete but should focus on bone, joint, muscle, and nerve status. Useful findings include rash (JRA, HSP, serum sickness, gonococcal infection, Lyme disease, Kawasaki disease, inflammatory conditions), hepatosplenomegaly, lymphadenopathy, eye changes on slit-lamp examination, and a positive joint examination.

   c. Laboratory studies: These studies should be based on the findings of the history and PE.
- (1) CBC: Leukocytosis favors an infectious or inflammatory cause.
- (2) ESR and CRP elevations favor an infectious or inflammatory cause. A highly elevated ESR is *not* usually seen in traumatic, mechanical orthopedic problems.
- (3) ANA and rheumatoid factor are not very sensitive or specific tests.
- (4) Synovial fluid examination and culture; blood, throat, and stool cultures; monospot test; and antibody titers (EBV, parvovirus, *Borrelia* organisms) are helpful in selected patients with suspected infection. In patients with acute monarticular arthritis, an elevated ESR or CRP, temperature greater than 38.5° C, and leukocytosis are independent predictors for the diagnosis of septic arthritis. In a patient whose symptoms exceed 2 weeks, a low CRP, absence of fever, and elevated IgG are independent predictors for the diagnosis of JRA.
- (5) Perform bone marrow aspiration in patients with suspected malignancy.
- (6) U/A: HSP.

   d. Imaging

(1) An x-ray examination is indicated in patients with suspected orthopedic problems (e.g., trauma, Legg-Calvé-Perthes disease, slipped capital femoral epiphysis), osteoid osteoma, and malignancy.

(2) Radionuclide joint and bone scans may be useful (e.g., malignancy, diskitis, osteoid osteoma, toddler's fracture, Legg-Calvé-Perthes disease). Bone scintigraphy is useful with occult bone and periosteal injuries (child abuse, sports injuries) and *may* differentiate among septic arthritis, cellulitis, and osteomyelitis in the rare cases in which this cannot be done clinically.

(3) Ultrasound of the hip is useful because absence of an effusion rules out transient synovitis and septic arthritis.

(4) CT scan may localize a foreign body in a patient with monarticular arthritis.

e. Arthroscopy: Useful for evaluating traumatic and mechanical joint problems.

4. Differential diagnosis

a. Trauma and orthopedic conditions
   (1) Child abuse
   (2) Femoral neck anteversion
   (3) Legg-Calvé-Perthes disease
   (4) Osgood-Schlatter disease
   (5) Osteochondritis dissecans
   (6) Osteoid osteoma
   (7) Slipped capital femoral epiphysis
   (8) Sports injuries
   (9) Subluxation or chondromalacia of patella (patella-femoral pain syndrome)

b. Inflammatory conditions
   (1) Acute rheumatic fever
   (2) Connective tissue disorders (e.g., SLE)
   (3) Inflammatory bowel disease
   (4) JRA
   (5) Psoriatic arthritis
   (6) Vasculitis: HSP, Kawasaki disease, periarteritis

c. Infectious and postinfectious
   (1) Antecedent enterobacterial infections (*Salmonella, Shigella,* and *Yersinia* organisms)
   (2) Gonococcal infection
   (3) Lyme disease
   (4) Osteomyelitis
   (5) Periarticular cellulitis
   (6) Septic arthritis
   (7) Viral infections (hepatitis, mononucleosis, parvovirus, rubella)

d. Miscellaneous

16

ORTHOPEDICS

(1) Foreign body synovitis, arthritis
(2) Hypermobility syndromes
(3) Inflammatory bowel disease
(4) Malignancy
(5) Neuropathic arthropathy
(6) Psychogenic conditions
(7) Sickle cell disease
(8) Transient synovitis of the hip
(9) Drug reaction

e. Diagnostic tips

(1) Fever and ESR or CRP are the most useful screening parameters. An elevation of either suggests an inflammatory or infectious origin.

(2) A normal ESR or CRP and the absence of fever are strongly *against* an inflammatory or infectious cause but may be seen in pauciarticular JRA.

(3) In monarticular disease, a positive joint examination in association with fever or an elevated ESR suggests septic arthritis or osteomyelitis.

(4) A positive joint examination *not* associated with fever or an elevated ESR suggests an orthopedic problem but may also occur with JRA, SLE, and psoriatic arthritis.

(5) A rash is predictive of inflammatory disorders.

5. Specific disorders

a. Gonococcal arthritis: There are two forms; GU infection is usually asymptomatic with both.

(1) Multiple large (knees, wrists, and ankles) and small joints are involved, often in association with fever, chills, and skin lesions. The blood culture may be positive.

(2) Monarticular arthritis with minimal systemic signs and symptoms: Blood culture is negative, but organisms may be recovered from a joint effusion and from skin lesions. It may initially appear as repeated episodes of tenosynovitis coincident with menses.

b. Hypermobility syndrome: May occur with a number of syndromes or as a distinct clinical entity. Along with evidence of hypermobility, the patient usually has recurrent episodes of self-limited arthralgias involving multiple joints. Episodes may last for several days to several weeks.

c. JRA: After excluding other possibilities, consider JRA in patients with arthritis that lasts more than 6 weeks. JRA may exhibit one of three forms as follows:

(1) Systemic: Multiple joints and prominent constitutional symptoms (rash, spiking fevers); 10% to 15% of patients.

(2) Polyarticular: More than four joints; often symmetric and often involves the hands; minor systemic manifestations; 15% of patients.

(3) Pauciarticular: Four or fewer joints; systemic involvement rare; young girls (less than 4 years of age) with pauciarticular disease and positive ANA are at high risk for uveitis; 70% of patients.

(4) Conditions often confused with JRA include soft-tissue pain resulting from myalgia, malignancy, hypermobility syndromes, infectious arthritis, "growing pains," and psychogenic pain. Misdiagnosis is especially common in patients with monarticular disease. ANA and rheumatoid factor screens are helpful if positive but are not very sensitive.

Note: The diagnosis of JRA should be considered in children with chronic joint swelling, even in the absence of pain; 25% of children with pauciarticular JRA report no pain.

d. Lyme disease

(1) Lyme disease is a tick-borne, immune-mediated, inflammatory response to the deer tick-borne spirochete, *Borrelia burgdorferi.* It is reported in most states, but distinct foci are in the Northeast, upper Midwest, and Mid-Atlantic regions. The onset of illness is generally from May to November, with the peak in June to July.

(2) Typically, clinical features occur in three stages, but there is considerable overlap, and features of late Lyme disease may develop without any history of early disease or rash. Only one third of patients remember a previous tick bite.

(a) Stage 1 (early localized infection): Occurs 2 to 30 days after the bite. Erythema migrans appears at the site of the bite; it starts as an erythematous papule or macule that develops into an expanding (at least 5 cm) erythematous annular lesion with central clearing. It is most common on the lower extremities but may occur on the face and axillae. It is often accompanied by fever and mild constitutional symptoms. Some children with Lyme disease have a history of an antecedent flu-like illness *without* erythema migrans.

(b) Stage 2 (early disseminated infection): Occurs 1 to 4 months after the bite; multiple erythema migrans-like cutaneous lesions; asymmetric oligoarthritis; neurologic involvement (cranial nerve palsies, aseptic meningitis, encephalitis); cardiac involvement (myocarditis, A-V block).

(c) Stage 3 (late persistent infection): Occurs weeks to 2 years after the bite; arthritis and encephalopathy with or without neuropathy occur. Arthritis often starts abruptly with swelling, mild-to-moderate pain and redness, with or without effusion, of large joints, especially the knee. A single joint, usually the knee, is involved in two thirds of cases; fewer than four joints are involved in almost all cases. It represents reactive arthritis, not an actual infection. The swelling is often out of proportion to the degree of pain. Attacks may last from days to months, with frequent recurrences (if untreated) during the

16

ORTHOPEDICS

first year after onset. Arthritis may be accompanied by fatigue, but fever and other systemic symptoms are unusual; ESR may be elevated. In patients with a joint effusion, the synovial fluid shows a neutrophil-predominant pleocytosis; WBC count is usually greater than 40,000/mL.

(3) Diagnosis

   (a) Most clinical manifestations of Lyme disease are nonspecific and may be present in a variety of other diseases. The condition is overdiagnosed, mostly as a result of the misuse and misinterpretation of serologic tests, especially in endemic areas.

   (b) The diagnosis should be based on a careful clinical and epidemiologic evaluation. Serologic testing should be performed *only* when the clinical evaluation suggests the diagnosis. Serologic test results should never be the sole criteria for the diagnosis of Lyme disease. In endemic areas there may be a high incidence of seropositive results among individuals who have never had clinically apparent disease.

   (c) Confirmation of the diagnosis is based on the demonstration of *Borrelia* antibodies by ELISA. Specific IgM antibodies appear 3 to 4 weeks after infection begins, peak after 6 to 8 weeks, and then decline. Specific IgG antibodies appear 6 to 8 weeks after the onset of infection, peak after 4 to 6 months, and may remain elevated indefinitely.

Note: Early treatment may blunt the antibody response. Once IgG antibody has developed, antimicrobial treatment may result in a decline in titer, but the antibody is usually detectable for several years.

   (d) Serologic testing performed in reference laboratories (CDC, State Health Department) is reliable. Commercially available serologic testing kits have poor sensitivity and specificity (high percentage of false-positive results because of cross-reacting antibodies) and are not reliable.

   (e) Immunoblotting (Western blot) is a useful way to validate positive or equivocal ELISA results.

   (f) Serologic testing is not indicated for patients with definite erythema migrans. The patient should be treated for Lyme disease irrespective of the serologic test results.

   (g) In patients with early disseminated disease and possible CNS involvement, an LP should be performed and the CSF should be tested for *Borrelia* antibodies.

   (h) Serologic confirmation should be obtained for patients with suspected late persistent infection. A negative result makes the diagnosis unlikely; a positive result does not definitively establish Lyme disease as the cause of the illness but merely establishes that the patient was at some time infected with *B. burgdorferi*.

(4) Treatment
    (a) Early localized infection, mild carditis or arthritis, isolated Bell's palsy
        (1) Patients less than 9 years of age: Amoxicillin 50 mg/kg/d in 3 divided doses (maximum 500 mg/dose).
        (2) Patients more than 9 years of age: Doxycycline 100 mg bid, or amoxicillin 50 mg/kg/d ÷ tid (maximum 500 mg/dose).
        (3) The duration of treatment is 21 to 30 days depending on manifestations and the clinical response.
        (4) Although it may be less effective, erythromycin 30 to 50 mg/kg/d (maximum 250 mg/dose) ÷ qid is an acceptable alternative for patients who are allergic to penicillin.
    (b) Severe carditis or persistent arthritis
        (1) Penicillin G 300,000 U/kg/d ÷ q4h (maximum 20 million U) IV × 14 to 30 days *or*
        (2) Ceftriaxone 75 to 100 mg/kg/d (maximum 2 g) IV × 14 to 30 days
    (c) Neurologic involvement: Ceftriaxone 75 to 100 mg/kg/d (maximum 2 g) IV × 14 to 30 days
    (d) Relapses can occur and require retreatment with the same or other antibiotics

Note: **In Lyme-endemic areas, patients who have fever and fatigue within a month after a deer-tick bite should be considered for empiric antimicrobial treatment.**

(5) Prognosis
    (a) Among untreated patients, 80% develop arthritis or neurologic or cardiac complications.
    (b) Most treated children are disease-free after a year of follow-up, irrespective of the stage of infection at the time of treatment. However, such patients may have subsequent episodes of erythema migrans.
(6) Prevention
    (a) In endemic areas, wear clothing with long sleeves and long pants. Inspect children and pets daily for ticks.
    (b) Remove ticks by grasping with a fine tweezer close to the skin and pulling gently after a tick bite.
    (c) Antibiotic prophylaxis is not indicated.
e. Malignancies: The patient may have localized or diffuse bone pain or "arthritis" as an early sign of unrecognized malignancy (leukemia, neuroblastoma). There may be true arthritis secondary to bony, capsular, or periosteal lesions. In acute leukemia, pain tends to involve few joints, is evanescent, and is often out of proportion to the findings of the examination. Night pain, pain without stiffness, nonarticular bone pain, and a refusal to walk should always raise suspicion of

16

ORTHOPEDICS

leukemia. X-ray studies, radionuclide scans, and bone marrow aspirates are eventually diagnostic but may not become positive for many months.

f. Mechanical problems: Complaints are often chronic, and the diagnosis is suggested by the history. In the absence of fever and an elevated ESR, a positive joint examination suggests an orthopedic disorder. An x-ray examination and MRI may be helpful.

g. Parvovirus-associated arthritis: In children, infection with human parvovirus B19 may be associated with arthritis.

(1) Patients have fever, anorexia, malaise, fatigue, pauciarticular or polyarticular arthritis/arthralgia; large joints (especially knee) more than small joints. Monoarticular involvement is rare. One third of the patients have a rash.

(2) The diagnosis is suggested by elevation of IgM anti-human parvovirus B19 antibody titer. ESR is usually normal; RA factor is not present. Imaging studies may show joint effusion or synovial thickening.

(3) The duration of joint symptoms is generally brief; most resolve within 4 months. However, some children may develop chronic arthritis and fulfill the criteria for JRA.

(4) NSAIDs can be used for pain relief.

h. Septic arthritis

(1) Usually monoarticular. Most often due to hematogenous spread but may also result from extension of metaphyseal osteomyelitis or direct innoculation of a joint from a puncture wound. The hip, knee, and ankle are most commonly affected.

(2) Beyond the neonatal period, signs and symptoms include: painful swollen joint, limited range of motion, fever, irritability, limp, refusal to walk, and toxic appearance. Neonates may be afebrile and manifest only irritability and decreased movement of an extremity. The diagnosis can also be difficult in the setting of recent antibiotic usage.

(3) Responsible organism:

(a) Neonate: Group B streptococcus, *S. aureus,* Gram negative rods

(b) From 2 months to 4 years of age: *S. aureus, H. influenzae* (in patients not immunized with HIB vaccine)

(c) Older than 4 years of age: *S. aureus,* Group A β *hemolytic streptococcus*

Note: **Think of salmonella in patients with a hemoglobinopathy, gonococcus in teenagers, and *P. aeruginosa* in foot infections.**

(4) Diagnostic studies:

(a) Laboratory findings include: leukocytosis; elevated ESR, elevated CRP and positive blood culture (one third to half of cases).

(b) Plain x-rays may show soft tissue swelling or an adjacent bone lesion (osteomyelitis, trauma), but are not generally helpful. Ultrasound is very sensitive in detecting a hip joint effusion. A bone scan is indicated if an adjacent osteomyelitis is suspected.

(c) Aspiration of the affected joint is the most important diagnostic procedure and is always indicated if there is clinical suspicion of an infected joint. There is an intense synovial leukocytosis (WBCs greater than 50,000, PMNs greater than 90%). Gram's stain is positive in 30% to 60% of cases, and synovial fluid culture is positive in more than 80% of cases.

Note: **The combination of joint pain, temperature higher than 38° C and ESR greater than 20 mm/h is highly sensitive and specific for the diagnosis of septic arthritis.**

(5) Treatment decisions are based on age, immunization status, and results of Gram's stain and cultures. Usually, antibiotics are given IV for 1 week followed by 2 weeks of oral therapy. An infected hip or knee can be surgically drained via arthroscopy or arthrotomy. Drainage is especially important for the hip joint, which is at high risk for the development of avascular necrosis.

(6) The prognosis is excellent if treatment is started within 4 days of the onset of symptoms.

E. KNOCK KNEES (GENU VALGUM)

1. Most children are slightly knock-kneed at 3 to 5 years of age; excessive knock knee may develop in late childhood or adolescence. With genu valgum, the medial malleoli cannot touch when the knees are touching. The child may walk and run awkwardly but does not experience pain.

2. Genu valgum may be any of the following:
a. Apparent: Fat thighs, hypotonia, lax joints
b. Pathologic: Paralytic disorders, JRA, rickets, trauma, bone infection
c. Physiologic (idiopathic): Accounts for the vast majority of cases

3. The assessment of idiopathic genu valgum may be made by an x-ray examination of the child's legs while he or she is standing (feet straight ahead). This examination excludes some of the pathologic causes of the disorder. It is not needed in mild cases.

4. Idiopathic genu valgum resolves spontaneously with growth. Fewer than 1% of children who are affected develop degenerative arthritis of the knee. Surgery may be needed in severe cases (i.e., more than 8 cm between medial malleoli) but this is rare.

F. LEGG-CALVÉ-PERTHES DISEASE

1. Legg-Calvé-Perthes disease is avascular necrosis of the femoral head with collapse and subsequent repair.

16

ORTHOPEDICS

a.   The male-to-female ratio is 6:1; 80% of cases occur between 4 to 10 years of age.

b.   The etiology is unknown, but some cases may be related to clotting abnormalities (increased clot formation or decreased clot breakdown).

c.   Affected children are slightly shorter than their peers and have delayed skeletal maturation.

d.   Routine childhood trauma may bring an asymptomatic child to attention.

2.   The disease is self-limited but may last 2 to 4 years. There are five stages, which are listed as follows:

a.   Prenecrosis, in which there is vascular compromise

b.   Necrosis (3 to 6 months), in which the affected section of bone dies with microfracture formation

c.   Revascularization (6 to 12 months), in which the dead bone is resorbed and replaced with cartilage

d.   Reossification (18 to 36 months), in which the deformed femoral head reossifies

e.   Remodeling, in which there is some improvement of the joint

3.   The affected child presents with a limp, with or without intermittent pain in the hip or thigh, and decreased hip motion (especially rotation and abduction). It is usually unilateral, but there is asymmetric bilateral disease in approximately 5% of cases. Laboratory studies are normal.

4.   The radiographic picture varies by the stage of the disease. On AP and frog-leg lateral radiographs, there may be a widened joint space (growth failure), a lucent crescent under the femoral head margin, distortion of the femoral neck and head (shortened neck, flattened head), and loss of density in the metaphysis. Bone scintigraphy may quantify the amount of avascularity, and MRI can provide additional anatomic detail.

Note: The process may be radiographically silent during the first 3 to 6 months.

5.   Treatment is based on chronologic age, bone age, and disease severity and can range from activity restriction, physical therapy, and traction to casting/bracing or surgical containment (proximal femoral varus osteotomy). Prognosis depends on age and extent of femoral head involvement. Most children under age 5 and with less than 50% femoral head involvement can be managed nonsurgically.

G. LIMP

1.   A limp can be painless or painful.

a.   The causes of *painless* limp include an alteration in muscle tone, strength, or joint function. Specifically, these alterations include the following:

   (1)   Neurologic problems: Flaccid paralysis, spasticity, ataxia, spinal diseases such as masses or herniated disks.

   (2)   Muscle disease: Muscular dystrophy, arthrogryposis.

   (3) Joint disorders: Contractures, hyperextensible joints, developmental dysplasia of the hip.

   (4) Bone disorders: Knock knees, leg-length discrepancies, Blount disease, tibial torsion, slipped capital femoral epiphysis, coxa vara, epiphyseal dysplasias, spondylolisthesis.

   (5) Hysteria or mimicry.

   (6) Generally, painless limps are insidious in onset. The child is not acutely ill. The cause is usually apparent from the PE, which must include a careful neurologic assessment to rule out intraspinal disorders.

b. Causes of *painful* limp include the following:

   (1) Trauma: Local, especially foot lesions or foreign bodies, toddler's fracture, ligamentous strains and sprains, tendonitis, tendon tears, muscle bruises, fractures, injections, or patellar subluxation in adolescent girls

   (2) Infections: Septic joint, osteomyelitis, pyomyositis, intervertebral disk inflammation or infection, epidural abscess

   (3) Intraabdominal processes: Appendicitis, retroperitoneal mass, ileal adenitis

   (4) Inflammatory disorders: Toxic synovitis, rheumatic fever, JRA, SLE, other collagen-vascular disorders

   (5) Aseptic necrosis, osteochondritis, other orthopedic conditions: Legg-Calvé-Perthes disease, Osgood-Schlatter disease, chondromalacia patellae, osteochondritis dissecans, SCFE

   (6) Neoplasms: Leukemia, malignant and benign bone tumors

   (7) Hematologic disorders: Hemophilia with hemarthrosis, sickle cell disease (hand-foot-and-mouth syndrome), phlebitis, scurvy

   (8) Miscellaneous: HSP, serum sickness, inflammatory bowel diseases

2. The painful limp may have an acute or gradual onset; the child may be febrile (infectious processes) or afebrile. Depending on the cause, the child may have GI symptoms or dermatologic findings.

a. The history should address all of these issues, with particular emphasis on the onset, progression, duration, aggravating factors, and measures to relieve the pain.

b. Other symptoms of illness should be elicited; ask about chronic conditions, medication use, previous orthopedic injury or surgery, recent fever or infection.

c. Do not forget child abuse.

3. The PE should be complete.

a. Observe gait.

b. The affected limb's appearance, joints, symmetry with mate, and range of motion (active and passive) should be assessed.

c. The limbs should be systematically palpated for tenderness because a minor buckle fracture may be subtle. The most commonly involved

16

ORTHOPEDICS

areas are the distal tibia and calcaneus. Palpation is also a good way to localize a possible osteomyelitis.

d. The skin, back, and other joints should be carefully examined.

e. An abdominal and rectal examination must be performed if an abdominal process (e.g., psoas abscess) is suspected.

4. Laboratory tests are dictated by the history and physical findings.

a. An x-ray examination of the entire limb may be useful to identify and localize the problem. An ultrasound may help identify an effusion and bone scintigraphy may be diagnostic.

b. If the child appears ill, a CBC with differential, ESR, and blood culture are in order.

c. A suspicious joint needs to be tapped. If abuse is suspected, a radiographic trauma series may be in order.

5. Treatment of the limp is directed at the underlying disorder, most of which are discussed elsewhere in this chapter.

H. METATARSUS ADDUCTUS

1. In metatarsus adductus, the bones of the forefoot are deviated medially on the bones of the midfoot at the tarsometatarsal joint; it is most prominent at the first joint. The sole of the foot is laterally convex and medially concave; the fifth metatarsal may be subject to excessive weight-bearing forces. When the child stands, the hindfoot may be in a valgus position. Metatarsus adductus may be supple or fixed. Genetic and intrauterine forces may play roles in its occurrence.

2. Supple metatarsus adductus implies that the deviation is easily correctable with passive manipulation of the foot.

a. Children with this variant usually require either no treatment or simple stretching exercises.

b. At diaper changes, the parent holds the heel in one hand and with the other hand gently exerts laterally directed pressure against the first metatarsal.

c. Straight-last or outflare shoes worn day and night may also be beneficial.

3. Rigid metatarsus adductus in children often does not correct spontaneously; passive correction is impossible. This condition may require a serial cast or brace correction; if begun in the first month through the sixth month of life, correction usually occurs in 1 to 2 months. Serial casting may be effective up to 1 to 2 years of age but is ineffective after 2 years. After the deformity has been corrected by casts, holding casts, straight-last shoes, or outflare shoes are used until there is no chance of recurrence. Symptomatic children older than 3 to 4 years of age usually require surgery to correct the defect.

I. OSGOOD-SCHLATTER DISEASE

1. Osgood-Schlatter disease consists of a painful enlargement of the tibial tuberosity as a result of a vigorous quadriceps pull in a growing child.

The inflammation at the patellar tendon insertion accounts for the symptom of pain below the kneecap, especially after physical activity or kneeling. The examiner can elicit this pain by pressing on the tibial tuberosity at the patellar tendon insertion. An x-ray examination is unnecessary if the presentation is classic. The x-ray examination shows soft-tissue swelling and an irregular, prominent tubercle; ossicles may be present in the tendon.

2. The disease is self-limited; symptoms cease when the proximal tibial epiphysis closes (14 to 16 years of age).

a. Mild cases can be managed by rest, quadriceps and hamstring stretching, restriction of activity, antiinflammatories, and ice packs. After the pain subsides, activity can be resumed gradually.

b. Crutches, knee immobilization, or casting may be necessary in more severe cases.

J. OSTEOMYELITIS

1. Acute osteomyelitis occurs either through hematogenous spread, from direct inoculation of bacteria, or via spread from a contiguous nidus of infection. Chronic osteomyelitis is a result of inadequately treated acute osteomyelitis.

2. If the spread is by bloodstream, the initial occult bacteremia occurred days to weeks before the onset of symptoms. There may be a history of trauma to the affected limb. Penetrating trauma can introduce bacteria from skin, clothing, shoes, or the instrument of trauma.

3. The femoral and tibial metaphyses are the most commonly involved bones, but any bone can be affected. Children younger than 2 years of age are more likely than older children to have a bone infection spread into the contiguous joint space.

4. *S. aureus* is the most common bacterial pathogen, followed by gram-negative rods, group A streptococcus, and *H. influenzae* (less likely now because of HIB immunization). *Pseudomonas aeruginosa* is an important cause of osteomyelitis of the foot, especially if a puncture wound occurred through a sneaker. *Salmonella* organisms are the most common cause of osteomyelitis in patients with a hemoglobinopathy.

5. Important historical information includes the nature of the bone/limb symptoms and a history of trauma, fever, or constitutional symptoms. Does the child limp or refuse to bear weight altogether (if the leg is involved)? Does the child refuse to use the limb (leg or arm)? What type of trauma occurred and when? Has the child been irritable? Does the child have a hemoglobinopathy?

6. The PE should be complete, but particular attention should be given to the affected limb. Is it swollen, bruised, red, hot, tender? Will the child actively use the extremity? Will he or she allow the examiner to passively move it? Is the child febrile?

7. Laboratory tests to assist in the diagnosis include a CBC with differential (WBC increased with shift to the left), ESR (usually

16

ORTHOPEDICS

increased), CRP (usually increased), and blood culture. Aspiration of material from the involved bone can identify the offending organism.

8. Radiographic studies of the affected bone may demonstrate only soft-tissue findings within 3 to 4 days of symptom(s) onset. These findings include swelling, edema, and alterations in fat lines and planes between muscles.

9. After 7 to 10 days of symptoms, the x-ray study shows periosteal elevation, lytic lesions, and sclerosis.

10. MRI is helpful in confirming the diagnosis, if the affected region can be localized.

11. A bone scan may show increased uptake at the involved site as early as 1 to 2 days into the illness. However, the incidence of false-negative findings is high (25%), and increased uptake is also seen in trauma, cellulitis, neoplasms, and septic arthritis. Its main role is for infections that are poorly localized.

12. Differential diagnosis
a. Cellulitis
b. Septic joint
c. Soft-tissue injury secondary to trauma
d. Fracture
e. Tumor

13. Treatment
a. Oxacillin 150 mg/kg/d IV ÷ q6h *or* (if penicillin allergy) cefazolin 50 to 100 mg/kg/d ÷ q8h *or* (if penicillin and cephalosporin allergy) clindamycin 25 to 40 mg/kg/d ÷ q8h. Remember, however, that there is cross-sensitivity to the cephalosporins among *some* individuals with "cillin" allergies (penicillin skin testing can be helpful). IV therapy is given for 3 to 7 days until clinical improvement is noted. After that, the patient's drug regimen can be changed to oral therapy: dicloxacillin 25 to 50 mg/kg/d ÷ q6h *or* cephalexin 100 mg/kg/d ÷ q6h *or* clindamycin 10 to 40 mg/kg/d ÷ q8h. Good compliance must be ensured. During oral therapy, serum bactericidal or antibiotic levels are monitored in difficult cases (slow responses or unusual host factors). A bactericidal titer of 1:8 or a β-lactam concentration of greater than 20 mcg/ml is desirable. Titers and levels are measured 45 to 60 minutes after a dose of oral suspension and 1.5 to 2 hours after ingestion of a capsule or tablet.

b. *Pseudomonas* organisms should be covered if the suspected infection is in the sole of the foot, especially if the patient had been wearing rubber-soled shoes at the time of the injury; treat with IV ticarcillin 200 to 300 mg/kg/d ÷ q4-6h and gentamicin 5 to 7.5 mg/kg/d ÷ q8h.

c. In a neonate or a patient with a hemoglobinopathy, *Salmonella* organisms may be the cause; treat with IV ampicillin 200 mg/kg/d ÷ q4h *and* gentamicin 7.5 mg/kg/d ÷ q8h. In neonates, nafcillin and cefotaxime can be used; in patients with sickle cell disease, cefotaxime or ceftriaxone can be used.

d. Failure to respond to IV antibiotics within 48 hours should prompt an investigation for a bone sequestrum or subperiosteal abscess that could require surgical debridement.

e. If the patient does not respond to IV staphylococcus coverage, consider other organisms and change therapy accordingly.

f. Total treatment (IV and PO) should be based on clinical response and decline in CRP. Waiting for normalization of the ESR is an overly conservative end point. Most patients with staphylococcal infection can be successfully treated with a 3 to 4 week course of antibiotics.

g. Involve an orthopedist early. The patient may also require physical therapy.

16

K. PULLED ELBOW (NURSEMAID'S ELBOW)

1. With a pulled elbow, the annular ligament surrounding the radial neck becomes partially interposed between joint surfaces (Fig. 16-8).

a. This series of events occurs when a young child's forearm or wrist is jerked with longitudinal and/or pronational forces. Do *not* make this diagnosis after a fall which is more likely to cause a subtle fracture.

b. The child holds his or her arm in extension and actively resists attempts to flex it.

c. X-ray studies are normal.

2. Treatment consists of hypersupination of the forearm with the elbow held in flexion; once the child's ligament is released, he or she begins to use the arm again. Some orthopedists recommend a posterior splint for 10 days to allow healing of the ligament, especially if the subluxation is recurrent. Parents and siblings should be educated about the mechanism of injury and discouraged from jerking the arm.

L. SCOLIOSIS

1. Scoliosis is a lateral curvature of the spine; 80% of cases are idiopathic, but there are also congenital and neuromuscular causes. On examination, there is lateral bending of the spine, but, as it curves, it also rotates producing a paravertebral rib hump.

a. Girls are more commonly affected than boys.

b. The usual onset is after 9 to 10 years of age for girls and after 11 to 12 years of age for boys.

2. Screening for scoliosis should begin at 6 to 7 years of age (Fig. 16-9).

a. Look at the standing child from behind for asymmetry of the arm/trunk angles, shoulder lines, and flank creases.

b. Place your hands on the iliac crests to detect differences in leg lengths.

c. Have the child bend at the waist as he or she extends the arms in front with the palms together (a diving position). As the child bends to touch the toes, observe the horizontal plane of each set of ribs to determine on which side an elevation occurs. The elevation is on the convex side of the curve, and the depression is on the concave side.

ORTHOPEDICS

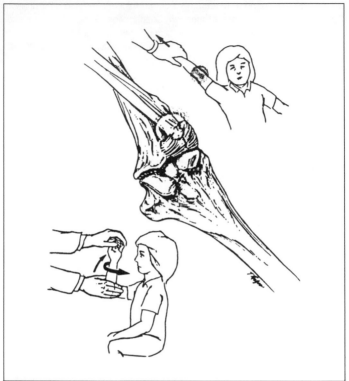

FIG. 16-8

A "pulled" or "nursemaid's" elbow is a partial tear of the annular ligament of the radial head; it can be reduced by flexion and supination.

d. Observe the patient from the side during the bending test to determine if there is kyphosis (an abnormal angling of the spine rather than a rounded contour).

e. In school screening programs, a scoliometer is used to identify scoliosis. If the angle of trunk rotation (ATR) is greater than 7 degrees, the child should be referred.

Note: **The presence of back pain, spinal stiffness, and limited range of motion is suggestive of an irritating lesion (e.g., tumor, spondylolysis, diskitis) in the spinal column: A careful neurologic evaluation, including MRI is indicated.**

3. Probability of worsening can be calculated using curve magnitude, chronologic age, and Risser grade (skeletal maturity). Worsening of scoliotic curves is associated with the following:

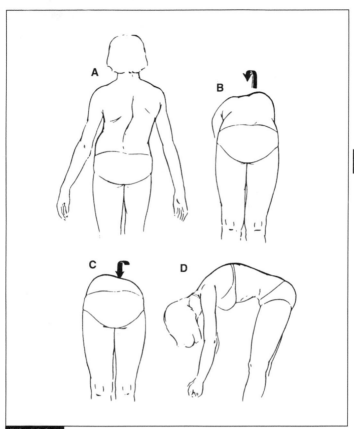

FIG. 16-9

Screening for spinal deformities. **A,** Scoliosis may be demonstrated by subtle or striking elevation of one shoulder, a trunk shift, and waistline asymmetry. **B,** Forward bending with the hands clasped and the knees straight may reveal a thoracic prominence on the convex side, even if the standing examination appears normal. **C,** Further forward bending shows any lumbar curve (usually opposite of the thoracic curve). **D,** Always look from the side to see a focal kyphosis.

a. Younger age (less than 12 years of age) at diagnosis, especially if the curve is severe.
b. Severity of the curve, with those greater than or equal to 30 to 40 degrees the most likely to progress. A patient who reaches maturity with a curve less than 40 degrees is unlikely to progress as an adult.

   c.   Skeletal immaturity, as measured by the ossification of the iliac apophysis.

   d.   Gender, with small curves in boys much less likely to progress.

4.   Refer the child for an x-ray examination or an orthopedic consult if the angle of trunk rotation (i.e., the angle between the horizontal plane and a plane across the posterior trunk at the point(s) of *maximum* deformity) is greater than 7 degrees or if the vertebral angulation (Cobb measurement) is greater than 20 to 25 degrees. If a smaller curve is present, the child should still be followed up with bend tests or x-ray examinations until growth ceases.

5.   Treatment

   a.   For the immature patient with a curve of 25 to 40 degrees, bracing is indicated (70% to 80% effective in preventing further progression).

   b.   Surgery is recommended for immature patients with a curve greater than 40 degrees and for mature patients with a curve greater than 50 degrees or documented progession.

M. SLIPPED CAPITAL FEMORAL EPIPHYSIS

1.   SCFE is an abrupt or gradual displacement of the proximal femoral head on the femoral neck.

   a.   The male-to-female ratio is 2:1, and it most commonly occurs during preadolescence or adolescence (mean age 11.5 years in girls; 13.0 years in boys). Patients are often tall and overweight. The cause is unknown, but the following factors have been implicated: growth spurts, hormonal factors, an intrinsically defective growth plate, genetic predisposition, and trauma.

2.   The child may have an acute limp; pain in the groin, thigh, or knee; and inability to bear weight. Hip motion (especially abduction and internal rotation) is painful and limited. Flexing the involved hip to 90 degrees causes external rotation. Alternatively, the child may have a gradual onset of intermittent pain and limping. Some 25% of cases are bilateral.

3.   The x-ray examination of SCFE may show a widened growth plate of the proximal femur on the affected side.

   a.   Because many slips are posterior, a frog-leg lateral x-ray examination is mandatory.

   b.   In true cases, the x-ray study demonstrates the altered position of the femoral head on the neck (Fig. 16-10).

   c.   Medial and posterior displacement of the femoral head with apparent loss of height can be seen, especially by drawing a line along the lateral aspect of the femoral neck.

4.   Treatment of SCFE is directed toward preventing further slippage, avascular necrosis, premature degenerative arthritis, and further gait deterioration. This is accomplished by stabilization of the epiphysis with a metallic screw or cortical bone graft, followed by use of crutches for partial weight bearing.

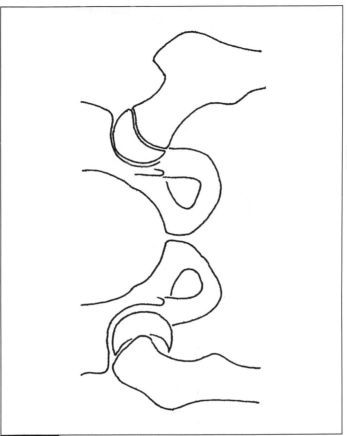

FIG. 16-10

In slipped capital femoral epiphysis, the femoral head is displaced inferiorly, posteriorly, and medially; at times this may be very subtle.

5. Delay in diagnosis and treatment puts the child at risk for premature degenerative arthritis.

N. TORTICOLLIS

1. Torticollis (wryneck, tilted neck) may be congenital (vertebral anomalies, intrauterine malposition, birth trauma) or acquired (vertebral column or spinal cord tumors, inflammatory disorders such as cervical adenitis or intervertebral diskitis, or trauma such as cervical subluxation or neck muscle strain). The most common cause is neck muscle strain

acquired during play, participation in sports, or an awkward sleeping position.

2. In a child with torticollis, the head is tilted toward the affected side and the chin is rotated to the contralateral side (Fig. 16-11). The sternocleidomastoid muscle is shortened as a result of muscle spasm.

3. Because torticollis may be secondary to subluxation or dislocation of the facets of the atlantoaxial joint, anteroposterior, lateral, and open-mouth odontoid x-ray studies should be obtained if suspicion is high.

4. Treatment of torticollis resulting from neck strain consists of warm soaks, analgesics, mild antiinflammatory agents, and a soft cervical collar. Treatment of torticollis resulting from atlantoaxial subluxation consists of rest and cervical traction; a soft collar may provide relief after reduction. Surgery is rarely necessary.

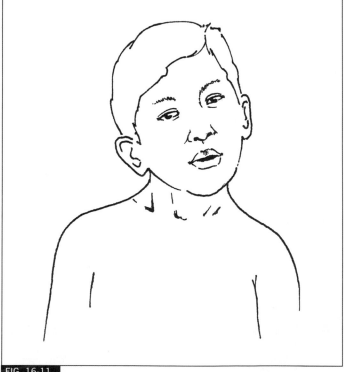

FIG. 16-11

In torticollis, the ear typically is tilted toward the affected side, and the chin rotated to the contralateral side.

O. TRANSIENT SYNOVITIS

1. Acute inflammatory synovitis with effusion of the hip joint. Peak incidence occurs at 3 to 6 years of age, and boys are more commonly affected than girls. The cause is unknown, but the episode may follow a URI or minor trauma.

2. The child with transient synovitis usually exhibits acute onset of limp and hip pain, but pain may be referred to the knee. The limp is characterized by a shortened stance on the affected side, with guarding or spasm of the muscles around the hip joint. Severely affected children may refuse to walk. On examination, the hip is held in flexion with slight abduction and external rotation and there is limited active and passive range of motion at the hip as a result of muscle guarding. There may be low grade fever and malaise. It is almost always unilateral.

Note: With septic arthritis, the child will not permit any range of motion, even if slowly and carefully performed.

3. Laboratory tests are indicated if the child is febrile or if there is suspicion that he or she has a septic joint. In toxic synovitis, the CBC with differential and ESR are normal or only mildly elevated; although the soft-tissue planes around the hip may be distorted, the hip x-ray examination is normal. Ultrasound may show a small amount of joint effusion. Aspiration of the joint should be performed unless the child has no fluid or is afebrile and has a normal ESR (less than 20 mm/h). With toxic synovitis, the joint fluid is sterile as opposed to the fluid from a septic joint, which shows an intense leukocystosis and may have organisms on Gram's stain.

4. Hospitalization may be necessary if the child has a high fever or severe symptoms.

a. If the child is not hospitalized, serial examinations of the hip should be performed every day or every few days because synovitis may herald septic arthritis, osteomyelitis, neoplasm, Legg-Calvé-Perthes disease, or SCFE.

b. Toxic synovitis usually resolves in 3 to 10 days; prolonged symptoms should prompt reconsideration of the diagnosis. A second episode occurs in 5% to 15% of cases, but there are no long-term sequelae.

c. Treatment consists of rest, analgesics, and restricted activity; severely affected patients may benefit from light traction.

16 ORTHOPEDICS

P. BIBLIOGRAPHY

General
Staheli LT: *Fundamentals of pediatric orthopedics,* Philadelphia, 1998, Lippincott-Raven Press.
Bowlegs
Staheli LT: *Fundamentals of pediatric orthopedics,* Philadelphia, 1998, Lippincott-Raven Press.
Developmental Dysplasia of the Hip
American Academy of Pediatrics: Clinical practice guidelines: early detection of developmental dysplasia of the hip, *Pediatrics* 105:876, 2000.
Aronsson D et al: Developmental dysplasia of the leg, *Pediatrics* 94:201, 1994.

Hennrikus WL: Developmental dysplasia of the hip; diagnosis and treatment in children younger than 6 months, *Pediatr Ann* 28:740, 1999.
Rosendahl D et al: Ultrasound screening for developmental dysplasia of the hip in the neonate, *Pediatrics* 94:47, 1994.
Staheli L: Management of congenital hip dysplasia, *Pediatr Ann* 18:24, 1989.

In-Toeing
Craig C, Goldberg M: Foot and leg problems, *Pediatr Rev* 14:395, 1993.
Rosman M: When parents ask about in-toeing, *Contemp Pediatr* 4:116, 1987.
Staheli LT: *Fundamentals of pediatric orthopedics,* Philadelphia, 1998, Lippincott-Raven Press.

Joint Pain and Joint Swelling
American Academy of Pediatrics: Treatment of Lyme borreliosis, *Pediatrics* 88:176, 1991.
Baltimore R, Shapiro E: Lyme disease, *Pediatr Rev* 15:167, 1994.
Barton LL, Dunkle LM, Habib FH: Septic arthritis in childhood: a 13-year review, *Am J Dis Child* 141:898, 1987.
Biro F, Gewanter HL, Baum J: The hypermobility syndrome, *Pediatrics* 72:701, 1983.
Brewer EJ, Jr: Pitfalls in the diagnosis of juvenile rheumatoid arthritis, *Pediatr Clin North Am* 33:1015, 1986.
Gerber MA, Shapiro ED: Diagnosis of Lyme disease in children, *J Pediatr* 121:157, 1992.
Kocher MS, Zurakowski D, Kasser JR: Differentiating between septic arthritis and transient synovitis of the hip in children: an evidenced-based clinical prediction algorithm, *J Bone Joint Surg* 81A:1662, 1999.
Matan AJ, Smith JT: Pediatric septic arthritis, *Orthopedics* 20:630, 1997.
Nocton JJ et al: Human parvovirus B19-associated arthritis in children, *J Pediatr* 122:186, 1993.
Ostrov BE: Differentiation of systemic juvenile rheumatoid arthritis from acute leukemia near the onset of disease, *J Pediatr* 122:595, 1993.
Rose CD et al: The overdiagnosis of Lyme disease in children residing in an endemic area, *Clin Pediatr* 33:663, 1994.
Salazar JC et al: Long-term outcome of Lyme disease in children given early treatment, *J Pediatr* 122:591, 1993.
Schaller JG: Arthritis as a presenting manifestation of malignancy in children, *J Pediatr* 81:793, 1972.
Schaller JG: Arthritis in children, *Pediatr Clin North Am* 33:1565, 1986.
Shapiro ED: Lyme disease, *Pediatr Rev* 19:147, 1998.
Sherry DD et al: Painless juvenile rheumatoid arthritis, *J Pediatr* 116:921, 1990.
Sood SK: Lyme disease, *Pediatr Infect Dis J* 18:913, 1999.
Welkon CJ et al: Pyogenic arthritis in infants and children, *Pediatr Infect Dis J* 5:669, 1986.

Knock Knees
Staheli LT: *Fundamentals of pediatric orthopedics,* Philadelphia, 1998, Lippincott-Raven Press.

Legg-Calvé-Perthes Disease
Bunnell W: Legg-Calvé-Perthes disease, *Pediatr Rev* 7:299, 1986.
Staheli LT: *Fundamentals of pediatric orthopedics,* Philadelphia, 1998, Lippincott-Raven Press.
Wall EJ: Legg-Calve-Perthes disease, *Curr Opin Pediatr* 11:76, 1999.

Limp
MacEwen G, Dehne R: The limping child, *Pediatr Rev* 12:268, 1991.
Renshaw T: The child who has a limp, *Pediatr Rev* 16:458, 1995.
Sherry D: Limb pain in childhood, *Pediatr Rev* 12:39, 1990.
Singer J: The cause of gait disturbance in 425 pediatric patients, *Pediatr Emerg Care* 1:7, 1985.
Tunnessen W: *Signs and symptoms in pediatrics,* Philadelphia, 1999, JB Lippincott.

Metatarsus Adductus
Craig C, Goldberg M: Foot and leg problems, *Pediatr Rev* 14:395, 1993.
Rosman M: When parents ask about in-toeing, *Contemp Pediatr* 4:116, 1987.
Staheli LT: *Fundamentals of pediatric orthopedics,* Philadelphia, 1998, Lippincott-Raven Press.

Osgood-Schlatter Disease
Staheli LT: *Fundamentals of pediatric orthopedics,* Philadelphia, 1998, Lippincott-Raven Press.

Osteomyelitis and Septic Arthritis

Barkin R, editor: *Emergency pediatrics,* ed 3, St Louis, 1990, Mosby.

Burnett MW, Bass JW, Cook BA: Etiology of osteomyelitis complicating sickle cell disease, *Pediatrics* 101:296, 1998.

Gold R: Diagnosis of osteomyelitis, *Pediatr Rev* 12:292, 1991.

Krugman S et al: *Infectious diseases of children,* ed 9, St Louis, 1992, Mosby.

Peltola H, Unkila-Kallic L, Kallic MJT et al: Simplified treatment of acute staphylococcal osteomyelitis of childhood, *Pediatrics* 99:846, 1997.

Pulled Elbow (Nursemaid's Elbow)

Nichols H: Nursemaid's elbow: reducing it to simple terms, *Contemp Pediatr* 5:50, 1988.

Quan L, Marcuse E: The epidemiology and treatment of radial head subluxation, *Am J Dis Child* 139:1194, 1985.

Skaggs DL, Mirzayan R: The posterior fat pad sign in association with occult fracture of the elbow in children, *J Bone Joint Surg* 81A:1429, 1999.

Scoliosis

Berweick D: Scoliosis screening, *Pediatr Rev* 5:238, 1984.

Marsh J: Screening for scoliosis, *Pediatr Rev* 14:297, 1993.

McLain R, Karol L: Conservative treatment of the scoliotic and kyphotic patient, *Arch Pediatr Adolesc Med* 148:646, 1994.

Roach JW: Adolescent idiopathic scoliosis, *Orthopedics Clin North Am* 30:353, 1999.

Staheli LT: *Fundamentals of pediatric orthopedics,* Philadelphia, 1998, Lippincott-Raven Press.

Slipped Capital Femoral Epiphysis

Ledwith C, Fleisher G: Slipped capital femoral epiphysis without hip pain leads to missed diagnosis, *Pediatrics* 89:660, 1992.

Staheli LT: *Fundamentals of pediatric orthopedics,* Philadelphia, 1998, Lippincott-Raven Press.

Torticollis

Caputo A et al: The sit-up test: an alternative clinical test for evaluating pediatric torticollis, *Pediatrics* 90:612, 1992.

Staheli LT: *Fundamentals of pediatric orthopedics,* Philadelphia, 1998, Lippincott-Raven Press.

Transient Synovitis

Do TT: Transient synovitis as a cause of painful limps in children, *Curr Opin Pediatr* 12:48, 2000.

Haueisen D et al: The characterization of "transient synovitis of the hip" in children, *J Pediatr Orthop* 6:11, 1986.

Kocher MS, Zurakowski D, Kasser JR: Differentiating between septic arthritis and transient synovitis of the hip: an evidence-based clinical prediction algorithm, *J Bone Joint Surg* 81A:1662, 1999.

OTOLARYNGOLOGY

A. ALLERGIC RHINITIS

1. Most common cause of chronic nasal symptoms in children. May be seasonal or perennial.
2. Seasonal
a. Due to outdoor allergens: Grass and tree pollens in the spring; weed pollens in the fall; mold spores.
b. Peak incidence in mid-adolescence; rare before 3 years of age.
3. Perennial
a. Due to indoor allergens: Dust mite; animal dander (especially cats); mold; cockroaches.
b. May occur at any age.
4. History
a. Nasal congestion and pruritus; paroxysmal sneezing; clear watery discharge; conjunctival erythema and pruritus; nasal speech; mouth-breathing; throat-clearing; disturbed sleep; fatigue.

Note: Chronic nasal congestion is hallmark of perennial rhinitis whereas nasal itching and sneezing predominates in seasonal rhinitis.

b. With seasonal rhinitis, there should be a history of typical symptoms for at least two consecutive years involving the same season.
c. Symptoms are often aggravated by passive smoke exposure, pollutants, and temperature and humidity changes.
d. Often a family history of atopy.
5. Physical examination
a. Pale, bluish boggy nasal mucosa and enlarged turbinates; nasal polyps; pharyngeal cobblestoning.
b. Allergic shiners, allergic salute, allergic nasal creases.
c. There may be associated sinusitis or middle ear effusion.
6. Diagnosis
a. Based on history (especially seasonal pattern), PE, allergy testing, and response to treatment.

Note: Nasal itching is the symptom that best distinguishes allergic rhinitis from other forms of rhinitis.

b. Allergy skin prick testing can be used to support the diagnosis and identify the offending allergen. Reliable anytime after patient reaches 1 year of age. RAST testing may also be helpful.
c. Documentation of eosinophils in a Hansel or Wright-Giemsa stain of nasal secretions is highly suggestive of allergic rhinitis or nonallergic rhinitis with eosinophilia (NARES).
7. Differential diagnosis
a. Foreign body: Unilateral purulent discharge with odor
b. Anatomic: Septal deviation; adenoidal hypertrophy
c. Chronic infection: Sinusitis (purulent nasal discharge, low-grade fever, malaise, anorexia)

17

d. Vasomotor (nonallergic, noninfectious): Thin discharge, negative history for atopy, negative skin tests; may be eosinophilic (NARES) or non-eosinophilic

e. Nasal polyposis: R/O cystic fibrosis

8. Treatment

a. Reduce allergen exposure by *environmental control measures;* effective but hard to achieve, especially when family pet is involved.

b. An *antihistamine* may be effective for watery eyes, itching, and rhinorrhea but less effective for nasal congestion. A number of nonsedating preparations, i.e., fexofenadine, loratadine, azelastine (also available as a nasal spray), and astemizole, are available. Can be used on a regular basis.

c. A *decongestant* such as pseudoephedrine can be effective for nasal congestion/obstruction and can be given as combination antihistamine preparation.

d. *Anticholinergic* (Ipratropium bromide) nasal spray for rhinorrhea.

e. An intranasal *mast cell stabilizer* (cromolyn sodium, nedocromil sodium) can be effective as prophylaxis for pruritus, sneezing, and rhinorrhea. Onset of action is 2 to 4 weeks and, because of short duration of action, must be used 4 to 6 times a day.

f. A variety of *intranasal corticosteroids* (beclomethasone, budesonide, flunisolide, fluticasone, triamcinolone) are available in aqueous or aerosol sprays that can be used on a qd or bid dosage schedule. Most are approved for use in children more than 6 years of age. They are the most effective form of therapy.

   (1) Response may be seen within 24 hours, but may take 2 weeks to reach maximal effect.

   (2) Side-effects include epistaxis and nasal drying; no systemic effects.

g. Immunotherapy

   (1) Indicated when there is incomplete symptom relief after avoidance measures and pharmacotherapy or patient cannot tolerate medications.

   (2) May take 12 months to be effective.

B. EPISTAXIS

1. Peak age 4 to 10 years of age; boys are affected more than girls; usually from anterior portion of nasal septum.

2. Cause

a. Young children: Trauma, inflammation.

b. Older children: Dryness, crusting, "picking".

Note: **In teenage girls, epistaxis may be associated with menses; in teenage boys, it may be associated with angiofibroma.**

c. Blood dyscrasia and clotting abnormalities are rare but need to be considered with chronic or recurrent episodes.

3. Diagnosis
a. Careful examination to identify bleeding point
b. CBC, clotting studies with recurrent episodes
4. Management
a. Compression of anterior nasal septum for approximately 10 minutes with gauze soaked with oxymetazoline (Afrin) or Neo-Synephrine may be helpful.
b. With persistent bleeding, use silver nitrate cautery and/or packing (Gelfoam, petrolatum gauze).
c. Consult an ENT specialist if the bleeding is profuse or if the site is not located.
d. In cases caused by dryness, crusting, or "picking," humidification, local petrolatum, and well-trimmed fingernails can be helpful.

17

OTOLARYNGOLOGY

C. FOREIGN BODIES

1. Ear
a. Foreign bodies in the ear can be almost anything, e.g., plastic toy parts, earring parts, beads, and erasers; insects, including cockroaches are frequently seen in older children.
b. Presentation: Pain, decreased hearing, discharge, "digging at ear"; unusual presentations include persistent cough and hiccups.
c. Management: Some 90% of objects can be removed in the office or ED by irrigation, suctioning, or instrumentation. Parents should be cautioned against trying to remove objects at home. Cooperation is essential. Sedation and a topical anesthetic (2% lidocaine spray) may be helpful.

Note: Irrigation should never be used for button batteries or vegetable matter.

   (1) If the object does not completely occlude the ear canal, use an ear loop, curette (friable objects), or forceps.
   (2) Two choices for insects.
       (a) Fill ear canal with microscope immersion oil or mineral oil. Once killed, the insect can be removed by irrigation or instrumentation.
       (b) Irrigate the ear canal with 2% lidocaine, which usually causes the insect to flee but may be associated with vertigo.
   (3) If there is inflammation or laceration of the external canal or tympanic membrane following FB removal, an antibiotic otic drop should be used.
d. Indications for ENT referral include:
   (1) Lack of instrumentation or lack of staff to restrain uncooperative child.
   (2) Failure to remove FB on initial attempt; multiple attempts increase the risk of trauma and increase the likelihood that general anesthesia will be needed.

(3) Obvious injury to the external auditory canal or tympanic membrane.

(4) Object wedged in medial portion of canal or up against tympanic membrane.

(5) Glass, other sharp-edged FB, button battery, or putty.

Note: A new hazard is the alkaline button battery, which can produce rapid tissue destruction on contact with moist tissue and can lead to perforation of the TM, destruction of ossicles, and ulceration of local tissues. Button batteries should be removed by an ENT specialist with the patient under sedation or general anesthesia.

2. Nose

a. Cause: Hair beads, toy parts, paper, food, crayons, erasers.

b. Presentation: Mucopurulent discharge, foul odor, bleeding. It can sometimes present as *generalized* body odor. Unilateral purulent or malodorous nasal discharge is *always* suggestive of a FB. A chronic foreign body can lead to a rhinolith or erosion into a contiguous structure.

c. Management: Most nasal FBs can be handled in the office or ED with simple equipment. Parents should be cautioned against trying to remove objects at home. Cooperation, a topical anesthetic (2% lidocaine), and vasoconstriction are helpful. It is important not to push objects into the nasopharynx, where they can be aspirated by a struggling child.

(1) Most objects can be removed with a small hook, loop, forceps, or nasal suction; best performed by ENT.

(2) A cooperative child can be asked to take a deep breath through the mouth and then forcefully exhale through the obstructed nostril with occlusion of the uninvolved nostril.

(3) An unesthetic but effective technique involves occluding the nonobstructed nostril with digital pressure and blowing into the patient's mouth with a tight seal. This technique should be reserved for relatives and close friends.

(4) Button batteries can rapidly cause tissue damage and need to be removed quickly!

3. Upper airway

a. Laryngotracheal

(1) Presentation: Dyspnea, cough, stridor, and wheezing. A choking episode is observed in 90% of cases. It is commonly confused with croup. FB should always be considered in the differential diagnosis of croup, especially in the absence of URI symptoms.

(2) Diagnosis: Lateral neck and high kV x-ray studies of the airway may be helpful. The CXR is usually normal. If suspicious of a FB in the upper airway, refer to an ENT specialist for endoscopy.

(3) Management: Remove the FB via a rigid endoscope.

b. Cricopharyngeal
  (1) Presentation: Dysphagia, excessive salivation, pain in throat, FB sensation, tenderness on palpation over trachea.

Note: There may be no clinical findings in many cases of cricopharyngeal FBs.
  (2) Diagnosis: An intraoral examination, laryngoscopy, and high kV x-ray study of the airway may be helpful; a normal x-ray study is not helpful.
  (3) Management: Remove the FB via a rigid endoscope.

4. Lower airway
a. Highest incidence occurs in children 1 to 3 years of age. Usually involves food items (nuts, seeds, beans) or small toy parts; right more than left (rarely bilateral).
b. Presentation
  (1) Acute: Choking, cough, cyanosis, hoarseness, respiratory distress
  (2) Chronic: Persistent cough, wheeze, pneumonia
c. Diagnosis
  (1) Often delayed because initial aspiration/choking episode not observed.
  (2) PE: Unilateral decreased breath sounds.
  (3) Chest radiograph: Atelectasis, infiltrate, emphysema. Fluoroscopy and lateral decubitus films useful to demonstrate air trapping. Only 20% of aspirated objects are radiopaque.

Note: Chest radiograph is normal in 20% of cases.
d. Management
  (1) If there is suspicion of a foreign body, endoscopic examination of the airway is mandatory, even in the absence of positive physical and radiographic findings. During bronchoscopy, the entire bronchial tree should be examined because there may be multiple foreign bodies.
    (a) For a patient with acute respiratory distress or evidence of a radiopaque object, unilateral decreased breath sounds, or radiographic evidence of obstructive emphysema, rigid bronchoscopy should be carried out.
    (b) Otherwise, the initial examination can be carried out with a flexible bronchoscope (by an operator also skilled in rigid bronchoscopy) and if a foreign body is found, removal is carried out by rigid bronchoscopy. This has the advantage of examining more distal smaller airways and decreasing the number of false-negative rigid bronchoscopies carried out under general anesthesia.

5. Esophagus
a. Causes: Mostly coins (especially pennies), followed by safety pins and straight pins; in 5% of cases there may be multiple FBs. Items usually lodge in the proximal esophagus at the level of the thoracic inlet.

17

OTOLARYNGOLOGY

b. Presentation: Symptoms include pain, FB sensation, coughing, choking, vomiting, dysphagia, and drooling.

c. Diagnosis: Metallic FBs are easily diagnosed by AP and lateral x-ray examinations of the neck and chest. However, wood, plastic, and glass objects may not be recognized on an x-ray. Hand-held metal detectors are also highly accurate and can be used as a screening alternative to x-ray studies.

d. Evaluation: All patients who come to the ED with a history of a metallic object ingestion should be screened by an x-ray examination or a metal detector.

e. Management

(1) Immediate removal is indicated if the child is symptomatic, the foreign body is a sharp object or button battery, there is a coin in the upper third of the esophagus, or there is a history of esophageal disease or surgery.

Note: A lodged esophageal foreign body may unmask a preexisting stricture or vascular ring.

(2) Asymptomatic patients with a coin in the distal esophagus should be observed and given nothing by mouth. The coin should be removed if a repeat x-ray examination shows that it has not passed.

(3) Methods of removal include rigid endoscopy with forceps extraction or flexible endoscopy with forceps extraction. The choice of technique depends on the location of the coin, duration of impaction, associated symptoms, and expertise of available personnel.

(a) Use rigid endoscopy if there is a history of prolonged impaction, impaction of a sharp or irregular object, respiratory compromise, or a history of esophageal disease or surgery.

(b) Use flexible endoscopy for recently impacted coins.

(c) During endoscopy, the patient should be anesthetized and intubated to protect the airway.

Note: A Foley catheter can be used for recently impacted coins in the proximal esophagus, and a dilating Bougie can be used for those in the distal esophagus. However, the use of these techniques is still controversial.

(4) Once a coin enters the stomach, it is almost always passed spontaneously (average 5 days). Surgery is indicated only if there is a history of previous GI surgery (e.g., pyloric stenosis) or if the patient becomes symptomatic (e.g., severe pain, vomiting).

(5) Button batteries

(a) Button batteries (most often from hearing aids, toys, or watches) can rapidly cause tissue injury secondary to liquefaction necrosis (alkali leakage) or electrochemical burns, especially if lodged in the esophagus. There is a risk of mercury absorption from fragmented mercuric oxide cells.

(b) Prompt radiographic evaluation is indicated to determine the location of all ingested button batteries.

(c) Esophageal batteries should be removed immediately via an endoscope and under direct observation. The Foley catheter technique is contraindicated because of the risk of perforation.

(d) Large batteries (larger than 15 mm) in the stomach can be observed safely for up to 48 hours; if not passed, endoscopic removal is indicated.

(e) Asymptomatic patients with small battery (smaller than 15 mm) ingestion do not require a follow-up x-ray examination once the battery is past the esophagus.

(f) Once beyond the pylorus, button batteries are usually passed without incident; passage can be confirmed by stool inspection. Surgery is indicated only if the patient develops signs of perforation or obstruction.

(g) Ipecac is contraindicated for button batteries in the stomach. The efficacy of antacids and H_2 blockers is unproven. Blood mercury levels are indicated only if it is observed that the mercuric oxide cell has split in the GI tract.

17

OTOLARYNGOLOGY

D. HOARSENESS

1. Acute: Sudden voice change that lasts only a few days
   a. Etiology: Acute inflammation of vocal cords secondary to viral URI or vocal abuse such as screaming, shouting, or singing
   b. Treatment: Humidification, gargles, hot/cold liquids
2. Chronic: Voice change that lasts several weeks
   a. Causes: Vocal abuse or misuse, "screamer's nodules" (nodules on vocal cords), tumors (rare) such as laryngeal papillomas, psychogenic condition, trauma (postintubation), allergic laryngitis, gastroesophageal reflux, hypothyroidism.

Note: **Hoarseness that is worse in the morning and frequent throat clearing are suggestive of gastroesophageal reflux.**

   b. Treatment: Symptomatic, voice therapy. Nodules usually resolve around puberty and surgical removal is rarely indicated. Referral to an ENT specialist and laryngoscopy are indicated if hoarseness persists beyond a few weeks, is recurrent, or is accompanied by stridor or increased respiratory effort. Depending on airway findings, a plain x-ray examination, CT scan, or MRI evaluation of the airway and surrounding structures may be helpful.

E. OTITIS

1. Acute otitis media
   a. Symptoms: Ear pain, pulling at ear. There may be nonspecific findings of irritability, poor feeding, vomiting, and diarrhea, with or without fever. AOM is usually associated with URI. Peak incidence is 6 to 18 months.

During the first year of life, approximately 50% of episodes of AOM may be clinically asymptomatic.

  b. Signs: The hallmark is tympanic immobility on pneumatic otoscopy.
- (1) Erythema of TM: May be an early sign (crying alone may cause mild injection of TM)
- (2) Absent or distorted landmarks: Thickened, inflamed TM, often bulging
- (3) Asymmetry of appearance of TMs
- (4) Otorrhea

  c. Cause
- (1) In children less than 3 months of age: Consider the usual pathogens *(Streptococcus pneumoniae, Haemophilus influenzae, Moraxella catarrhalis)* plus gram-negative organisms, *Staphylococcus aureus,* and *Chlamydia trachomatis* (in infants with otitis and afebrile pneumonia).
- (2) In children older than 3 months of age: 30% to 45% *S. pneumoniae,* 20% nontypable *H. influenzae,* 20% *M. catarrhalis.* The remainder of instances result from a variety of bacteria, including group A streptococcus, viruses, and (?)mycoplasma; 15% to 30% of *H. influenzae* strains and 90% to 100% of *M. catarrhalis* strains isolated from middle ear fluid are beta-lactamase producers. A high percentage of *S. pneumoniae* isolates are now penicillin and multidrug resistant. Young age, day-care attendance, hospitalization, and prior antibiotic exposure are risk factors for colonization and infection with resistant strains.
- (3) *H. influenzae* is the usual pathogen in the "otitis-conjunctivitis syndrome."
- (4) Bullous myringitis: Bullae on TM, often hemorrhagic and painful. Causes include bacterial, viral, and (uncommonly) mycoplasma. Treat as acute bacterial otitis media.
- (5) Viral agents have been identified in approximately 40% of cases of AOM.

  d. Laboratory studies
- (1) With acute otorrhea, the drainage culture usually identifies the middle ear bacterial pathogen; however, the culture may also grow canal flora.
- (2) NP culture *does not* predict middle ear bacteriology.
- (3) TC is indicated in a child with accompanying exudative pharyngitis.
- (4) Tympanocentesis to obtain middle ear fluid for Gram's stain and C&S is indicated for neonates, patients with severe otalgia and toxicity, those who fail to respond to appropriate antimicrobial therapy, those with suppurative complications, and selected patients with immunodeficiency.

e. Treatment
  (1) Neonates: Consider a full sepsis workup and admission because of the risk of sepsis and meningitis. Broad-spectrum IV antibiotic coverage with ampicillin plus gentamicin, or ampicillin plus cefotaxime is indicated. Preferably, tympanocentesis for C&S should be performed before initiating therapy.
  (2) Children more than 3 months of age (several approaches to therapy): Although many cases of AOM resolve spontaneously, a clear-cut advantage for antimicrobial therapy has been demonstrated. The choice of antibiotic should be individualized on the basis of the patient's age, recent history of otitis, drug treatment history, associated illness, and community bacterial susceptibility patterns.
    (a) For most patients, amoxicillin 40 mg/kg/d ÷ bid or tid × 10 days remains the first-line drug for the initial treatment of AOM. Patients at increased risk for infection with drug-resistant *S. pneumoniae* should be treated with high-dose amoxicillin (80 mg/kg/day ÷ bid or tid).
    (b) Patients allergic to penicillin can be treated with erythromycin-sulfisoxazole (Pediazole) 40 to 50 mg/kg/day ÷ tid × 10 days; azithromycin (Zithromax) 10 mg/kg on day 1 followed by 5 mg/kg on days 2 through 5; or clarithromycin (Biaxin) 15 mg/kg/day ÷ bid × 10 days.
    (c) If there is no response within 48 to 72 hours, switch to a second-line drug effective against beta-lactamase producers: amoxicillin plus clavulanate potassium (Augmentin) 80 to 90 mg/kg/d ÷ bid × 10 days; cefuroxime axetil (Ceftin) 125 mg bid (for patients less than 2 years of age) or 250 mg bid (for patients more than 2 years of age) × 10 days; cefprozil (Cefzil) 30 mg/kg/day ÷ bid × 10 days; or cefpodoxime proxetil (Vantin) 10 mg/kg/day ÷ bid × 10 days. Patients with severe disease or anticipated noncompliance can be treated with IM ceftriaxone 50 mg/kg × 3 consecutive daily doses.
    (d) Patients who fail treatment with a second-line drug should be referred to ENT.

Note: In some situations (older child, mild episode, relatively otitis-free past history, prompt symptomatic improvement), a shorter (i.e., 5- to 7-day) course of antimicrobial therapy may be adequate.

  (3) Do not use erythromycin, first-generation cephalosporins, sulfonamides, or penicillin; these drugs are not effective against *H. influenzae.*
  (4) In infants with otitis and afebrile pneumonia, consider erythromycin and sulfisoxazole (Pediazole) to cover *C. trachomatis.*

       (5)   In children with otitis and purulent conjunctivitis, consider a beta-lactamase–resistant antibiotic to cover beta-lactamase–producing *H. influenzae.*

       (6)   Antihistamines/decongestants: No evidence of efficacy.

       (7)   Analgesics/antipyretics: Use prn for fever, pain. Auralgan otic drops (antipyrine, benzocaine, glycerin) may be effective as a local anesthetic for the ear canal or TM. Do not use if the TM has perforated or if there is discharge in the canal.

       (8)   A topical antibiotic suspension can be added for AOM with tympanostomy tubes or perforation and drainage.

f.   Follow-up: A recheck is indicated in the following situations:

       (1)   Lack of clinical response

       (2)   History of otitis media with effusion

       (3)   History of recurrent otitis media

       (4)   Children less than 3 years of age

2.   Recurrent acute otitis media

a.   Recurrent AOM is defined as three episodes of AOM within 6 months or four episodes within 1 year; it often results from different pathogens, but drug resistant *S. pneumoniae* (DRSP) is the predominant organism.

b.   Evaluate for an underlying problem (e.g., allergy, immune defect, chronic sinusitis, adenoidal hypertrophy, anatomic defect in upper airway). Passive smoke exposure, episode of AOM before 6 months, sibling with a history of recurrent AOM, lack of breast-feeding, craniofacial abnormalities, day-care attendance, and bedtime bottle propping may be predisposing factors.

c.   Management: Antimicrobial prophylaxis with amoxicillin (20 mg/kg hs) or sulfisoxazole (50 to 75 mg/kg hs) × 6 months or through the winter-spring season. Continuous prophylaxis is probably more effective than intermittent prophylaxis; if this technique fails, referral to an ENT specialist is indicated for probable tympanostomy tube placement. Adenoidectomy may be indicated for patients who fail after the use of tympanostomy tubes, and for patients older than 4 years of age with persistent middle ear effusion.

Note: An episode of AOM occurring during chemoprophylaxis should be treated with a second-line antibiotic.

3.   Otitis media with effusion: Also referred to as serous otitis, secretory otitis, "glue ear," nonsuppurative otitis media, or mucoid otitis media. It is defined as fluid in the middle ear *without* signs or symptoms of ear infection.

a.   Following treatment of AOM, middle ear effusion is present in 70% of patients at the 2-week follow-up, in 40% at 1 month, in 20% at 2 months, and in 10% after 3 months; it may also be picked up as an incidental finding in an asymptomatic patient. In approximately 50% of cases, pathogenic bacteria are recovered from middle ear fluid.

Note: Pneumatic otoscopy should always be used when evaluating the middle ear. Tympanometry can be used for confirmation.

b. Predisposing factors: Mechanical obstruction (adenoidal hypertrophy, cleft palate), allergy, ciliary dyskinesia, barotrauma (diving, flying), passive smoke exposure, attendance at day-care.

c. Symptoms: Decreased hearing, ear fullness, ear popping. Fever and ear pain are usually absent.

d. Signs: Opaque, gray, thickened TM with decreased mobility; may be bulging (early) or retracted (late); with or without air bubbles or air-fluid level behind TM; abnormal tympanogram; conductive hearing deficit.

e. Course: Most cases resolve spontaneously over several weeks to months but may be associated with a significant conductive hearing loss. Every child who has had fluid in both middle ears for a total of 3 months should undergo a hearing evaluation.

f. Treatment
    (1) Antibiotics: For patients with OME, a course of antibiotic with an agent effective against beta-lactamase producers is indicated in the following circumstances:
        (a) Unfavorable past history of otitis media
        (b) Associated chronic URI (longer than 2 weeks) that is not improving
        (c) Tube placement being considered because of chronic OME (longer than 3 months)
    (2) Antihistamines, decongestants: No evidence of efficacy.
    (3) Steroids: The use of oral steroids is controversial. There are conflicting data on efficacy. Steroids may be indicated in selected patients before surgical approaches.
    (4) Myringotomy and tympanostomy tube placement: Somewhat controversial but probably indicated if effusion persists longer than 4 to 6 months in spite of medical therapy and if significant hearing loss (greater than 20 dB in the better-hearing ear) is present. Myringotomy alone *is not* helpful. The main indication for tubes is to improve hearing.

Note: Tympanostomy tubes are not benign. Complications include persistent otorrhea, tympanosclerosis, atrophy, residual perforation of TM, and cholesteatoma.

    (5) Adenoidectomy: This approach may be indicated in a patient who fails tympanostomy tube placement, a patient with evidence of obstructing adenoidal hypertrophy, or a child older than 4 years of age who has persistent OME.

Note: Adenoidectomy is contraindicated in patients with a cleft palate.

4. Chronic otitis media

a. Chronic otitis media exhibits intermittent/chronic foul-smelling otorrhea, hearing loss, or an abnormal otoscopic examination (granulation tissue, cholesteatoma) in patients with a history of recurrent AOM. This condition requires ENT consultation.

17

OTOLARYNGOLOGY

Note: Consider the possibility of ciliary dyskinesia in patients with recurrent or chronic draining otitis and evidence of lung infection. Only 50% of cases have situs inversus.

b. Fluid aspirated through the perforated membrane may be helpful and should be sent for Gram's, potassium hydroxide, and acid-fast stains, as well as bacterial, fungal, and mycobacterial cultures. *Pseudomonas* and *S. aureus* are common pathogens.

c. Treatment: A topical ophthalmic or otic suspension containing neomycin or polymyxins may be helpful, but parenteral antibiotics may be needed on the basis of C&S results. Definitive therapy involves surgical debridement of the middle ear space.

5. Otitis externa

a. Otitis externa involves inflammation of the skin lining the auditory canal and is often secondary to trauma (e.g., from cotton swabs, bobby pins) or infection. It is also known as "swimmer's ear."

b. Symptoms: Pain on pulling the pinna or tragus, itching, discharge.

c. Signs: Edematous, erythematous auditory canal with discharge.

d. Treatment

   (1) Steroid-antibiotic (ciprofloxacin HC otic suspension 3 drops or ofloxacin otic solution 5 drops) in affected ear bid × 5 to 7 days. Use suspension, not solution, if PE tubes are in place; a solution may cause pain on contact with the middle ear. A cotton wick can be moistened with antibiotic drops and inserted in the auditory canal bid.

   (2) Avoid swimming until the problem resolves.

F. PHARYNGITIS (INCLUDING TONSILLITIS AND TONSILLOPHARYNGITIS)

1. Clinical features

a. Signs and symptoms: Abrupt onset of fever, sore throat, malaise, headache, abdominal pain, and sandpapery rash (scarlet fever). Pharynx is at least erythematous, with or without tonsillar hypertrophy, with or without exudate, with or without ulcerations, with or without membranous covering, with or without palatal petechiae, and anterior cervical adenitis. Antibody rise against group A β-*hemolytic streptococcus* correlates best with enlarged, tender anterior cervical nodes.

b. Pharyngitis usually occurs in the winter-spring months.

c. The peak age is 5 to 15 years, but diagnosis needs to be considered even in infants and toddlers.

2. Etiology

a. Bacterial

   (1) Group A β-*hemolytic streptococcus:* GABHS pharyngitis cannot be diagnosed on clinical grounds in most patients. However, patients with strep throat typically have acute onset of fever (often very high), sore throat, headache, abdominal pain, and vomiting.

The pharynx may appear erythematous or exudative; palatal petechiae and tender anterior cervical lymph nodes may be present. Diagnosis of strep throat is based on a positive culture or direct antigen screen and evidence of pharyngitis.

    (2) Other bacteria: GC (high index of suspicion, positive clinical history, and PE), diphtheria (membranous pharyngitis, myocarditis); check immunization history.

b. Viral

    (1) Coxsackie virus (herpangina): Usually seen in summer and autumn; ulcers on soft palate, tonsils, pharynx. Also check soles and palms for vesicular lesions (hand-foot-and-mouth syndrome).

    (2) Epstein-Barr virus (infectious mononucleosis): May be associated with exudative or membranous pharyngitis, generalized lymphadenopathy, hepatosplenomegaly, rash, malaise, tender posterior cervical nodes, edema of the eyelids, and a nasal "twang" to the voice.

    (3) Adenovirus: Most common cause of nonstreptococcal pharyngitis; may be associated with abdominal pain, diarrhea, otitis media, rash (duration less than 3 days).

    (4) Herpes simplex virus: Both types I and II may produce pharyngitis with or without tonsillar exudate. Ulcerations may appear 1 to 2 days after onset. The probable cause is herpes if signs of glossitis or gingivostomatitis are present.

    (5) Other viruses: Enterocytopathogenic human orphan, parainfluenza, influenza, RSV.

Note: The presence of rhinorrhea, cough, hoarseness, and diarrhea favors a viral etiology.

c. Other organisms such as *Mycoplasma, Chlamydia*

3. Laboratory evaluation

a. A TC is the mainstay of diagnosis.

    (1) A single TC is 90% to 97% sensitive. The swab should make contact with both tonsillar regions and with the posterior pharyngeal wall.

    (2) Inoculate the swab on a 5% sheep-blood agar plate; it is helpful to place a 0.04 unit bacitracin disk on the plate (95% of GABHS demonstrate a large zone of inhibition around the disk).

    (3) Anaerobic incubation may slightly increase the yield of GABHS, but its routine use is not justified or necessary.

Note: Approximately 15% to 18% of children with infectious mononucleosis also have group A β-*hemolytic streptococcus* on TC.

b. A direct antigen screen (enzyme immunoassay) may be helpful. The test is very specific (few false-positive results), but false-negative results may be seen in up to 15% to 25% of streptococcal infections. The usual strategy is to treat if the antigen screen is positive; perform a TC if the screen is negative.

17

OTOLARYNGOLOGY

    c. CBC plus differential plus smear (lymphocytosis with atypical lymphs may be seen in approximately 80% of patients with infectious mononucleosis). Platelets are decreased with some viral syndromes. Consider infectious mononucleosis when the TC is negative and severe pharyngitis persists. Perform a heterophile monospot test (may be negative before 5 years of age or during the first weeks of illness) or a specific serologic test for EBV antibodies.

4. Treatment
   a. Antibiotics
   (1) Penicillin remains the drug of choice; a penicillin-resistant strain of GABHS has never been identified. Response to treatment should be rapid.
   (2) Treatment of GABHS pharyngitis decreases the risk of rheumatic fever but does not prevent poststreptococcal glomerulonephritis. Antibiotics shorten the duration and severity of symptoms if given early in the course. Although data are conflicting, immediate initiation of antibiotic therapy appears to increase the relapse or recurrence rate.
       (a) To ensure compliance: IM penicillin G benzathine as Bicillin C-R 900/300. It contains 900,000 U penicillin G benzathine and 300,000 U penicillin G procaine in a single-dose 2-ml injection.
       (b) For patients who will be compliant: PO penicillin V potassium × 10 days; 250 mg bid (for patients younger than 12 years of age) or 500 mg bid (for patients older than 12 years of age). No benefit is shown for a tid or qid schedule (decreases compliance). A full 10-day course is mandatory.

Note: There is evidence that a 6-day course of amoxicillin given once a day or a 5-day course of cefpodoxime proxetil is as effective as a 10-day course of PO penicillin.

       (c) For patients allergic to penicillin: Erythromycin ethylsuccinate 40 mg/kg/d ÷ qid × 10 days, or azithromycin 10 mg/kg as a single daily dose × 5 days. Tetracyclines and sulfonamides (including TMP/SMZ) are ineffective against GABHS infection.

Note: GABHS resistance to erythromycin is common in some countries (Japan, Finland) and is becoming more common in the United States.

       (d) If the patient has classic streptococcal symptoms, begin treatment while the TC is pending. If the patient is not highly symptomatic, it is best to withhold treatment until TC results are available (unless the patient is unlikely to return for follow-up).
       (e) The child may return to day-care or school 24 hours after beginning the antibiotic.
   b. Symptomatic treatment
   (1) Analgesics/antipyretics (ibuprofen more effective than acetaminophen)

      (2)   Throat lozenges, throat spray
c.   Posttreatment clinical and/or bacteriologic failure occurs in 10% to 20% of all cases.
      (1)   Failures may result from the presence of beta-lactamase–producing organisms in the oropharynx, lack of compliance, or a GABHS carrier state (the most common explanation). Some posttreatment failures may actually represent reinfection with the same or different serotypes.
      (2)   The most difficult dilemma for the clinician is to determine whether a patient is having repeated episodes of acute GABHS pharyngitis or is a streptococcus carrier experiencing repeated episodes of viral illness. The streptococcus carrier state is likely if any of the following are true:
          (a) Clinical findings and season (summer) suggest a viral etiology
          (b) Lack of immediate clinical response to antibiotic therapy
          (c) Presence of GABHS between episodes
          (d) No serologic response to GABHS extracellular antigens
          (e) Same serotype for all isolates

Note: It is best to avoid culturing patients whose clinical findings suggest a viral etiology and who are likely to be streptococcus carriers.

      (3)   Effective regimens for the patient with repeated episodes of GABHS pharyngitis include the following:
          (a) Clindamycin 20 mg/kg/d ÷ tid × 10 days
          (b) Cefuroxime axetil 250 mg bid × 10 days
          (c) Penicillin G benzathine IM and rifampin 10 mg/kg (maximum 600 mg/d) q24h × 8 doses
          (d) Rifampin 20 mg/kg (maximum 600 mg/d) q24h × 4 doses during the last 4 days of a 10-day course of oral penicillin V potassium
      (4)   Prophylaxis with daily penicillin or sulfonamide may be considered for the otherwise normal child who has had "true" recurrent episodes of GABHS pharyngitis, but the efficacy of this technique has not yet been documented in clinical trials.
      (5)   Indications for tonsillectomy include more than 6 GABHS episodes within 1 year, 4 episodes within each of 2 years, or 3 episodes within each of 3 years, with all episodes consisting of specific clinical findings.
5. Miscellaneous
a.   Culture any symptomatic family members of patients with streptococcal pharyngitis.
b.   A culture of asymptomatic family members generally is not necessary.
c.   In the winter-spring months, as many as 20% of asymptomatic schoolchildren are GABHS carriers.
d.   A routine posttreatment culture is not indicated. Indications include recurring symptoms, a family history of rheumatic fever, "ping-ponging"

17

OTOLARYNGOLOGY

of streptococcal infections in the family, outbreak in a closed community, and a patient who is being considered for T&A.

G. SINUSITIS

1. Some 5% to 10% of URIs in early childhood are complicated by acute sinusitis, which is suggested by the failure of the URI to improve after 10 days. It results from obstruction of the sinus ostia along with an alteration in mucociliary clearance.
2. Predisposing conditions
   a. Anatomic: Nasoseptal deformity, polyps, large adenoids, cleft palate, choanal atresia, intranasal FB
   b. Cystic fibrosis
   c. Immunodeficiency
   d. Ciliary dyskinesia
   e. Allergy
   f. Diving, flying

Note: In a teenager with maxillary sinusitis, consider a dental origin.

3. Presentations
   a. Cough (occurring during the night more than the day), malodorous breath, with or without low-grade fever, painless periorbital swelling in the morning, anterior/posterior rhinorrhea
   b. High fever, purulent nasal discharge, with or without facial pain, with or without headache, with or without periorbital edema
   c. PE: Boggy, erythematous nasal mucosa; facial tenderness (in older children and adolescents)
4. Bacteriology
   a. Same as otitis media: *S. pneumoniae* (40%), *H. influenzae* (20%), *M. (Branhamella) catarrhalis* (20%). In children with chronic sinusitis, up to 50% of isolates may be beta-lactamase producers.
   b. *S. pneumoniae* strains that are relatively resistant to penicillin have been recovered from young children with chronic sinusitis.
   c. Anaerobes and *S. aureus* may play a role in chronic infections, especially in older patients.
   d. An NP culture and TC *do not* correlate with sinus aspirate cultures.
5. Diagnosis
   a. Usually based on clinical picture. It is not the severity of symptoms, but their persistence that suggests the diagnosis.
   b. Transillumination: Not helpful if the patient is less than 10 years of age.
   c. Sinus x-ray studies: Usually sufficient to exclude or confirm the diagnosis in patients with signs and symptoms of acute sinusitis, but not indicated in uncomplicated sinusitis. Findings consistent with sinusitis include:
      (1) Mucosal thickening greater than 4 mm
      (2) Air-fluid level
      (3) Diffuse opacification

d.   CT scan: Imaging procedure of choice for recurrent, chronic, or complicated cases.
e.   Sinus aspiration: "Gold standard," but not routine.
     (1) Bacterial density equal to or greater than 10^4 CFU/ml or greater than 1 organism/HPF on a Gram's stain represents a true infection.
     (2) Reserve this technique for treatment failure, immunocompromised patients, those with severe facial pain, and those with orbital and intracranial complications.

Note: For patients with chronic/recurrent sinusitis, the workup may include allergy/ENT consultation, a sweat test (CF), serum immunoglobulin determinations, and nasal mucosal biopsy (ciliary dyskinesia).

6.   Treatment
a.   Acute sinusitis: Amoxicillin 40 mg/kg/day ÷ bid × 14 days is adequate for most cases. For hospitalized patients with severe sinusitis, IV cefotaxime 300 mg/kg/day ÷ q6h with or without vancomycin 60 mg/kg/day ÷ q6h should be considered for initial treatment to cover highly resistant pneumococcal strains.
b.   Patients allergic to penicillin can be treated with azithromycin 10 mg/kg on day 1 followed by 5 mg/kg on days 2 through 5, clarithromycin 15 mg/kg/day ÷ bid or trimethoprim-sulfamethoxazole 8 mg TMP/kg/day ÷ bid.

Note: There is evidence that clinically diagnosed, uncomplicated acute sinusitis is usually a self-limited illness of short duration. Delaying initiation of antibiotic therapy for 3 weeks after onset of symptoms will result in spontaneous resolution in at least 80% of untreated patients and will decrease unnecessary antimicrobial use.

c.   A second-line agent such as amoxicillin-clavulanate, cefuroxime axetil, cefprozil, or cefpodoxime proxetil (see acute otitis media for dosages) × 2 to 6 weeks is indicated for the following:
     (1) Failure to improve on amoxicillin.
     (2) Recent (within 1 month) treatment with amoxicillin.
     (3) Residence in an area with a high prevalence of DRSP or beta-lactamase producing organisms.
     (4) Frontal, sphenoidal or complicated ethmoidal sinusitis.
     (5) Subacute or chronic sinusitis (symptoms present more than 30 days).
d.   In patients with recurrent sinusitis (3 or more episodes in 6 months), a trial of antimicrobial prophylaxis should be considered.
e.   Topical decongestants and topical steroids (3 to 7 days) may reduce mucosal edema and promote patency of ostia. Antihistamines might help a patient with underlying atopy.
f.   Surgery (functional endoscopic sinus surgery) is reserved for complicated sinusitis and for patients with chronic or recurrent sinusitis

17

OTOLARYNGOLOGY

who fail trials of prolonged medical therapy (including antimicrobial prophylaxis). Surgery should be preceded by a CT scan.

H. UPPER RESPIRATORY INFECTION

1. Often begins as a sore or scratchy throat followed by rhinorrhea, sneezing, and nasal congestion. Bothersome cough develops in roughly 30% of occurrences. Usual duration is 7 to 10 days, although 25% of episodes may last up to 2 weeks. Average of 5 to 7 episodes per year in young children.
2. Treatment
a. Supportive measures are the mainstay of therapy
   (1) Rest and fluids.
   (2) Humidification (cool-mist vaporizer) may soothe inflamed, scratchy nasal and pharyngeal mucosa. Avoid passive smoke exposure and other environmental irritants.
   (3) Infants: Buffered saline nose drops with bulb syringe, 2 gtt in each nostril to loosen secretions, then aspirate with nasal aspirator. Use before feeding, bedtime, and prn.
   (4) Analgesics/antipyretics for malaise and fever prn.
b. Antihistamines and sympathomimetics: Efficacy has not been demonstrated in controlled studies, but they are often used. They should not be used in children less than 18 months of age because of hypersensitivity to antihistamine and sympathomimetic effects. Warn patients about drowsiness with antihistamines.
c. Topical decongestants: 0.25% phenylephrine (Neo-Synephrine) and ipratropium bromide (Atrovent) decrease mucosal swelling and rhinorrhea. Do not use more than 3 to 5 days (tachyphylaxis and rhinitis medicamentosa) or in children less than 6 months of age.
d. Cough medications
   (1) Guaifenesin (e.g., plain Robitussin) does not work.
   (2) Dextromethorphan is a short-acting cough suppressant and may help, especially with troublesome nighttime coughing.
e. Oral zinc has been recommended as a cold remedy but results in children have not been positive.

I. BIBLIOGRAPHY

Allergic Rhinitis
Estelle F, Simons R: Allergic rhinitis: recent advances, *Pediatr Clin North Am* 35:1053, 1988.
Meltzer EO: Treatment options for the child with allergic rhinitis, *Clin Pediatr* 37:1, 1998.
Naclerio RM: Allergic rhinitis, *N Engl J Med* 325:860, 1991.
Nash DR: Allergic rhinitis, *Pediatr Ann* 27:799, 1998.
Virant PS: Allergic rhinitis, *Pediatr Rev* 13:323, 1992.

Epistaxis
Culbertson M: Epistaxis. In Bluestone CD, Stool SE, editors: *Pediatric otolaryngology,* vol 1, Philadelphia, 1983, WB Saunders.

Foreign Bodies

Ansley JF, Cunningham MJ: Treatment of aural foreign bodies in children, *Pediatrics* 101:638, 1998.

Caravati EM et al: Pediatric coin ingestion: a prospective study on the utility of routine roentgenograms, *Am J Dis Child* 143:549, 1989.

Donnelley LF, Frush DP, Bissett GS: The multiple presentations of foreign bodies in children, *AJR* 170:471, 1998.

Kalan A, Tariq M: Foreign bodies in the nasal cavities: comprehensive review of the aetiology, diagnostic pointers and therapeutic measures, *Postgrad Med J* 76:484, 2000.

Litovitz T, Schmitz BF: Ingestion of cylindrical and button batteries: an analysis of 2382 cases, *Pediatrics* 89:747, 1992.

Martinot A, Closset M, Marquette CH, et al: Indications for flexible versus rigid bronchoscopy in children with suspected foreign body aspiration, *Am J Respir Crit Care Med* 155:1676, 1997.

McGahren ED: Esophageal foreign bodies, *Pediatr Rev* 20:129, 1999.

Schunk JE et al: Fluoroscopic Foley catheter removal of esophageal foreign bodies in children: experience with 415 episodes, *Pediatrics* 94:709, 1994.

Schweich PJ: Management of coin ingestion, *Pediatr Emerg Care* 11:37, 1995.

Seikel K, Primm PA, Elizondo BJ et al: Handheld metal detector localization of ingested metallic foreign bodies, *Arch Pediatr Adolesc Med* 153:853, 1999.

Sheikh A: Button battery ingestions in children, *Pediatr Emerg Care* 9:224, 1993.

Skoulakis CE, Doxas PG, Papadakis CE et al: Bronchoscopy for foreign body removal in children, *Int J Pediatr Otorhinolaryngol* 53:143, 2000.

Hoarseness

Kenna MA: Hoarseness, *Pediatr Rev* 16:69, 1982.

McMurry JS: Medical and surgical treatment of pediatric dysphonia, *Orolaryngol Clin North Am* 33:1111, 2000.

Otitis Media

Aranovitz GH: Antimicrobial therapy of acute otitis media: review of treatment recommendations, *Clin Ther* 22:29, 2000.

Barnett ED, Klein JO: The problem of resistant bacteria for the management of acute otitis media, *Pediatr Clin North Am* 42:509, 1995.

Bernard PAM et al: Randomized, controlled trial comparing long-term sulfonamide therapy to ventilation tubes for otitis media with effusion, *Pediatrics* 88:215, 1991.

Cantekin EI et al: Lack of efficacy of a decongestant: antihistamine combination for otitis media with effusion ("secretory" otitis media) in children, *N Engl J Med* 308:297, 1983.

Chang MG et al: *Chlamydia trachomatis* in otitis media in children, *Pediatr Infect Dis J* 1:95, 1982.

Del Beccaro MA et al: Bacteriology of acute otitis media: a new perspective, *J Pediatr* 120:81, 1992.

Hathaway TJ et al: Acute otitis media: who needs posttreatment follow-up? *Pediatrics* 94:143, 1994.

Institute for clinical systems improvement: Otitis media in children, *Postgrad Med* 107:239, 2000.

Kempthorne J, Giebink GS: Pediatric approach to the diagnosis and management of otitis media, *Otolaryngol Clin North Am* 24:905, 1991.

Klein JO: Nonimmune strategies for prevention of otitis media, *Pediatr Inf Dis J* 19:589, 2000.

Le CT et al: Evaluation of ventilating tubes and myringotomy in the treatment of recurrent or persistent otitis media, *Pediatr Infect Dis J* 10:2, 1991.

Mandel EM et al: Efficacy of amoxicillin with and without decongestant-antihistamine for otitis media with effusion in children: results of a double-blind, randomized trial, *N Engl J Med* 316:432, 1987.

Otitis media guideline panel: Managing otitis media with effusion in young children, *Pediatrics* 94:766, 1994.

Pichichero ME, Reiner SA, Brook I et al: Controversies in the medical management of persistent and recurrent acute otitis media, *Ann Otol Rhinol Laryngol* 109:2, 2000.

Rosenfeld RM et al: Clinical efficacy of antimicrobial drugs for acute otitis media: metaanalysis of 5400 children from thirty-three randomized trials, *J Pediatr* 124:355, 1994.

Schwartz RH et al: Use of a short course of prednisone for treating middle ear effusion: a double-blind crossover study, *Ann Otol Rhinol Laryngol* 89:296, 1980.

Shurin PA et al: Bacterial etiology of otitis media in first 6 weeks of life, *J Pediatr* 92:893, 1978.

17

OTOLARYNGOLOGY

Pharyngitis

Adam D, Scholz H, Helmerking M: Short-course antibiotic treatment of 4782 culture-proven cases of Group A streptococcal tonsillopharyngitis and incidence of poststreptococcal sequelae, *J Inf Dis* 182:509, 2000.

Bass JW, Person DA, Chan DS: Twice-daily oral penicillin for treatment of streptococcal pharyngitis: less is best, *Pediatrics* 105:423, 2000.

Berkovitch M, Vaida A, Zhovtis D et al: Group A streptococcal pharyngotonsillitis in children less than 2 years of age—more common than is thought, *Clin Pediatr* 38:361, 1999.

Chaudhary S et al: Penicillin V and rifampin for the treatment of group A streptococcal pharyngitis: a randomized trial of 10 days of penicillin vs 10 days penicillin with rifampin during the final 4 days of therapy, *J Pediatr* 106:481, 1985.

Fries SM: Diagnosis of group A streptococcal pharyngitis in a private clinic: comparative evaluation of an optical immunoassay method and culture, *J Pediatr* 126:933, 1995.

Gerber MA et al: Lack of impact of early antibiotic therapy for streptococcal pharyngitis on recurrence rates, *J Pediatr* 117:853, 1990.

Klein JO: Management of streptococcal pharyngitis, *Pediatr Infect Dis J* 13:572, 1994.

Markowitz M et al: Treatment of streptococcal pharyngotonsillitis: reports of penicillin's demise are premature, *J Pediatr* 123:679, 1993.

Pichichero ME: Group A beta-hemolytic streptococcal infections, *Pediatr Rev* 19:291, 1998.

Pichichero ME, Hoeger W, Marsocci SM et al: Variables influencing pencillin treatment outcome in streptococcal tonsillopharyngitis, *Arch Pediatr Adolesc Med* 153:565, 1999.

Pichichero ME, Margolis PA: A comparison of cephalosporins and penicillins in the treatment of group A beta-hemolytic streptococcal pharyngitis: a metaanalysis supporting the concept of copathogenicity, *Pediatr Infect Dis J* 10:275, 1991.

Shulman ST: Streptococcal pharyngitis: diagnostic considerations, *Pediatr Infect Dis J* 13:567, 1994.

Sumaya CU, Ench Y: Epstein-Barr virus infectious mononucleosis in children: clinical and general laboratory findings, *Pediatrics* 75:1003, 1985.

Sinusitis

Duplechain JK, White JA, Miller RH: Pediatric sinusitis, *Arch Otolaryngol Head Neck Surg* 117:422, 1991.

Garbutt JM, Goldstein M, Gellman E et al: A randomized, placebo-controlled trial of antimicrobial treatment for children with clinically diagnosed acute sinusitis, *Pediatrics* 107:619, 2001.

Lazar RH, Younis RT: The management of recurrent sinusitis in children, *Clin Pediatr* 31:30, 1992.

Nash D, Wald E: Sinusitis, *Pediatr Rev* 22:111, 2001.

Tinkelman DG, Silk HJ: Clinical and bacteriologic features of chronic sinusitis in children, *Am J Dis Child* 143:938, 1989.

Uri

Turner RB: The common cold, *Pediatr Ann* 27:790, 1998.

PULMONARY DISEASES

A. APNEA AND APPARENT LIFE-THREATENING EVENTS (ALTEs)

1. Apnea is defined as the cessation of respiratory airflow, which may result from the following:
a. Absence of respiratory effort (central)
b. Absence of nasal airflow despite respiratory effort (obstructive)
c. Combination of both (mixed)
2. Occasional respiratory pauses of 20 seconds or less may be a normal finding at any age. Apnea that lasts more than 20 seconds or is accompanied by bradycardia, pallor, hypotonia, or cyanosis is pathologic and warrants evaluation.
3. An increased frequency of mixed and obstructive apnea occurs in infants diagnosed with an ALTE. However, there is no evidence that apnea alone progresses to ALTEs or increases the risk for SIDS.
a. An ALTE is defined as an episode that is frightening to the observer and is characterized by some combination of color change (cyanosis, pallor, plethora), limpness, choking, and gagging. In most cases, either vigorous stimulation or CPR has been instituted.
b. The etiology of ALTEs includes acute infection (sepsis, pneumonia, RSV, meningitis), dysfunctional swallowing, GER, seizures, CNS disease, disorders of respiratory control, undetected hypoxia (especially in premature infants), anemia, poisoning, metabolic disorders, hypercalcemia, and upper airway obstruction. A treatable etiology is found in approximately 30% of cases.

Note: **In infants with ALTEs and with episodes of apnea there is a high incidence of GER and pH monitoring should be considered. However, a cause and effect relationship has not been proven. There is evidence that apnea usually precedes GER rather than the opposite.**

c. The infant who has had an ALTE is at significantly increased risk for SIDS, but such cases probably account for only 10% of SIDS deaths.
d. The infant who has had an ALTE should be hospitalized for observation, monitoring, and evaluation. Unless there is evidence to suggest otherwise, the parents' or caretakers' observations must be accepted as valid and accurate. Parental anxiety should not be minimized. The evaluation includes the following:
   (1) Careful history: Focus on circumstances of the event, perinatal history, family history. Awake apnea suggests seizures or GER/aspiration.
   (2) PE: Focus on upper airway, cardiac, pulmonary, and neurologic examinations. Observe feeding and sleeping patterns.

    (3) Laboratory studies: Minimum workup includes CBC, blood glucose, electrolytes, calcium, bicarbonate, ammonia, and SaO_2 while asleep.

    (4) Based on the initial evaluation, additional workup may include ABGs, LP, barium swallow, CXR, ECG, EEG, esophageal pH monitoring, metabolic screening, polysomnography, a head CT scan, and upper airway evaluation. The child with evidence of airway obstruction should be referred for polysomnography and ENT evaluation.

Note: Data obtained from polysomnography are not useful in identifying the infant at risk for SIDS and should not be used to determine the need for home monitoring.

    (5) Provide cardiorespiratory monitoring and parental CPR instruction.

Note: A normal evaluation and laboratory workup does not indicate that a significant event did not occur or that it will not happen again. If no treatable cause is found, the infant requires home monitoring.

    (6) Be supportive of the family, answer questions patiently, and ensure adequate follow-up. Parents should be included in the decision-making process.

4. Home monitoring

a. Indications include the following:

    (1) ALTE requiring vigorous stimulation or resuscitation (milder ALTE is a relative indication)

    (2) Sibling of two or more SIDS victims (monitoring the sibling of one SIDS victim is not officially recommended but is generally unavoidable)

    (3) Surviving twin of a SIDS victim

    (4) Infant with hypoventilation syndrome

    (5) Infant with tracheostomy or O_2-dependent BPD

    (6) Apnea and bradycardia associated with dysfunctional swallowing or GER, unless the GER is controlled by medical or surgical treatment

b. The monitor alarm should be set to sound for a respiratory pause longer than 20 seconds or for the following HR: less than 1 month of age, 80 bpm; 1 to 3 months of age, 70 bpm; 4 to 6 months of age, 60 bpm; more than 6 months of age, 50 bpm.

c. A documented ("smart") monitor with a built-in event recorder can be helpful in distinguishing "true" events from insignificant (e.g., loose lead) events. The monitor also provides information on compliance with monitor use.

d. Use of the monitor can be discontinued if the infant has gone 3 months without a significant event and has demonstrated an ability to tolerate stresses such as infection and immunizations without apnea or bradycardia alarms.

Note: It is recommended that all infants (except those with GER and craniofacial abnormalities) be placed in the crib to sleep in the supine position.

5. "Factitious" apnea

a. There is evidence that recurrent episodes of apnea may be related to child abuse (Munchausen by proxy) (see Chapter 12).

b. Clues to factitious apnea include the following:

    (1) Episodes that begin only in the presence of the parent (caretaker) but are witnessed by other persons called for assistance (often in the hospital setting); may need to be confirmed by covert video surveillance.

    (2) Evidence of physical abuse.

    (3) Previous SIDS death in the family.

    (4) Simultaneous death of twins.

    (5) History of unexplained disorders in the victim (symptoms do not make sense medically).

    (6) Death at an unusual age for SIDS.

    (7) One of the parents (usually the mother) is medically sophisticated and shows exemplary behavior in the medical setting; may be a discrepancy between family's and medical team's level of concern.

B. ASTHMA

1. Diagnosis

a. In children, recurrent episodes of coughing, wheezing, and dyspnea are almost always a result of asthma. Some children have only chronic/recurrent coughing (cough-variant asthma); others have cough, wheeze, and/or dyspnea only in association with exercise (exercise-induced asthma).

b. Features suggestive of asthma are periodicity of symptoms, nocturnal attacks, seasonal variation, and the relation of symptoms to allergen exposure or exertion. There is often a personal or family history of atopy.

c. Pulmonary function testing, including bronchodilator responsiveness, is helpful. Most important is the clinical response to anti-asthma therapy.

d. Airway inflammation is present in almost all patients with asthma, even during clinical remission; anti-inflammatory drugs are the cornerstone of asthma management. A number of triggers such as viral infection, cold air, exercise, allergens, and pollutants (e.g., cigarette smoke) can increase airway responsiveness and trigger acute attacks.

e. If the response to treatment is poor or if the patient has a productive cough, failure to thrive, choking episodes, or focal lung findings, consider other diagnoses such as FB, vascular ring, laryngeal web, CF, GER, aspiration, laryngotracheomalacia, ciliary dyskinesia, immunodeficiency, enlarged mediastinal nodes or tumor, or congenital lobar emphysema.

18

PULMONARY DISEASES

Note: Early childhood asthma is often underdiagnosed and under-treated; may lead to accelerated loss of pulmonary function over time.

2. Chronic asthma

a. The key to chronic asthma management is the long-term control of airway inflammation which is associated with decreased airway reactivity, partial or complete reversal of airway pathology, and improved clinical outcome.

b. Treatment regimens are based on assessment of disease severity (Table 18-1).

(1) Mild intermittent asthma: Symptomatic episodes are brief and resolve spontaneously or with the use of a short-acting beta-2-agonist delivered by MDI or small volume nebulizer. Between episodes, patients are asymptomatic and have normal pulmonary function. There are no ED visits and daily functioning is normal, including good exercise tolerance and no asthma-related school absenteeism.

(2) Mild persistent asthma: The patient should be on a daily asthma controller such as inhaled cromolyn sodium or nedocromil, low-dose inhaled corticosteroid (ICS), or a leukotriene modifier. Theophylline is less desirable because of side-effects and the need to monitor serum levels.

(3) Moderate persistent asthma: The cornerstone of therapy is the long-term use of ICS. Comparative daily doses are shown in Tables 18-2 and 18-3. A long-acting beta-2-agonist (e.g., salmeterol) and/or leukotriene modifier (montelukast, zafirlukast) can be added to the ICS to decrease the daily steroid dose required to maintain optimal control.

(4) Severe persistent asthma: A high-dose ICS usually will be needed. A long-acting beta-2-agonist and leukotriene modifier can be used as add-on therapy. Systemic corticosteroids may be needed on a short-term or long-term basis. If used on a long-term basis, weaning to alternate-day dosing will decrease the risk of side effects.

c. Asthma medications

(1) Inhaled corticosteroids: Once symptoms are controlled, it is important to maintain an effective dose of ICS for 1 to 3 months and to then wean slowly. Patients on long-term use of an ICS need to have their linear growth closely monitored. Long-term use, especially at high doses (greater than 400 mcg/day), is associated with decreased growth velocity, but there is no evidence that final adult height is affected. Fluticasone at dosages of 100 to 200 mcg/day is *not* associated with slowing of growth.

(2) Long-acting beta-2-agonists: These agonists have no anti-inflammatory properties and may mask increasing airway inflammation. They should never be used alone but should always be combined with an anti-inflammatory agent (e.g., ICS).

TABLE 18-1

CLASSIFICATION OF ASTHMA SEVERITY AND MANAGEMENT IN ADULTS AND CHILDREN

Severity of Asthma	Clinical Features Before Treatment	Long-Term* Medication (>5 Y)	Long-Term* Medication (<5 Y)
Intermittent	Daytime symptoms ≤2 times a week Nighttime symptoms ≤2 times a month FEV_1 or PEF ≥80% predicted PEF variability <20%	No anti-inflammatory agents needed	No anti-inflammatory agents needed
Mild persistent	Daytime symptoms >2 times a week Nighttime symptoms >2 times a month FEV_1 or PEF ≥80% predicted PEF variability 20% to 30%	Cromolyn or nedocromil or ICS low dose or Leukotriene modifier or Theophylline (not preferred)	Cromolyn or nedocromil or ICS low dose
Moderate persistent	Daily symptoms Nighttime symptoms >1 time a week FEV_1 or PEF >60% and <80% predicted PEF variability >30%	ICS medium dose or ICS medium-low dose + long-acting BD if needed ICS medium-high dose + long-acting BD	ICS medium dose or ICS medium dose + nedocromil or ICS medium-high dose + long-acting BD
Severe persistent	Continuous symptoms Frequent nighttime symptoms FEV_1 or PEF ≤60% predicted PEF variability >30%	ICS high dose + long-acting BD + systemic cortico-steroids long-term	ICS high dose + systemic cortico-steroids long-term if needed

*In addition to long-term medications, all patients should receive short-acting bronchodilator agents for quick relief of symptoms. FEV_1 = forced expiratory volume in 1 second; PEF = peak expiratory flow; ICS = Inhaled corticosteroids; BD = Bronchodilators. Adapted from: National Institutes of Health, National Heart, Lung and Blood Institute. *Guidelines for the Diagnosis and Management of Asthma, Expert Panel Report 2.* NIH Publication No. 97-4051, April 1997.

18

PULMONARY DISEASES

Chronic use may lead to tolerance, including cross-tolerance to short-acting beta-2-agonists. While their use may be helpful in patients with hard-to-control symptoms (including nighttime cough and wheeze), they probably do not provide significant *additional* benefit when added to an ICS.

Note: An DPI (Advair) containing both fluticasone and salmeterol is available.

TABLE 18-2

ESTIMATED COMPARATIVE DAILY DOSES FOR INHALED CORTICOSTEROIDS (Adults and Children ≥12 Y)

Drug	Low Dose	Medium Dose	High Dose
Beclomethasone dipropionate 42 mcg/puff 84 mcg/puff	168 to 504 mcg (4 to 12 puffs = 42 mcg) (2 to 6 puffs = 84 mcg)	504 to 840 mcg (12 to 20 puffs = 42 mcg) (6 to 10 puffs = 84 mcg)	>840 mcg (>20 puffs = 42 mcg) (>10 puffs = 84 mcg)
Budesonide turbuhaler 200 mcg/puff	200 to 400 mcg (1 to 2 inhalations)	400 to 600 mcg (2 to 3 inhalations)	>600 mcg (>3 inhalations)
Flunisolide 250 mcg/puff	500 to 1,000 mcg (2 to 4 puffs)	1,000 to 2,000 mcg (2 to 4 puffs)	>2,000 mcg (>8 puffs)
Fluticasone MDI: 44, 110, 220 mcg/puff DPI: 50, 100, 250 mcg/dose	88 to 264 mcg (2 to 6 puffs = 44 mcg) (2 puffs = 110 mcg) (2 to 6 inhalations = 50 mcg)	264 to 660 mcg (2 to 6 puffs = 110 mcg) (3 to 6 inhalations = 100 mcg)	>660 mcg (>6 puffs = 110 mcg) (>3 puffs = 220 mcg) (>6 inhalations = 100 mcg) (>2 inhalations = 250 mcg)
Triamcinolone acetonide 100 mcg/puff	400 to 1,000 mcg (4 to 10 puffs)	1,000 to 2,000 mcg (10 to 20 puffs)	>2,000 mcg (>20 puffs)

Source: National Institutes of Health, National Heart, Lung and Blood Institute. *Guidelines for the Diagnosis and Management of Asthma Expert Panel Report 2.* NIH Publication No. 97-4051, April 1997.

TABLE 18-3
ESTIMATED COMPARATIVE DAILY DOSES FOR INHALED CORTICOSTEROIDS (Children <12 Y)

Drug	Low Dose	Medium Dose	High Dose
Beclomethasone dipropionate 42 mcg/puff 84 mcg/puff	84 to 336 mcg (2 to 8 puffs = 42 mcg) (1 to 4 puffs = 84 mcg)	336 to 672 mcg (8 to 16 puffs = 42 mcg) (4 to 8 puffs = 84 mcg)	>672 mcg (>16 puffs = 42 mcg) (>8 puffs = 84 mcg)
Budesonide turbuhaler 200 mcg/puff	100 to 200 mcg (1 to 2 inhalations)	200 to 400 mcg (1 to 2 inhalations)	>400 mcg (>2 inhalations)
Flunisolide 250 mcg/puff	500 to 750 mcg (2 to 3 puffs)	1,000 to 1,250 mcg (4 to 5 puffs)	>1,250 mcg (>5 puffs)
Fluticasone MDI: 44, 110, 220 mcg/puff DPI: 50, 100, 250 mcg/dose	88 to 176 mcg (2 to 4 puffs = 44 mcg) (2 to 4 inhalations = 50 mcg)	176 to 440 mcg (4 to 10 puffs = 44 mcg) (2 to 4 puffs = 110 mcg) (2 to 4 inhalations = 100 mcg)	>440 mcg (>4 puffs = 110 mcg) (>2 puffs = 220 mcg) (>4 inhalations = 100 mcg) (>2 inhalations = 250 mcg)
Triamcinolone acetonide 100 mcg/puff	400 to 800 mcg (4 to 8 puffs)	800 to 1,200 mcg (8 to 12 puffs)	>1,200 mcg (>12 puffs)

Source: National Institutes of Health, National Heart, Lung and Blood Institute. *Guidelines for the Diagnosis and Management of Asthma, Expert Panel Report 2.* NIH Publication No. 97-4051, April 1997.

18

PULMONARY DISEASES

    (3) Leukotriene (LT) modifiers:

        (a) These medications represent the first mediator-specific therapy for asthma.

        (b) Available drugs include:

            (i)   Montelukast (Singulair), an LT receptor antagonist approved for children 2 years of age and older. The usual dose is a 4 mg chewable tablet for children 2 to 5 years, a 5 mg chewable tablet for children 6 to 14 years of age and a 10 mg tablet for adolescents over 14 years of age administered at bedtime.

            (ii) Zafirlukast (Accolate), an LT receptor antagonist approved for use in children 7 years of age and older. The usual dose is 10 mg bid for children 7 to 11 years of age and 20 mg bid for children 12 years of age and older.

            (iii) Zileuton (Zyflo), an inhibitor of LT synthesis approved for use in children 12 years of age and older. The usual dose is 600 mg qid. Its use is hampered by the qid dosage regimen and the need to monitor liver enzymes.

        (c) LT modifiers have some anti-inflammatory effects but not to the same extent as corticosteroids; they should not be used in place of corticosteroids for anti-inflammatory control. Improvement in airway function occurs within the first treatment day, but onset of action is slow, and they should never substitute for beta-agonists as rescue therapy.

        (d) The safety profile of LT modifiers is very good. There is no apparent tolerance after prolonged usage.

        (e) Potential uses of LT modifiers include:

            (i)   First-line treatment of young (2 to 5 years) wheezing children with mild, recurrent symptoms.

            (ii) They have a complementary effect in children treated with inhaled corticosteroids and can be used as add-on therapy in patients who remain symptomatic despite moderate use of inhaled corticosteroids. Also, they may facilitate tapering from high-dose corticosteroid therapy.

            (iii) They may have a role in providing long-term protection against EIA.

    (4) Levalbuterol: In the patient who cannot tolerate inhaled albuterol (racemic mixture of (S) and (R) albuterol), levalbuterol (R component) can be substituted.

  d. Treatment responses

    (1) If a patient does not respond to high-dose ICS or a systemic corticosteroid, the diagnosis of asthma should be questioned and another diagnosis such as CF or allergic bronchopulmonary aspergillosis (ABPA) should be considered.

    (2) For poor responders, look at adherence with the prescribed treatment program, including correct use of inhalers. Also look for

associated conditions such as allergic rhinitis, sinusitis, and GER that can exacerbate asthma.

(3) Atopic features, parental asthma, and maternal smoking may be risk factors for the development of persistent asthma.

e. Adjuncts to pharmacologic therapy

  (1) Environmental control

    (a) Obtain a careful history of the relationship between attacks and allergen exposure. Skin tests and RASTs may be helpful.

    (b) If sensitive, avoid outdoor allergens (ragweed, trees, grass, molds) and stay indoors with the windows closed in an air-conditioned environment. Air purifiers and ventilation systems may be helpful.

    (c) Control indoor allergens, primarily dust mites (Table 18-4) and molds; control roaches; remove animals from the home or at least from the patient's bedroom.

    (d) Avoid tobacco smoke exposure, pollutants, wood stoves, and chemicals.

  (2) Allergen-specific immunotherapy: Indicated in highly selected patients when one or more allergic triggers have been identified and the patient's symptoms cannot be controlled by medication and environmental measures. The most common antigen used is dust-mite extract.

  (3) Education: Probably *the most* important component of successful asthma management; every patient and family should be provided with the following:

    (a) An understanding of asthma

    (b) A program to monitor symptoms, peak flow, and medication usage

    (c) A prearranged action plan for exacerbations

    (d) Written guidelines

Note: A number of educational materials are now available on the Internet and CD ROM-based computer games.

18

PULMONARY DISEASES

TABLE 18-4
HOUSE DUST MITE CONTROL MEASURES
ESSENTIAL
Encase mattress in an airtight cover.
Either encase pillow or wash it weekly.
Wash bedding in 48.8° C water weekly.
Avoid sleeping or lying on upholstered furniture.
Remove carpets that are laid on concrete.
DESIRABLE
Reduce indoor humidity to <50%.
Remove carpeting from bedroom.
Chemical agents to kill mites or alter mite antigens.

3. Acute asthma

a. Asthma action plan: Every family should have a plan to monitor their child's course and manage flare-ups. Daily home peak flow monitoring can be helpful in the early recognition of worsening airway obstruction. Young children can be monitored by close observation of signs and symptoms.

b. Home treatment: Mild to moderate acute exacerbations can often be treated by initiating or increasing the frequency (q 20 minutes up to 1 hour) of short-acting beta-2-agonist therapy delivered by MDI or small-volume nebulizer. For patients using an ICS, the dose can be increased. Based on the patient's prior history and response to therapy, a 5- to 7-day course of oral prednisone (1 to 2 mg/kg/d) may be started. Patients who show a good clinical response can be gradually weaned back to their prior treatment regimen. Those who have a partial response need additional medical follow-up, and those who have a poor response should be referred to the emergency department.

Note: For infants and young children who have virally triggered asthma attacks, an oral corticosteroid started at the onset of URI symptoms may reduce the frequency and severity of acute attacks.

c. Treatment in the Emergency Department:

(1) The severity of the exacerbation should be assessed (Table 18-5).

(a) History: If the patient is in acute distress, obtain a brief, pertinent history. When did wheezing begin? Precipitating event (e.g., URI, allergen, irritant, exercise, weather change)? Is the child a known asthmatic, or is this a "first-time" wheezer? Any associated illness? Medications? Last dose? Course of previous episodes? Previous hospitalizations? What type of ED or inpatient treatment has usually reversed acute attacks? Consider other diagnoses if this is the first wheezing episode, especially if wheezing is atypical or not responding to therapy or if there is no family history for atopy.

(b) PE: Check all vital signs. Assess the degree of severity; supraclavicular retractions correlate well with the degree of obstruction. Cyanosis? Tightness? (Some patients may have such poor air movement that no wheezing is heard.) Measure pulsus paradoxus (significant bronchospasm produces pulsus paradoxus greater than 15 mm Hg). Evaluate the state of hydration and mental status. Look for a focus of infection.

(c) Laboratory tests: If a patient is taking theophylline, obtain a serum theophylline level. In a cooperative child more than 6 years of age, measure PEFR; a flow rate less than 30% often predicts a need for admission. Measure O_2 saturation by pulse oximetry. ABGs should be obtained in a patient with evidence of severe obstruction, a change in mental status, or clinical worsening. Po_2 less than 50 mm Hg or Pco_2 greater

(3) A leukotriene receptor antagonist (e.g., montelukast [Singulair]) may be effective for up to 24 hours in protecting against EIA.

(4) Inhaled steroids have little effect on EIA unless they are used for several weeks, but they may help overall control by reducing inflammation.

(5) Teachers and coaches should be alerted to the child's problem and management.

C. BRONCHIOLITIS

1. Bronchiolitis is an acute, viral-induced inflammatory process of the small airways that causes airway hyperreactivity, edema, and inflammation. Most cases occur prior to 2 years of age (peak 6 months) and greatest severity is prior to 1 year of age. Peak incidence is from November to March.

2. Cause: The majority of cases are secondary to RSV infection, but may also be caused by parainfluenza, adenovirus, influenza and rhinovirus infection. RSV infection can be documented by ELISA and immunofluorescence assays, but not routinely indicated.

3. Clinical presentation: Two- to three-day prodrome of URI symptoms, followed by acute onset of respiratory distress with coughing, wheezing, tachypnea, retractions, rales, irritability, and variable fever. Apnea may occur in young infants.

4. PE: Assess the degree of respiratory distress. Tachypnea? Flaring? Retractions? Cyanosis? Hydration? Decreased air entry, lethargy, and cyanosis are *bad* signs. There is good correlation between the severity of retractions and the degree of hypoxemia.

5. Laboratory tests: Not usually helpful. CXR shows hyperinflation and bronchial wall edema. Pulse oximetry is useful in assessing disease severity. ABGs are indicated in patients with severe distress or evidence of incipient respiratory failure.

6. Predictors of severe disease include the following:

a. Toxic appearance

b. History of prematurity (less than 34 weeks gestation), chronic cardiorespiratory disease

c. O_2 saturation less than 95% (single best predictor of severity)

d. Age less than 3 months

e. Atelectasis on CXR

f. Respiratory rate greater than 70

7. Treatment

a. Most patients without underlying risk factors or severe disease and with normal oxygen saturation can be managed at home.

(1) Treatment is symptomatic (fluids, antipyretics).

(2) Oral or inhaled albuterol can be tried, but, in most cases, is not beneficial. It is probably more likely to be helpful in patients with a family history of asthma.

18

PULMONARY DISEASES

b. Indications for hospitalization: Severe respiratory distress; hypoxemia; dehydration; age less than 2 months, and underlying cardiopulmonary disease.
   (1) Maintenance IV fluids.
   (2) Humidified oxygen by nasal cannula or oxygen hood to maintain O_2 saturation greater than 95%.
   (3) There is no documented acute or long-term benefit from the use of aerosol ribavirin (even in very severe cases), nebulized albuterol, or systemic or nebulized corticosteroids.
   (4) CPAP administered nasally or by endotracheal tube can help correct severe hypoxemia; mechanical ventilation is indicated in patients with respiratory failure.
   (5) Strict isolation precautions are mandatory in the hospital setting.
8. Course
a. Major symptoms last 2 to 3 days and are followed by slow resolution over 10 to 14 days.
b. Up to 70% of episodes of bronchiolitis are followed by recurrent cough and wheeze. However, 5 years postinfection, there is no increased incidence of recurrent wheezing, and bronchiolitis is probably not a cause of atopic asthma in later life.

D. CHRONIC COUGH

A chronic cough is defined as a cough that persists for more than 1 month. A prolonged cough is abnormal at any age but is of particular concern in a young infant.
1. Cause varies by age group, but there is much overlap.
a. Infants: Congenital malformations (TEF, vascular ring, laryngeal cleft), dysfunctional swallowing, reflux/aspiration, bronchial hyperreactivity (especially postviral infection), pertussis, *Pneumocystis* organisms, *Chlamydia* organisms, CF, interstitial pneumonia
b. Toddlers and preschool-age children: FB aspiration, cough-variant asthma, recurrent viral URIs/sinusitis
c. Adolescents: Smoking, psychogenic (habitual) cough (loud, brassy "honking" cough only during waking hours in an otherwise well-appearing adolescent)
d. All ages: Cough-variant asthma, sinusitis/postnasal drip, allergy, infection (TB, pertussis, mycoplasma), CF, passive smoke exposure, recurrent viral URIs, ciliary dyskinesia
2. History: Often the best clue to diagnosis. Duration? Timing (season, day, night, feedings)? Degree of illness? Associated features? Character (Table 18-6)? Precipitating events? Family history? Sputum production? Wheezing? Growth pattern? Exercise tolerance? Immunizations? Environmental exposures? Allergies?
3. PE: General health, growth parameters, evidence of atopy, chest wall deformity, rales, wheezing, decreased breath sounds (localized findings with FB), digital clubbing (CF, bronchiectasis).

TABLE 18-6

CLUES TO ETIOLOGY FROM CHARACTERISTICS OF COUGH

Paroxysmal with cyanosis or choking: Pertussis, *Chlamydia* organisms, *Mycoplasma* organisms, CF

Short, dry, wheezing: Cough-variant asthma, lower respiratory tract infection

Harsh, barking: Tracheal irritation, compression of intrathoracic airways

Wet, productive: Resolving infection, suppurative lung disease, CF

Bizarre, barking: Psychogenic (habit)

4. Laboratory studies: Guided by results of the history and PE. Watchful waiting and reevaluation are often indicated before embarking on costly laboratory/radiographic workups.
   a. X-ray examination
      (1) CXR: Infection, anomalies, CF, FB
      (2) Barium esophagram: Vascular ring, GER
      (3) Sinus CT scan: Sinusitis
      (4) Fluoroscopy: FB
   b. PPD, serologic tests, cultures: Infection
   c. Sweat test: CF
   d. Immunoglobulins, T-cell studies, HIV testing: Immunodeficiency
   e. Cineradiographic swallowing study: Dysfunctional swallow, aspiration
   f. Pulmonary function tests (including bronchoprovocation): Reactive airway disease
   g. Bronchoscopy: Diagnostic procedure of choice for FB
5. Treatment is directed at the specific cause.
   a. Cough-variant asthma, often in the absence of wheezing, is the most common cause of chronic cough in children. It may be precipitated by viral illness, cold air, exercise, irritants, and allergens and is often worse at night. With high suspicion of cough-variant asthma, a trial of bronchodilator is useful.
   b. Psychogenic cough is often related to secondary gain or school phobia and is a therapeutic challenge. Options include suggestion, sheet-wrapping of the chest, hypnosis, behavior modification, and lidocaine nebulizations.
   c. There is little role for cough suppressants; codeine and dextromethorphan have been shown to be ineffective in children.

E. CROUP

1. Viral laryngotracheobronchitis is the most common cause of acute stridor in young children. There is an acute onset of biphasic or inspiratory stridor, a "barking" cough, hoarseness, retractions, variable fever, and variable respiratory distress; it usually follows a URI. The child often appears well between coughing episodes. The usual course is 3 to 7 days.
   a. Etiology: Parainfluenza, RSV, adenovirus, influenza A, rhinovirus, mycoplasma.

b. Usually occurs in fall-winter; peak age 6 months to 3 years.
c. PE: Assess the degree of distress, hydration, general activity, air entry, retractions, mental status (agitation, restlessness), tachycardia out of proportion to fever, and cyanosis.
d. Laboratory tests: Not usually helpful. An AP neck x-ray study may show subglottic narrowing (steeple sign) but is not usually indicated. ABGs are indicated only with clinical deterioration. Respiratory rate is the best predictor of hypoxemia. Pulse oximetry may be helpful but is not as reliable as careful, serial clinical assessments.
e. Differential diagnosis: Epiglottitis, peritonsillar abscess, bacterial tracheitis, FB, retropharyngeal abscess, subglottic stenosis, infectious mononucleosis, angioneurotic edema.
f. Management:
   (1) Calm the child (and family); avoid painful procedures. If supplemental oxygen is indicated (based on oximetry results) it is best delivered with the child sitting in the parent's lap.
   (2) For mild to moderate croup, give a single dose of IM or PO dexamethasone 0.6 mg/kg (maximum 10 mg). The PO route is more convenient and just as effective. Improvement may not be seen for 6 hours.
   (3) For moderate to severe croup seen in the ED:
      (a) Nebulize racemic ephinehprine (0.25 to 0.75 ml of 2.25% solution in 2.5 ml normal saline) or l-epinephrine (5 ml of 1:1000 solution). They are equally effective. Onset of action is 10 minutes, but duration is short (30 to 60 minutes) and may need to repeat q2h.
      (b) In addition, the child should receive a dose of PO or IM dexamethasone or nebulized budesonide (2 mg).
      (c) The child should be observed for at least 3 hours after the use of nebulized ephinephrine and prior to discharge home. Discharge criteria include: absence of stridor at rest, normal air entry, normal color, and alert.

Note: Although humidified air and "croup tents" are commonly used, there are no data to support their usefulness.

   (4) Indications for admission include evidence of respiratory compromise (e.g., cyanosis, fatigue, hypotonia, Pco_2 greater than 45, Po_2 less than 70), and dehydration.
   (5) Intubation (nasotracheal) or tracheostomy is rarely necessary. Indications include: hypercarbia, impending respiratory failure; increasing stridor, respiratory rate, heart rate, retractions; and cyanosis, exhaustion, or change in mental status.
   (6) Endoscopy is indicated for atypical, severe, or recurrent cases of LTB and for the child who fails extubation. In infants, the differential diagnosis includes airway hemangiomas, papillomas, and so forth.

2. Spasmodic croup

Spasmodic croup is the acute onset of a "barking" cough and inspiratory stridor with or without a preceding URI in a previously well afebrile child. It often occurs at night. Symptoms usually abate promptly but may recur for several nights.

a. Cause: Probably viral, but may represent an "allergic" response to a viral agent.

b. Management: Reassurance; IM or PO dexamethasone may be helpful but is seldom necessary.

3. Bacterial tracheitis

Bacterial tracheitis is also known as pseudomembranous croup or membranous laryngotracheitis. URI/cough is followed by the abrupt onset of fever, stridor, barking cough, toxic appearance, and respiratory distress. There is leukocytosis with a shift to the left; there is accompanying pneumonia in 50% of the cases.

a. Cause: *Staphylococcus aureus* (most common), *Haemophilus influenzae* (now uncommon).

b. Diagnosis: Established at laryngoscopy/bronchoscopy; airway obstruction secondary to thick, tracheal secretions; adherent membrane over inflamed, friable mucosa. An x-ray examination of the airway may show irregular tracheal densities with scalloping and narrowing of the trachea.

c. Management
   (1) Continuous monitoring in intensive care unit
   (2) Endoscopic removal of thick tracheal secretions and membranous exudate
   (3) Appropriate parenteral antibiotic therapy (e.g., IV cefuroxime)
   (4) Respiratory support; intubation often necessary

F. EPIGLOTTITIS

Now uncommon (HIB immunization) but a true pediatric emergency! The initial goal is to establish and maintain a good airway. A physician skilled in airway management *must* accompany the patient *at all times*.

1. Classic presentation
a. Fulminant course in a previously well child.
b. Stridor, respiratory distress (within hours of onset), sore throat, muffled voice, dysphagia (refuses to drink), high fever. The typical appearance is a child in a toxic condition who prefers to sit (do not make the patient lie down!), head forward (tripod position), open mouth, drooling, anxious appearance; *coughing is not a prominent feature.*
Note: Many children with epiglottitis will present *without* all of these signs and symptoms.
c. Age at onset: Ranges from 7 months to 10 years (average age 3 years). Infants less than 2 years of age may have a less fulminant course that may be confused with viral croup.

18

PULMONARY DISEASES

TABLE 18-7

CLINICAL GUIDELINES: EPIGLOTTITIS VS. CROUP (LARYNGOTRACHEOBRONCHITIS)

	Epiglottitis	Croup
Age	May affect all ages, peak 3-5 yr	Younger children, 3 mo-3 yr
Etiology	Bacterial (H. influenzae)	Viral (parainfluenza)
Site of inflammation	Supraglottic	Subglottic
Onset of respiratory symptoms	Usually rapid (30 min-6 hr)	Slow (1-4 days)
Symptoms		
Appearance	Anxious, ill, toxic	Often nontoxic
Position	Upright, forward	Variable
Temperature	Usually high (>39° C)	Normal to high
Respiratory distress	Usually present	Variable
Retractions	Usually late finding	Progressive
Voice/cough	Muffled/often absent	Hoarse/"seal bark"
Mouth	Open, jaw forward, may drool	Closed, nasal flaring

TABLE 18-8

FREQUENCY OF SYMPTOMS IN COMBINED SERIES OF EPIGLOTTITIS PATIENTS

Symptom	Frequency (%)	Symptom	Frequency (%)
Fever	85	Dysphagia	40
Respiratory distress	80	Drooling	37
Retractions	59	Cyanosis	33
Stridor	54	Cough	25
Sore throat	46	Hoarseness	23

d. Cause: Prior to HIB immunization, *H. influenzae* type B; the blood culture is positive in 80% of the cases. At present, common causes include GABHS infection, caustic agents, and thermal burns.

e. Differential diagnosis: Croup, pharyngitis, bacterial tracheitis, retropharyngeal abscess, angioneurotic edema. Croup does *not* have such a rapid evolution and has more coughing and hoarseness; stridor may be similar to epiglottitis. Although croup may be severe, the child is not usually in the degree of distress that is seen with epiglottitis (Tables 18-7 and 18-8).

2. Initial management: Minimize disturbance, keep child calm, and avoid attempts to visualize the pharynx or epiglottis. Laboratory tests are not usually helpful or indicated.

a. If the child has the classic presentation, ENT and/or anesthesiology should be notified and the child transported to the OR for direct inspection of the supraglottic larynx and nasotracheal intubation. A tracheostomy is rarely needed.

b. If the presentation is not straightforward and if the child is not in severe distress, immediately obtain an x-ray examination (*lateral view*) of the neck with the patient *erect* (*not* supine) and call ENT and/or anesthesiology.

Note: The lateral neck x-ray study is normal in 20% of cases of epiglottitis.

c.   *All* patients with documented epiglottitis need an artificial airway regardless of the degree of distress at the time of evaluation because they can decompensate quickly; the airway should be placed in the OR.

d.   If a patient is clinically *suspected* of having epiglottitis, the following protocol is followed:

(1)   *Examination of the pharynx is prohibited once epiglottitis is suspected.* Minimize disturbance; keep the patient upright; unobtrusively administer facial O_2 (blow-by); *do not* draw blood or place IV lines; do not give PO fluids.

(2)   The patient should never be left without a physician in attendance. Parents often are helpful in relieving the child's anxiety. *Do not* crowd the child.

(3)   When the child is transported for any reason, he or she should be accompanied by a parent and a physician capable of securing an airway. Airway equipment should be on hand (resuscitation bag, laryngoscope, ETT, and 14-gauge angiocatheter for emergency tracheotomy). The patient should be transported in the *upright* position, with *minimum disturbance,* and with oxygen unobtrusively administered.

e.   Treatment should include an antibiotic effective against GABHS and beta-lactamase–producing strains of *H. influenzae* (e.g., IV cefotaxime, ceftriaxone); there is no role for steroids.

Note: Do not forget rifampin prophylaxis for appropriate family members/contacts.

G. FOREIGN-BODY ASPIRATION

1.   Presentation of lower airway FB

a.   Signs and symptoms include acute choking episode, wheezing, coughing, stridor, dyspnea, and evidence of chest infection; there may be hemoptysis. A choking episode is observed in only 50% to 80% of cases, which often leads to a delay in diagnosis.

b.   The usual age is 6 months to 3 years. Males are affected twice as often as females.

c.   The most common object is a peanut; hot dogs, balloons, toy parts, and balls are also common.

d.   Always suspect a FB if pneumonia does not resolve completely or recurs after antibiotic therapy is stopped.

2.   Diagnosis

a.   The history is crucial but is often not obtained or appreciated. There may be a long latent period between aspiration and the signs and symptoms of infection.

18

PULMONARY DISEASES

b. The diagnostic triad includes coughing, localized wheezing, and locally diminished or absent breath sounds but is not present in up to 50% of patients.

c. CXR may show air trapping, mediastinal shift, atelectasis, or pneumonia but is normal in up to one third of all cases; a radiopaque object is seen in approximately 15% of cases.

Note: Left-sided aspiration is almost as common as right-sided aspiration.

d. Inspiratory and expiratory x-ray studies, left and right lateral decubitus films, and fluoroscopy may be helpful. However, if suspicious of FB and the initial evaluation results are normal, refer the patient for bronchoscopy.

3. Management

a. Bronchoscopy is the procedure of choice (see Chapter 17).

b. Because of the possibility of airway obstruction, chest physiotherapy should *not* be performed before endoscopy.

Note: There may be more than one FB. The endoscopist needs to look on both sides.

H. HEMOPTYSIS

1. Although a rare event, hemoptysis can be life threatening; it may be confused with hematemesis (Table 18-9).

Note: Always think of a pulmonary source of bleeding in children with unexplained hematemesis.

2. Differential diagnosis

a. In children, the most likely causes are infection and aspirated FBs.

b. In infants and young children, also consider tumors, autoimmune disease, bronchiectasis, AV malformations, cysts, child abuse, and hemosiderosis (hemoptysis, infiltrates, iron deficiency anemia).

3. Evaluation

a. Obtain a careful history of underlying illness, fever, coughing, sputum, stridor, wheezing, joint pain, weight loss, family illness, trauma, choking episodes, medication use, exposure to toxins, and travel.

b. Always start the examination at the top; the nasopharynx or oral cavity is often the source of bleeding.

c. Check skin for hemangiomata, telangiectases, and signs of trauma.

TABLE 18-9		
COMPARISON OF HEMOPTYSIS WITH HEMATEMESIS		
	Hemoptysis	Hematemesis
Color	Bright red	Dark red
pH	Alkaline	Acid
Appearance	Frothy	± Food particles
Symptoms	Cough	Nausea, retching

d. CXR is the procedure with the highest yield. However, a normal x-ray study does not rule out a pulmonary source of bleeding. Except in cases of blood-tinged sputum or mild bleeding, a patient with hemoptysis should be admitted. Bronchoscopy is necessary if initial evaluation results are normal.
4. Treatment of hemoptysis is management of the underlying disorder.

I. PNEUMONIA

1. History: May be *acute* or *subacute* onset, fever with or without chills, coughing, difficult or rapid breathing with or without pain on inspiration, toxic appearance, malaise. Ask about exposure to TB, immunization status, previous pneumonia, and HIV risk factors.
2. PE: All vital signs
a. Tachypnea is a very sensitive clinical sign but may be associated with other disorders (e.g., DKA, salicylate poisoning, FB, bronchiolitis, asthma).
b. Rales are often present but may be absent depending on the type of pneumonic process.
c. Sputum production is rare in young children (i.e., less than 6 years of age).
d. Shallow breathing and splinting occurs secondary to pleuritic pain.
e. There may be localized findings of decreased breath sounds and dullness to percussion.
f. Right lower lobe pneumonia may present as right-side abdominal pain.
g. Look for other sites of infection (e.g., OM, conjunctivitis).
3. Laboratory
a. CXR: Infiltrate may not be present early in illness. Infiltrates may be lobar, segmental, nodular, miliary, interstitial, or perihilar. Other significant findings include pleural effusion, pneumatoceles (can be seen with many bacteria, not just *S. aureus*), and cavitations. In most cases the CXR cannot differentiate among bacterial, viral, mycoplasma, and chlamydia pneumonias. A CXR is not indicated in all patients with suspected pneumonia; most are diagnosed clinically.
b. TB skin test: Indicated in patients with chronic or complicated pneumonia, those with a positive family history, and for other high-risk groups (e.g., immigrants from Russia and southeast Asia).
c. CBC: WBC count may be higher in bacterial vs. viral pneumonias, but there is a great deal of overlap, and the results do not usually alter treatment. Moderate eosinophilia may be present in chlamydia, parasitic, allergic, and hypersensitivity pneumonias.
d. Blood culture: Not obtained routinely. It is positive in only 10% to 15% of hospitalized patients with presumed bacterial pneumonia. Consider the clinical setting (e.g., age, fever, WBC count, toxic appearance).
e. Cold agglutinins: Used as a screening test for *Mycoplasma pneumoniae* but does not discriminate well between mycoplasma and viral infections; rarely positive in patients less than 5 years of age.

18

PULMONARY DISEASES

f.   Antigen detection tests: Serum or urine CIE or latex agglutination tests for pneumococcal, Group B streptococcal, and *H. influenzae* antigens can help establish a bacterial etiology but are not practical in most outpatient settings.

g.   Chlamydia studies: Conjunctival scraping or NP swab may be Giemsa stained or cultured (special media required) for *Chlamydia* organisms. Fluorescent antibody microscopy of NP secretions correlates well with culture results.

h.   Cultures: In most cases an NP or throat culture is worthless; a culture and Gram's stain may be helpful if a good sputum (not saliva) specimen is obtained.

i.   Tracheal aspirate: Rarely used in children; probably better than sputum but still may be contaminated with upper respiratory secretions.

j.   Pleural effusions: Should be tapped. The fluid should be sent for culture, AFB, Gram's stain, chemistry studies, and cytologic tests.

k.   A lung puncture, open-lung biopsy, and bronchoalveolar lavage may be helpful in highly select, complicated cases.

l.   CRP: In general, an elevated CRP is indicative of bacterial infection, but there is considerable overlap with other conditions.

4.   Etiology: Conclusive evidence is difficult to obtain in children. Etiology may be suspected on the basis of age, clinical presentation and community outbreaks. Among pediatric outpatients with pneumonia, approximately 10% to 20% result from a bacterial agent; most result from viral agents such as influenza, parainfluenza, adenovirus, and RSV (especially in infants). In approximately 10% of children there is coexistent viral and bacterial infection. In older children (older than 8 years of age) and adolescents, *M. pneumoniae* and *Chlamydia pneumoniae* are common etiologic agents. Most neonatal pneumonias are bacterial.

a.   Bacterial: Acute onset of symptoms with significant fever and lobar consolidation suggests bacterial pneumonia. Most common organism (based on lung punctures and blood culture) is *Streptococcus pneumoniae*. *S. aureus* should be considered in young or debilitated infants, especially if effusions or pneumatoceles are present. Streptococcal pneumonia may be associated with a scarlatiniform rash; the blood culture and pleural fluid cultures may be positive, but TC is often negative. It may run a fulminant course.

Note: Immunization with *Haemophilus influenzae* type B vaccine eliminates the possibility of HIB as the etiologic pathogen.

b.   Viral: Viral causes include adenovirus, influenza, parainfluenza, and RSV. In older children there is usually a nonproductive cough and systemic symptoms such as myalgias, headache, coryza, fatigue, and general malaise. In infants, wheezing and rales are often prominent features.

c.   *Chlamydia* organisms: *Chlamydia trachomatis* may be responsible for 15% to 30% of afebrile pneumonias in early infancy. The typical patient is afebrile with a staccato cough, peripheral eosinophilia, and diffuse interstitial infiltrates. Half of the patients have conjunctivitis.

d. *Mycoplasma* organisms: Common in school-age children and young adults. Infection is characterized by a gradual onset, low-grade or absent fever, interstitial infiltrates, and greater severity of symptoms.

e. Fungal, protozoal, and TB infections must be considered in chronic pneumonia.

f. In general, viral and bacterial causes cannot be reliably distinguished on the basis of the clinical picture, laboratory results, or radiographic findings. In addition to investigating the cause, consider an underlying disease process predisposing the patient to chronic, persistent, or recurrent pneumonias, such as immune compromise (congenital, AIDS-related, iatrogenic), CF, TEF, BPD, GER, FB, dysfunctional swallow, lobar emphysema, and bronchogenic cysts. Remember that not all infiltrates are infectious (e.g., metastases, lymphoma).

5. Treatment

a. Infants less than 2 months of age should be hospitalized and treated IV with ampicillin and an aminoglycoside such as gentamicin, after an appropriate sepsis workup. Need to cover *Group B streptococcus, H. influenzae, S. pneumoniae, S. aureus,* and *E. coli.* For infants with suspected chlamydia infection (afebrile, staccato cough), treat with erythromycin 50 mg/kg/day ÷ q6h alone or in combination with sulfisoxazole.

b. Children age 3 months to 8 years with mild to moderate symptoms can usually be treated as outpatients. Prudent clinical practice involves treating pneumonia as if it were bacterial and not performing an extensive laboratory evaluation. Initial therapy with high-dose amoxicillin 80 to 100 mg/kg/day ÷ tid or amoxicillin plus clavulanate potassium (augmentin) 40 mg/kg/day ÷ bid is appropriate. The patient with moderate to severe symptoms or who fails to respond after 48 hours of outpatient therapy should be hospitalized and treated IV with a third-generation cephalosporin such as cefotaxime or ceftriaxone.

c. For children older than 8 years of age with mild to moderate symptoms, a macrolide such as clarithromycin (Biaxin) 15 mg/kg/day + bid or azithromycin (Zithromax) 500 mg on day 1, followed by 250 mg once daily on days 2 through 5 is appropriate.

d. An ongoing problem involves *S. pneumoniae* isolates that show intermediate or high-level resistance to penicillin. Many of these strains may show a pattern of multiple drug resistance. Vancomycin remains uniformly effective. For severe community-acquired pneumonia in an area with a high incidence of penicillin-resistant *S. pneumoniae,* IV therapy with a third-generation cephalosporin (e.g., ceftriaxone or cefotaxime) plus clindamycin or vancomycin is appropriate pending culture and sensitivity results.

18

PULMONARY DISEASES

e. Antiviral agents, ribavirin, amantadine, acyclovir, and ganciclovir should be considered for highly select patients, especially those with an immunodeficiency.

f. General supportive care: Rest, antipyretics as necessary, hydration. Cough suppressants are not recommended for pneumonia; expectorants do not work.

g. Patient follow-up in 1 to 2 days.

   (1) If improved, see patient again at the completion of therapy. Uncomplicated bacterial pneumonia should improve in 24 to 48 hours.

   (2) Consider inadequate therapy, incorrect diagnosis (possibly FB), or noncompliance if no improvement or progression of the process occurs.

   (3) Follow-up CXR: Usually not necessary unless patient has persistent symptoms, recurrent pneumonia, or FTT. In one study, 20% of children had residual infiltrates 3 to 4 weeks after acute pneumonia (although clinically better), whereas 100% had a negative x-ray study within 3 months.

   (4) Remember to perform a TB skin test on the patient if one has not recently been placed.

J. BIBLIOGRAPHY

Apnea

Arad-Cohen N, Cohen A, Tirosh E: The relationship between gastroesophageal reflux and apnea in infants, *J Pediatr* 137:321, 2000.

Bruhn FW et al: Apnea associated with respiratory syncytial virus infection in young infants, *J Pediatr* 90:382, 1977.

Keens TG, Ward SLD: Apnea spells, sudden death, and the role of the apnea monitor, *Pediatr Clin North Am* 40:897, 1993.

Kravitz RM, Wilmott RW: Munchausen syndrome by proxy presenting as factitious apnea, *Clin Pediatr* 29:587, 1990.

NIH consensus development conference on infantile apnea and home monitoring, *Pediatrics* 79:292, 1987.

See CC et al: Gastroesophageal reflux-induced hypoxemia in infants with apparent life-threatening event(s), *Am J Dis Child* 143:951, 1989.

Asthma

Becker A: Clinical evidence with montelukast in the management of chronic childhood asthma, *Drugs* 59(suppl 1):29, 2000.

Bisgaard H: Leukotriene modifiers in pediatric asthma management, *Pediatrics* 107:381, 2001.

Bisgaard H: Long-acting beta-2-agonists in management of childhood asthma: a critical review of the literature, *Pediatr Pulmonol* 29:221, 2000.

Boulet L-P: Long- versus short-acting beta-2-agonists: implications for drug therapy, *Drugs* 47:207, 1994.

Edwards AM, Stevens MT: The clinical efficacy of inhaled nedocromil sodium (Tilade) in the treatment of asthma, *Eur Respir J* 6:35, 1993.

Gelber LE et al: Sensitization and exposure to indoor allergens as risk factors for asthma among patients presenting to the hospital, *Am Rev Resp Dis* 147:573, 1993.

Helms PJ: Corticosteroid-sparing options in the treatment of childhood asthma, *Drugs* 59(suppl 1):15, 2000.

Inman MD, O'Bryne PM: Anti-inflammatory therapy in the treatment of asthma, *Curr Opin Pulm Med* 1:50, 1995.

Kercsmar CM: Aerosol treatment of acute asthma: and the winner is . . ., *J Pediatr* 136:428, 2000.

Kwong KYC, Jones CA: Chronic asthma therapy, *Pediatr Rev* 20:327, 1999.

Larsen GL: Asthma in children, *N Engl J Med* 326:1540, 1992.

McFadden ER, Jr: Management of patients with acute asthma: what do we know? What do we need to know? *Ann Allergy* 72:385, 1994.

National Heart, Lung, and Blood Institute: Guidelines for the diagnosis and management of asthma, Pub No 91-3042A, Bethesda, MD, June 1991, National Institutes of Health.

National Heart, Lung and Blood Institute: Guidelines for the diagnosis and management of asthma, Expert Panel Report 2, NIH Publication No. 97-4051, Bethesda, MD, April, 1997, National Institutes of Health.

Osmond MH, Klassen TP: Efficacy of ipratropium bromide in acute childhood asthma: a meta analysis, *Acad Emerg Med* 2:651, 1995.

Papo MC et al: A prospective, randomized study of continuous versus intermittent nebulized albuterol for severe status asthmaticus in children, *Crit Care Med* 21:1479, 1993.

Ross RN, Nelson HS, Finegold I: Effectiveness of specific immunotherapy in the treatment of asthma: a meta-analysis of prospective, randomized, double-blind, placebo-controlled studies, *Clin Ther* 22:351, 2000.

Rowe B, Bretzlaff JA, Bourdon C et al: Intravenous magnesium sulfate treatment for acute asthma in the emergency department: a systematic review of the literature, *Ann Emerg Med* 36:181, 2000.

Warner JO: The beta-2-agonist controversy: another relevance to the treatment of children, *Eur Respir Rev* 4:21, 1994.

Bronchiolitis

Baron ME, Zanga JR: Bronchiolitis, *Primary Care* 23:805, 1996.

Berger I, Argaman Z, Schwartz SB et al: Efficacy of corticosteroids in acute bronchiolitis: short-term and long-term follow-up, *Pediatr Pulmonol* 26:162, 1998.

Cade A, Brownlee KG, Conway SP et al: Randomized placebo-controlled trial of nebulized corticosteroids in acute respiratory syncytial viral bronchiolitis, *Arch Dis Child* 82:126, 2000.

De Boeck K, Van derAa N, Van Lièrde S et al: Respiratory syncytial virus bronchiolitis: a double-blind dexamethasone efficacy study, *J Pediatr* 131:919, 1997.

Guerguerian A-M, Gauthier M, Lebel MH et al: Ribavirin in ventilated respiratory syncytial virus bronchiolitis: a randomized, placebo-controlled trial, *Am J Respir Crit Care Med* 160:829, 1999.

Klassen TP: Recent advances in the treatment of bronchiolitis and laryngitis, *Pediatr Clin North Am* 44:249, 1997.

Klassen TP et al: Randomized trial of salbutamol in acute bronchiolitis, *J Pediatr* 118:807, 1991.

Kneyber McJ, Steyerberg EW, DeGroot R et al: Long-term effects of respiratory syncytial virus (RSV) bronchiolitis in infants and young children: a quantitative review, *Acta Paediatr* 89:654, 2000.

Shaw KH et al: Outpatient assessment of infants with bronchiolitis, *Am J Dis Child* 145:151, 1991.

Wohl ME: Bronchiolitis, *Pediatr Ann* 15:307, 1986.

Chronic Cough

Cloutier MM, Loughlin GM: Chronic cough in children: a manifestation of airway hyperreactivity, *Pediatrics* 67:6, 1981.

Ewig JM: Chronic cough, *Pediatr Rev* 16:72, 1995.

Kamel RK: Chronic cough in children, *Pediatr Clin North Am* 38:593, 1991.

Lavigne JV et al: Behavioral management of psychogenic cough: alternative to the "bedsheet" and other aversive techniques, *Pediatrics* 87:532, 1991.

Meyer AA, Aitken PV Jr: Evaluation of persistent cough in children, *Primary Care* 23:883, 1996.

Taylor JA et al: Efficacy of cough suppressants in children, *J Pediatr* 122:799, 1993.

Croup and Epiglottitis

Ausejo M, Saenz A, Pham B et al: The effectiveness of glucocorticoids in treating croup: meta-analysis, *BMJ* 319:595, 1999.

Cressman WR, Myer CM, III: Diagnosis and management of croup and epiglottitis, *Pediatr Clin North Am* 41:265, 1994.

Custer JR: Croup and related disorders, *Pediatr Rev* 14:19, 1993.

Gorelick MH, Baker MD: Epiglottitis in children, 1979 through 1992: effects of Haemophilus influenzae *type b* immunization, *Arch Pediatr Adolesc Med* 148:47, 1994.

18

PULMONARY DISEASES

Griffin S, Ellis S, Fitzgerald-Baron A et al: Nebulized steroid in the treatment of croup: a systematic review of randomized controlled trials, *Br J Gen Pract* 50:135, 2000.

Klassen TP: Croup: a current perspective, *Pediatr Clin North Am* 46:1167, 1999.

Kunkel NC, Baker MD: Use of racemic epinephrine, dexamethasone, and mist in the outpatient management of croup, *Pediatr Emerg Care* 12:156, 1996.

Losek JD et al: Epiglottitis: comparison of signs and symptoms in children less than 2 years old and older, *Ann Emerg Med* 19:55, 1990.

Malhotra A, Krilov LR: Viral croup, *Pediatr Rev* 22:2, 2001.

Rittichier KK, Ledwith CA: Outpatient treatment of moderate croup with dexamethasone: intramuscular vs oral dosing, *Pediatrics* 106:1344, 2000.

Super DM, Cartelli NA, Brooks LJ et al: A prospective randomized double-blind study to evaluate the effect of dexamethasone in acute laryngotracheitis, *J Pediatr* 115:323, 1989.

Waisman Y et al: Prospective randomized double-blind study comparing l-epinephrine and racemic epinephrine aerosols in the treatment of laryngotracheitis (croup), *Pediatrics* 898:302, 1992.

Foreign-Body Aspiration

Gay BB et al: Subglottic foreign bodies in pediatric patients, *Am J Dis Child* 140:165, 1986.

Healy GB: Management of tracheobronchial foreign bodies in children: an update, *Ann Otol Rhinol Laryngol* 99:889, 1990.

Laks Y, Barzilay A: Foreign body aspiration in childhood, *Pediatr Emerg Care* 4:102, 1988.

Puhakka H et al: Tracheobronchial foreign bodies, *Am J Dis Child* 143:543, 1989.

Rovin JD, Rodgers BM: Pediatric foreign body aspiration, *Pediatr Rev* 21:86, 2000.

Hemoptysis

Beckerman RC et al: Familial idiopathic pulmonary hemosiderosis, *Am J Dis Child* 133:609, 1979.

Metz SJ, Rosenstein BJ: Uncovering the cause of hemoptysis in children, *J Respir Dis* 5:43, 1984.

Pyman C: Inhaled foreign bodies in childhood, *Med J Aust* 1:62, 1971.

Tom LWC et al: Hemoptysis in children, *Ann Otolaryngol* 89:419, 1980.

Pneumonia

Broughton RA: Infections due to *Mycoplasma pneumoniae* in childhood, *Pediatr Infect Dis J* 5:71, 1986.

Cherian T et al: Simple clinical signs of acute lower respiratory tract infection, *Lancet* 2:125, 1988.

Churgay CA: The diagnosis and management of bacterial pneumonias in infants and children, *Primary Care* 23:821, 1996.

Denny FW: Acute respiratory infections in children: etiology and epidemiology, *Pediatr Rev* 9:135, 1987.

McCarthy PL et al: Radiographic findings and etiologic diagnosis in ambulatory childhood pneumonias, *Clin Pediatr* 20:686, 1981.

McCracken GH: Diagnosis and management of pneumonia in children, *Pediatr Infect Dis* 19:924, 2000.

Paisley JW et al: Pathogens associated with acute lower respiratory tract infections in young children, *Pediatr Infect Dis J* 3:14, 1984.

Ramsey BWS et al: Use of bacterial antigen detection in the diagnosis of pediatric lower respiratory tract infections, *Pediatrics* 78:1, 1986.

Schutze GE, Jacobs RF: Management of community-acquired bacterial pneumonia in hospitalized children, *Pediatr Infect Dis J* 11:160, 1992.

Turner RB et al: Etiologic diagnosis of pneumonia in pediatric outpatients by counterimmunoelectrophoresis of urine, *Pediatrics* 71:780, 1983.

SCHOOL HEALTH ISSUES

A. PHILOSOPHY

1. Children who attend group child care, Head Start, preschool, or formal school merit special attention because they and the staff at these facilities are affected by their presence in groups. Children are likely to acquire a number of viral and bacterial infections from each other. The staff is also challenged by the numerous infections that circulate and by the accommodations they must make for children with special needs.

2. Before entering into group care or school, a child should receive a thorough health assessment by his or her regular medical provider. If performed properly, this assessment is one of the most important that any child will receive; it is meant to detect potential problems that might interfere with learning or participating in group activities. Especially important are assessments of hearing, vision, language, and development. Any detected abnormalities should be noted and, *if significant,* reported to the caregiver and school.

3. Other important information includes a history of allergies (e.g., allergen, if known; usual symptoms and severity; measures to be taken if an exposure occurs); chronic medical conditions, especially those that might require treatment at child care or school; *all* medications, but especially those that might need to be given while the child is in child care or at school; and any emergency procedures that must be followed.

4. It is also a good idea to include certain screening tests during the preenrollment visit. Screening tests for anemia, lead poisoning, and tuberculosis are helpful if a child has not recently had these tests; in some jurisdictions they are mandated by law.

5. Once the child is in child care or in school, there needs to be a free flow of information between the medical provider and the child care provider or teacher. An "us vs. them" attitude is not in the best interest of the child or family. If the medical provider detects a problem that will need to be dealt with by a child-care provider or teacher, he or she should communicate the information in a timely fashion. Parents are to be involved in this process. When a child-care provider or teacher detects a new problem or has a question, he or she should discuss it with the parent and, if necessary, contact the medical provider.

6. When children are in group situations, whether child care or school, the medical provider must be careful to consider the public health implications of a given disease in a child of a given age and in a given situation. A child may need to be excluded from care or school depending on the period of contagiousness of a given disease and the age and developmental level of the child.

B. SPECIFIC ISSUES

1. Abuse
a. Child-care providers and teachers sometimes are reluctant to report suspected abuse because they fear that they lack expertise. They therefore defer to the medical provider. This strategy is not optimal, especially if there is a time lapse between the caregiver or teacher's initial observation and the assessment by the medical provider.
b. Medical providers should do their best to cooperate with any initiative taken by the child-care facility or school to safeguard a child or clear up any concerns about marks on a child's body.

2. Behavior problems
a. A full discussion of behavior problems is provided in Chapter 4.
b. It is important to remember that the behaviors manifested by a child in a child-care facility or school might not be the behaviors that he or she demonstrates in the medical provider's office or at home. For example, a child with school phobia generally has symptoms only at school. An only child who has trouble getting along with other children may have problems at the child-care facility but not at home, where he or she does not need to deal with competition.

3. Chronic conditions
a. Asthma, seizures, sickle cell disease, hemophilia, HIV infection, diabetes, and allergies are discussed elsewhere in this text. Child-care providers and school personnel should be aware of the signs and symptoms of a chronic condition, the precipitating events (e.g., specific allergen exposure), and routine/emergency procedures to be followed in the event of an exacerbation. All information and instructions should be in writing, with one copy in the child's medical records and one copy at the child-care facility or school.
b. When a chronic condition warrants medication, try to space the doses so that they are not needed in school if at all possible. Many child-care providers are not permitted under state regulations to dispense medications, and many school personnel are uncomfortable doing so. Remember, not all schools and certainly not all child-care facilities have a nurse on site each day; therefore try to keep medications to a minimum in such settings. Always provide written instructions, including dosage, route, and time of administration on the forms required by the child-care facility or school. Keep a copy in the child's medical records.
c. If a child has very special needs (e.g., tube feedings, respiratory treatments, catheterizations), be sure to be as explicit as possible when documenting when and how to perform such procedures. Specify the type of treatment, the time of administration, and what should be done if it is unsuccessful. For tube feedings, specify the type of formula, dilution (if warranted), rate of feed (especially if gravity- or pump-driven), and measures to be taken if the feeding cannot proceed (e.g., obstruction to fluid inflow, vomiting, abdominal distension, tube

extrusion). Such orders must arrive before the child because many schools will not permit a child to remain if the proper orders are not on file.

d. Specify explicitly what the school or child-care facility needs to do in an emergency. For example, should 911 be called immediately, or should other measures be instituted before the 911 call? Remember, there may not be a health professional on site to make a medical decision; therefore try to anticipate questions. If a child has a seizure disorder, do all seizures or only certain ones warrant a 911 call? If the latter, which ones are they? If a child has asthma, which attacks warrant a 911 call and which warrant other therapies first? Does the staff know the signs of severe respiratory distress? If a child is at risk to experience a respiratory arrest, for whatever reason, what should the staff do while waiting for emergency treatment? If a child has diabetes, which reactions warrant a 911 call and which warrant a call to the parent? Does the staff know the signs and symptoms of hypoglycemia, hyperglycemia, and DKA? If the child has severe allergic reactions or anaphylaxis in response to an allergen, does the child-care facility or school have an EpiPen on hand, and do they know how to use it? Take nothing for granted! When writing directives for nonmedical personnel, make sure that they both have the recommended equipment and know how to use it. Be as explicit in your instructions as possible, and always encourage questions.

e. If a child has a chronic, terminal condition, do not assume that he or she will die at home or in a hospital. Many children have struggled to attend school for as long as possible, and therefore it is quite possible that such children could die at school. Make sure you know the laws in your state regarding advanced directives (also known as DNR orders). Document the parents' (and patient's, if applicable) wishes and your orders on any legal forms required. Give guidelines for what *can* be done and what should *not* be done. For example, if a child can receive "blow-by" oxygen but not intubation or CPR, state this. In many jurisdictions, if an ambulance is called the paramedics *will* begin CPR unless the patient is accompanied by advanced directive documentation. If this procedure is followed in your state, obtain the necessary documentation so that a needless resuscitation is not instituted. For information regarding the laws in your state, call your local Emergency Medical Services or hospice organization.

4. Day-care issues

a. Many infants and preschool-age children are in substitute care during part of every workday. A child's day-care arrangements should be part of every history.

b. Day-care attendance (e.g., Who cares for the child? Where? For how many hours each day? Are there other children present?) should be documented for the following presenting complaints/diagnoses:

(1) Sepsis (contacts may need prophylaxis)

(2)   Meningitis (contacts may need prophylaxis)
(3)   Epiglottitis (contacts may need prophylaxis)
(4)   Streptococcal pharyngitis (contacts with pharyngitis need evaluation)
(5)   Otitis media (recurrent)
(6)   Bacterial diarrhea (contacts may need evaluation)
(7)   Food poisoning (ill contacts need evaluation)
(8)   Hepatitis (contacts may need prophylaxis)
(9)   Lice (contacts need observation)
(10) Scabies (contacts need observation)
(11) Pinworms (contacts need observation)
(12) HSV-1 (contacts with skin lesions need evaluation)
(13) Impetigo (contacts with skin lesions need evaluation)
(14) Tinea (contacts with skin lesions need evaluation)
(15) Chicken pox (contacts with skin lesions need evaluation)
(16) Conjunctivitis (symptomatic contacts need evaluation)
(17) Injury that is poorly explained or does not fit the description given
(18) Question of abuse (physical, sexual, emotional)

Note: In items 1 through 16, contacts include infants, children, teens, and adults.

c.   Entities such as pneumonia, sinusitis, croup, and bronchiolitis may also be related to day-care attendance. URI and GE are common in day-care settings.

5.   Dermatologic conditions

a.   If a child has an acute or chronic skin condition that is infectious, provide this information in writing to the child-care facility or school. Because child-care and school personnel encounter many children with undefined rashes, they often err on the conservative side and exclude any child with a rash until they are reassured that it is not contagious.

b.   Although skin conditions have been discussed in Chapter 5, the common conditions listed in Table 19-1 may warrant exclusion from school.

6.   Giftedness

a.   The definition of *giftedness* includes general intellectual ability, specific academic aptitude, the ability for creative thinking, leadership ability, psychomotor ability, and the ability to excel in the visual or performing arts. Obviously, few individuals possess all of these gifts. However, the definition is important because it highlights the fact that giftedness is not merely having a high IQ.

b.   When parents perceive that their children are gifted, they may knowingly or unknowingly place demands on them. Some parents may be overly critical, overly dominating, overly conscientious, or overly directive.

c.   The parental behaviors listed in Point b may cause a gifted child to become perfectionistic (fear of failure), overly controlling, overly frustrated with his or her own abilities, or overly demanding of others to

TABLE 19-1			
COMMON DERMATOLOGIC CONDITIONS			
Spread	Incubation	Infectious Period	Exclusion
HEAD LICE			
Head-to-head	17-25 days	When viable nits are present	Until 24 hr after therapy or as long as viable ova remain
HERPES			
Direct contact	3-5 days	Up to 3 wk (without acyclovir)	Until all cutaneous lesions are scabbed
IMPETIGO			
Direct contact, fomites	1-10 days	As long as draining/weepy lesions are present	As long as draining lesions are present or until 24 hr of therapy (streptococcus) or 48 hr of therapy (staphylococcus)
SCABIES			
Human-to-human	14-17 days	As long as mites are present	Until 24 hr after therapy
TINEA			
Direct contact, fomites	2-3 wk for obvious lesions	Months to years if untreated	None once therapy is started; remember, scalp lesions require *oral* therapy
WARTS			
Direct contact	1-20 mo (usually 4 mo)	Months to years	None, but try to cover warts

       meet his or her expectations. If they are bored, gifted children may also act out in class and disrupt other students who are trying to learn at their own pace.

d.   Medical providers should encourage the parent(s) of a child who appears gifted to discuss class placement with the teacher. If the child becomes disruptive when bored, additional challenging assignments can perhaps be provided. Medical providers should caution parents to treat their gifted children age appropriately and not as small adults. Just because a child is gifted intellectually or artistically does not mean that he or she is emotionally mature for his or her age. Although parents should be encouraged to stimulate their children's abilities, every activity need not be stimulating. Gifted children need to relax too.

e.   Referral for counseling might be in a gifted child's best interest if the child appears to be under enormous stress to succeed (whether imposed internally or externally), disruptive, or without friends.

7.   Immunizations

a.   All children should be current-for-age on their immunizations at the time they enter child care or school. This information should be documented on the proper form for their jurisdiction. Any religious exemption or medical contraindication for one or more immunizations should be clearly documented.

b. Some jurisdictions require a second MMR upon entry into elementary school; others require it upon entry to middle school. Follow the laws in your area when considering when to immunize your patients.

8. Infectious illnesses

a. Most of the conditions listed in Table 19-2 are discussed in greater detail elsewhere in this book.

b. Special considerations should be taken when an ill child is in child care, preschool, or the early elementary grades, or if the child lacks control of body secretions/excretions.

9. Learning problems

A number of reasons determine why some children do not succeed in school or do not work to their capacity. Some of these reasons are outlined as follows:

a. School readiness

(1) Although most children are ready to begin kindergarten at age 5, others are ready at age 4, and still others are not ready until 6 or 7 years of age. The result of starting a child in school too early may be sub-par performance or outright failure, which leads to retention in a given grade. Reasons such as poor grade achievement, young chronologic age, social immaturity, behavior problems, delayed physical development, and parental wishes are given for a student's failure to be promoted. Generally, retained students are more likely to be younger for their grade, male, and of lower socioeconomic status. Children who were of low birth weight, malnourished in early life, or exposed to drugs, alcohol, or cigarettes in utero are more likely to fail a grade. Children whose families are not supportive of education are also less likely to succeed in school.

(2) Helpful information for the medical provider includes observations from the child's preschool experience. For example, how does the child compare with his or her peers in child care? Can the child attend to tasks well, or is he or she easily distracted? How does the child get along with other children? How does he or she handle frustrations or learn new tasks? Medical providers can also screen a child by using the Denver Developmental Screening Test, Preschool Readiness Experimental Screening Scale, or Sprigle School Readiness Screening Test. If on these screens a child does not demonstrate the skills needed for school success, he or she should receive a full evaluation by a psychologist or developmental pediatrician. If a specific disability is detected (e.g., speech delay), a referral should be made to a specialist in that area (e.g., speech therapist). Remedial and developmentally appropriate approaches are preferable to retention in the hope that another year will help the child "catch on."

Text continued on p. 335

TABLE 19-2

INFECTIOUS ILLNESSES

Spread	Incubation	Infectious Period	Exclusion
ADENOVIRAL INFECTIONS			
Respiratory droplets, fecal-oral	2-14 days	Respiratory illness, 2-8 days; GI illness, 0-8 days; conjunctivitis, 14 days	Respiratory illness, none; diarrheal illness, until no further diarrhea; conjunctivitis, 14 days
CAMPYLOBACTER ORGANISMS			
Fecal-oral, contaminated water	1-7 days, usually 2-4 days	2-3 days after onset of therapy; if no therapy, 5-7 wk	Until 2 days after initiation of antibiotics or until no longer symptomatic
CHLAMYDIA TRACHOMATIS			
Vertical only	5-14 days (conjunctivitis), 14-60 days (pneumonia)	None (no horizontal transmission)	None
CORONAVIRUS			
Respiratory, aerosols	2-3 days	Several days	None
COXSACKIEVIRUS A16 (HAND-FOOT-AND-MOUTH DISEASE)			
Fecal-oral, oral-oral	4-6 days	Weeks	None
CRYPTOSPORIDIA			
Fecal-oral, including fomites and contaminated water	5-10 days	2-5 wk or 2 wk after cessation of therapy	Until asymptomatic
CYTOMEGALOVIRUS			
Contact with urine or saliva	1 mo	6-24 mo	None
ENTEROBIUS VERMICULARIS (PINWORM)			
Ingestion of eggs	2-8 wk	As long as adult worms are present	Until properly treated

Continued

19

SCHOOL HEALTH ISSUES

TABLE 19-2—cont'd

INFECTIOUS ILLNESSES—cont'd

Spread	Incubation	Infectious Period	Exclusion
ENTEROVIRUS			
Fecal-oral, oral-oral	7-14 days	Weeks	None, except children with poliovirus, who should be excluded until no further symptoms are present
GIARDIA LAMBLIA			
Fecal-oral, including fomites	1-4wk	Up to 12-14 mo (as long as cysts are excreted)	With completion of therapy and when no further diarrhea is present
HAEMOPHILUS INFLUENZAE			
Respiratory	Within 60 days (classroom)	Until 24 hr after initiation of parenteral therapy (invasive disease)	Until well and after receiving oral rifampin
HEPATITIS A			
Fecal-oral	15-50 days	Until 10 days after onset of dark urine	At least 10 days after onset of dark urine
HEPATITIS B			
Percutaneous, permucosal	6-24 mo	As long as surface antigen-positive	None
INFECTIOUS MONONUCLEOSIS			
Oral-oral, saliva	5-7 wk	Weeks-months	1-2 wk or longer depending on child's degree of illness
INFLUENZA (FLU)			
Respiratory	1-3 days	1-10 days	Until asymptomatic
MENINGOCOCCUS			
Respiratory, oral-oral	2 days to several weeks	Until at least 1 day after initiation of therapy; remember carrier state	Until asymptomatic

MUMPS			
Respiratory	12-25 days (usually 16-18 days)	From 1 week before to 9 days after symptoms	Until 9 days after onset of parotid swelling
MYCOPLASMA PNEUMONIAE			
Respiratory	2-3 wk	As long as cough is present	Until child is no longer ill
PARAINFLUENZA VIRUSES			
Respiratory, direct contact	3-6 days	3-16 days	Until child is no longer ill
HUMAN PARVOVIRUS B19 (FIFTH DISEASE)			
Respiratory, direct contact	4-14 days	1-3 days before onset of rash	None
PNEUMOCOCCAL DISEASE			
Respiratory	Up to 1 mo	Carrier state	Until child is no longer ill
RESPIRATORY SYNCYTIAL VIRUS			
Respiratory, including fomites	3-7 days	Before symptoms and for 1-3 wk; older children 3-7 days	Until child is no longer ill
RHINOVIRUSES (COMMON COLD)			
Respiratory, including fomites; direct contact	1-2 days	3 wk or as long as nasal symptoms are present	None
ROSEOLA			
Not fully known	5-15 days	Not fully known	Until rash is resolved and child is well
ROTAVIRAL INFECTION			
Fecal-oral, including fomites	1-3 days	Usually 4-5 days	Until no longer vomiting or having diarrhea
RUBELLA			
Respiratory, direct contact	14-21 days	From 5 days before to 7 days after onset of illness	At least 7 days after onset of rash

Continued

19

SCHOOL HEALTH ISSUES

TABLE 19-2—cont'd

INFECTIOUS ILLNESSES—cont'd

Spread	Incubation	Infectious Period	Exclusion
RUBEOLA			
Respiratory, direct contact	10-12 days	Until onset of rash	Until 5 days after onset of rash
SALMONELLA ORGANISMS			
Contaminated food	6-72 hr	Months	Until no further diarrhea
SHIGELLA ORGANISMS			
Fecal-oral, including fomites	12-48 hr (usually)	1-4 days (treated), 7-30 days without treatment	Until 5 days of antibiotics or two successive negative stool cultures
STAPHYLOCOCCAL DISEASE			
Direct contact, fomites	1-10 days (usually)	As long as lesions drain	As long as lesions drain or until at least 48 hr of antibiotics
STREPTOCOCCAL DISEASE			
Direct contact, respiratory spread	12-96 hr (pharyngitis), 10 days (impetigo)	Up to 2 wk	Until at least 24 hr after start of antibiotics and afebrile
TUBERCULOSIS			
Respiratory	2-10 wk	None in young children	None, unless draining wounds; however, children need to be receiving therapy
VARICELLA			
Respiratory, direct contact	10-21 days	Until all skin lesions have crusted or until 7 days after onset	Until pox are scabbed; if zoster, exclude if lesions cannot be covered; otherwise child can attend school
YERSINIA ORGANISMS			
Fecal-oral, contaminated food or water	2-11 days (usually)	Weeks, even with antibiotic therapy	As long as child has diarrhea

b. School placement
  (1) Public law 94-142 mandates that children be educated in the least restrictive environment. For many children with disabilities, this goal is realistic. Sometimes it is in a child's best interest to be educated in a facility that is somewhat more restrictive if that degree of restriction helps him or her to learn and interact with others.
  (2) Some children who have less severe problems might be able to remain in a regular classroom; sometimes special seating is all that is needed for the child to work more optimally toward his or her potential. Other children can remain in a regular classroom with the understanding that they will receive special instruction geared to their disability once or twice a week. Other students might remain in their regular classes but require daily special instruction.
  (3) Children with ADD/ADHD may benefit from special seating, special instruction, medication, behavioral modification, or a combination of these four techniques. Children with physical impairments should be handled on a case-by-case basis; some are best served in regular schools, whereas the physical impairments of others are so severe that they require special environments. The same is true of children with chronic medical conditions who experience periodic exacerbations. Placement in regular classes is generally preferred, but such children may need home (or hospital) teaching during periods of exacerbation. Also falling under this classification would be children with infectious conditions such as TB, AIDS, and hepatitis, especially if the child has oozing skin lesions or biting behaviors (AIDS and hepatitis B).
  (4) Children with severe emotional problems may benefit from inclusion in schools developed especially for them, where the staff is trained to manage such children optimally, and environments are planned to minimize the occurrence of physical injuries when the children lose control.
c. School failure
  (1) Even the best of efforts does not permit all children to smoothly progress from one grade to another. Sometimes it is in the child's best interest to remain in a grade.
  (2) The medical provider should fully evaluate every child who fails a grade, especially if the child previously was a good or adequate student. In this evaluation, the usual histories (perinatal, medical, developmental, family, and social) are solicited. The child's academic history is also reviewed (e.g., academic achievement, global or specific problem areas, classroom behavior, school attendance, special school services provided, and any psychoeducational testing).

19

SCHOOL HEALTH ISSUES

(3) The examination should be complete and should particularly highlight the child's emotional state, intellectual functioning (with the examiner), neurologic examination, and sensory examination. Vision and hearing should be tested. Any skin markings that might indicate an underlying neurologic abnormality (e.g., café au lait spots, hypopigmented macules) should be noted in addition to the child's level of puberty. A simple mental status examination (e.g., asking the child for three wishes or asking the child to draw himself or herself or his or her family) may yield useful information about the child's mental state.

(4) Neurodevelopmental testing such as the Pediatric Early Elementary Examination test may disclose problems in the way a child functions in different areas of development. Neurodevelopmental testing is best performed by a pediatrician with expertise in this area. A full psychoeducational evaluation is crucial in understanding the interplay of emotions, intellect, and learning style/problems in a particular child.

(5) The child who fails usually experiences a diminution in self-esteem; family members may contribute to this feeling. Consideration should be given to individual or family counseling if the medical provider senses that the child and/or family is coping poorly with the school failure.

d. Language disorders
   (1) Language disorders include difficulty in word comprehension, difficulty in oral language production and use, and difficulty in expression or sound production (e.g., stuttering).
   (2) Referral to a speech pathologist as soon as a disability is discovered gives the child the best chance for optimal learning and coping with his or her deficit.

e. Mathematical disabilities
   (1) In this society the ability to use numbers meaningfully is important, not only for scientists and computer operators but also for all individuals who must handle their finances or shop wisely in a store. Hence, children who are "no good at math" are at a serious disadvantage for learning to operate optimally in society. Depending on the severity of the disability, such students may require the services of a number of professionals or only math tutoring. To optimize the child's educational potential, such assistance should be provided as soon as the disability is discovered.
   (2) It is important not to accept parental explanations for poor math performance such as "I've never been any good at math; why should she be any different?" or "Girls are not supposed to be good at math." Parents should be counseled not to encourage self-fulfilling prophecies for their child's educational failure. The fact that a parent did not excel at a given subject does not mean

that his or her child will share the same fate. The gender of the child does not necessarily predict the subjects in which a child will excel or fail.

f. Dyslexia

    (1) Even more critical than the ability to compute is the ability to read. Between 5% and 15% of school-aged children have dyslexia (reading disability), with boys outnumbering girls by a ratio of 2:1. Although a complete review of the literature on dyslexia is beyond the scope of this text, it is important to note that a variety of etiologies are suggested. A variety of neuropsychological tests are used to assess dyslexia and are usually performed by a specialist in the field, who should be consulted as early as possible.

    (2) It is important for the medical provider to perform a PE, with special attention given to the neurologic examination. "Soft" neurologic signs, as well as the "hard" signs of deficiencies or asymmetries of appearance or function, must be noted and reported.

g. Attention deficit disorder/attention deficit hyperactivity disorder

    (1) *ADD* implies a short attention span, whereas *ADHD* implies a degree of hyperactivity in association with the short attention span. Between 3% and 5% of children have ADD; 80% of boys and 50% of girls with ADD are hyperactive.

    (2) The hallmarks of ADD/ADHD are inattention, impulsivity, and hyperactivity. The 14 historical criteria listed in Table 19-3 are used to assess whether a child truly has ADD/ADHD; to meet these diagnoses, a child must have 8 of the 14 symptoms for at least 6 months.

TABLE 19-3

CRITERIA FOR ADD/ADHD

1. Often fidgets with hands or feet or squirms in seat
2. Has difficulty remaining seated when required to do so
3. Easily distracted by external stimuli
4. Has difficulty waiting for his or her turn
5. Blurts out answer before the question is completed
6. Has difficulty following through on instructions
7. Has difficulty sustaining attention in tasks or play
8. Shifts from one uncompleted activity to another
9. Has difficulty playing quietly
10. Talks excessively
11. Interrupts or intrudes on others' activities
12. Does not listen to what is said to him or her
13. Loses things necessary for tasks or activities
14. Engages in physically dangerous activities without considering the possible consequences

SCHOOL HEALTH ISSUES

19

TABLE 19-4
NEUROLOGIC SIGNS OF ADD/ADHD
1. Arms drop or spread when extended
2. Arms drop or spread when head is rotated
3. Hopping or one-foot stand that is too short
4. Finger- or foot-tapping that is too slow
5. Choreiform movements
6. Excessive associated and mirror movements
7. Finger-nose-finger dysmetria
8. Inadequate or sloppy tandem gait
9. Disdiadochokinesia
10. Inadequate ability to imitate finger movements
11. Finger agnosia
12. Double simultaneous stimulation-extinction
13. Head movement with extraocular muscle movement
14. Strabismus or inability to converge
15. Inadequate hold of lateral gaze
16. Grimace/inability to raise brow
17. Irregular tongue waggle
18. Slow speed of speech repeating

(3) The PE may be normal except for the neurologic component; especially important is the detection of certain neurologic signs (Table 19-4). Although these signs may be normal in a younger child, they are not normal as a child matures. Not every child with ADD/ADHD has all of these signs, but most have a majority of them when carefully evaluated.

(4) Several interventions can be tried if the history and PE point to a diagnosis of ADD or ADHD and include special educational interventions, behavior therapies, individual and family counseling, and medication. Medications should be used *only* in those children whose history and/or physical parameters meet the criteria of ADD/ADHD.

(a) Stimulants are the most widely used medications for ADD/ADHD in the United States; they are effective for at least 75% of the children who meet the diagnostic criteria for ADD or ADHD. They improve most levels of functioning but may be associated with a number of side-effects such as anorexia/weight loss, insomnia/nightmares, irritability or moodiness/agitation, growth impairment, and others. An alteration of the dose or its timing (especially in response to meals) or a switch to an intermediate-acting or long-acting rather than a short-acting preparation usually resolves most of these side-effects. In some cases, however, a medication may need to be discontinued. Medications used in the treatment of attention-deficit/hyperactivity disorder are shown in Table 19-5.

TABLE 19-5
MEDICATIONS USED IN THE TREATMENT OF ATTENTION-DEFICIT/HYPERACTIVITY DISORDER

Generic Class (Brand Name)	Daily Dosage Schedule	Duration	Prescribing Schedule
STIMULANTS (FIRST-LINE TREATMENT)			
Methylphenidate			
Short-acting (Ritalin, Methylin)	Twice a day (BID) to 3 times a day (TID)	3-5 hr	5-20 mg BID to TID
Intermediate-acting (Ritalin SR, Metadate ER, Methylin ER)	Once a day (QD) to BID	3-8 hr	20-40 mg QD or 40 mg in the morning and 20 mg early afternoon
Long-acting (Concerta, Metadate CD, Ritalin LA*)	QD	8-12 hr	18-72 mg QD
Amphetamine			
Short-acting (Dexedrine, Dextrostat)	BID to TID	4-6 hr	5-15 mg BID or 5-10 mg TID
Intermediate-acting (Adderall, Dexedrine spansule)	QD to BID	6-8 hr	5-30 mg QD or 5-15 mg BID
Long-acting (Adderall-XR*)	QD		10-30 mg QD
ANTIDEPRESSANTS (SECOND-LINE TREATMENT)			
Tricyclics (TCAs) Imipramine, Desipramine	BID to TID		2-5 mg/kg/day+
Bupropion (Wellbutrin)	QD to TID		50-100 mg TID
(Wellbutrin SR)	BID		100-150 mg BID

*Not FDA approved at time of publication.
+Prescribing and monitoring information in *Physicians' Desk Reference.*

19

SCHOOL HEALTH ISSUES

(b) All drugs should be increased, when necessary, in careful increments. Look for *any* side-effects with a clear understanding among parents, school, and the medical provider that there may be a tradeoff between an "acceptable" effect and the side-effects of the drug. If a lower dose is better tolerated but does not quite produce "perfect" results, all concerned may need to live with such results. Children who fail to show positive effects or who experience intolerable side effects on one stimulant medication should be tried on another of the recommended stimulant medications. Lack of response should also lead the clinician to assess the accuracy of the diagnosis and the possibility of undiagnosed coexisting conditions.

h. School phobia

(1) School phobia, also known as school refusal or school avoidance, is defined as a child's refusal to go to school or a refusal to stay in school for emotional reasons. Approximately 5% of elementary school students and 2% of middle school students have this disorder.

(2) There are two types of school phobia

(a) Anxiety-related type: The child is worried about something at home or school. There is a persistence of the separation anxiety that most children master by 3 to 4 years of age. There is overdependence on the parent(s), who tend(s) to be child oriented and concerned about the child experiencing too much stress in life. The children are excellent students. Girls outnumber boys.

(b) Secondary-gain type: There are few anxiety symptoms. Children with this type of school phobia tend to have had an illness for which they had to stay home and for which they received much sympathy and attention. The parent of this type of student is often lenient and does not value education. The children are average-to-poor students. Boys outnumber girls.

(3) Although *any* symptom can be associated with this disorder, the most common ones are headaches (real or feigned), abdominal pain, diarrhea, vomiting, chest pains, palpitations, dizziness, hyperventilation, and a "sore throat." The child with the anxiety-related type tends to have physiologic symptoms such as diarrhea, whereas the child with the secondary-gain type has a "sore throat," "fever" (often self-induced), or other symptoms that are hard to verify objectively.

(4) The following criteria are essential when faced with a student in whom a diagnosis of school phobia is being considered:

(a) Recurrent, often vague, physical symptoms

(b) No physical cause found on careful (sometimes repeated) examinations

(c) Symptoms that predominate in the mornings of school days and are virtually absent on weekends, school holidays, and summer vacation

(d) More than 5 days of school missed because of *this* problem

(5) A complete history is essential and requires not just the usual items. Also investigate events that may be precipitating the phobia such as a change of school, family stress (parental discord, separation, divorce, death, remarriage, birth of sibling, death of sibling), a recent move, academic stress (fear of "failure," even in a bright child), or stress at school (teacher-child mismatch, difficulties with peers, unsafe school environment, or unsafe journey to school). The following items are essential for an adequate evaluation:

(a) Type, duration, frequency, timetable of symptoms; age of onset; parent's idea of cause; feared medical diagnosis (e.g., "What is the worst thing this could be?"); previous evaluation or treatment

(b) Days absent this year and last year, days late, days sent home, parental attitudes about staying home from school, what the child does and where he or she stays when absent

(c) Change in school; difficulties with school work, teacher(s), classmates, other students; problems on school bus or with traveling to school

(d) Peer relations, both at and outside of school

(e) Family relations, stresses, illnesses

(f) Impressions from school nurse (if present) and teacher regarding the child's difficulties/absenteeism

(6) The PE should be complete; except for minor abnormalities, it is invariably normal. The normalcy of the examination should be highlighted for the parent(s) *and* child.

(7) Keep laboratory tests to a minimum; order only those that will contribute to your impression. A "million dollar" workup is unnecessary and leads both the parent and child into thinking that there is a real physical problem present.

(8) In considering the diagnosis of school phobia, keep in mind that there are other reasons for school absenteeism, such as parental overresponse to minor illnesses, chronic physical disease or learning disability with poor adaptation, truancy, depression, psychosis, substance abuse (child or parent), pregnancy, family dysfunction, child abuse (child must stay home until bruises are healed), and the need for one child to "baby-sit" a younger child while the parent works or runs errands.

(9) When fairly certain of the diagnosis of school phobia, explain to the parent(s) what the condition is (and is not), that it is not associated with a hidden physical disease, that the child has normal physical findings and laboratory tests (if ordered), that school phobia occurs in normal children with normal parents, and that the condition can be treated.

(10) Treatment consists of enlisting parental support in handling the matter firmly (e.g., insisting that if the child is ill enough to stay home from school, he or she needs to be seen by the medical provider, who will send the child to school if the examination is normal). The medical provider should also spend time with the child, sympathizing when appropriate (with the anxious child) and being firm when appropriate (with the secondary-gain child). Children must be told that it is the law that they attend school and that it is the responsibility of parents and medical providers to help them adjust to and thrive in school. The child's teacher, principal, and school nurse (if available) need to be part of the process. In general, drug therapy has no role in the treatment of school phobia.

(11) The following children should be referred to a child psychiatrist or psychologist:
   (a) Psychotic children
   (b) Depressed children
   (c) Children incapacitated by fear
   (d) Children of parents who exhibit symbiotic parent-child relations
   (e) Children requiring psychoactive drug therapy
   (f) Adolescents
   (g) Children whose physical disease has necessitated prolonged bed rest
   (h) Children/families unresponsive to counseling

(12) If parents deliberately keep children out of school, a referral to child protective services is in order.

10. Sports
   a. There are two main issues facing the medical provider in terms of school-related sports activities: the preparticipation physical assessment and the treatment of sports-related injuries.
   b. In considering the suitability of a given sport for a given student, considerations of the type of sport and the student's health history are crucial. Sports are classified into contact/collision (e.g., football), limited contact (e.g., baseball), and noncontact (e.g., swimming). Noncontact sports can be further subdivided into strenuous (e.g., aerobics), moderately strenuous (e.g., table tennis), and nonstrenuous (e.g., golf).
   c. Some students should not be permitted to engage in collision or strenuous sports because of their health history. For example, a child

with psychomotor seizures should not be permitted to engage in contact or strenuous sports; a child with an enlarged liver or spleen should not be permitted to engage in contact/collision/impact sports; a child with a history of two or more concussions (or even one depending on its severity) should avoid contact/collision/impact sports. The American Academy of Pediatrics has produced an exhaustive list of medical conditions and acceptable sports participation (see Bibliography).

d. The history obtained at the preparticipation assessment should ascertain whether any of the following are present: chronic or recurrent illness; illnesses lasting more than 1 week; hospitalizations/surgeries; missing or enlarged organs; cardiovascular problems; allergies; chest pain or dizziness with exercise; problems with heat; concussion, unconsciousness, or seizure either associated or unassociated with exercise or sports activity; medication use; eyeglasses use; dental appliance in place; history of injuries such as neck, knee, ankle, back, and shoulder; and a family history of early death or early heart attack.

e. The preparticipation examination should be complete and should particularly highlight the following areas: vision, hearing, chest examination with particular attention to adventitial breath sounds and cardiac sounds and rhythms, neurologic examination, and musculoskeletal examination. The examiner is looking for current and potential "trouble spots" that could lead to the disability or death of the young athlete.

f. Once the student begins his or her athletic career, the best way to prevent injuries is through proper conditioning, proper management of injuries, use of protective equipment, and matching of athletes. Proper nutrition must be stressed; inappropriate dieting must be avoided. The use of anabolic steroids must be strongly discouraged. Students with a history of heat-related illnesses should not compete or practice outdoors during hot weather.

g. The management of moderate to severe sports injuries should be left to specialists. Unfortunately, it is sometimes difficult to separate minor injuries from more serious ones. The classic RICE (Rest, Ice, Compression, Elevation) is a useful therapy for the first 72 hours.

(1) Resting the injured area is important because movement can encourage further bleeding into the tissue. It is very difficult for a young athlete to "lay off" a leg or not use an arm, because he or she really wants to participate. If an injured athlete must get around (e.g., to class), crutches or inflatable splints can be used, but rest is preferable. Further evaluation and treatment may be needed if pain, swelling, or tenderness persists after 3 days.

(2) Ice therapy is excellent and needs to be applied as soon as possible after the injury. It causes diminution of pain by slowing down nerve impulses and muscle spasms in the area. It causes vasoconstriction, which leads to decreased bleeding into the

tissue and less edema. Finally, fewer cells break down because of lessened oxygen demand. Ice needs to be applied during the first 48 hours after an injury for approximately 20 minutes tid or qid.

(3) Compression is used to decrease edema. Edema prevents cold therapy from reaching deeper levels, interferes with normal joint movement (and thus increases the need for rehabilitation), and can keep torn tissue ends apart so that scar tissue replaces the injured tissue. Elastic bandage compression is an excellent means of limiting edema.

(4) Elevation of an injured limb reduces the hydrostatic pressure that drives plasma into the interstitium and decreases the amount of edema by encouraging lymphatic drainage.

(5) Analgesics may be needed if pain is moderate or severe. Aspirin should be avoided because it prolongs bleeding time, which makes it more likely that further bleeding into the injured area will occur. Acetaminophen and ibuprofen are better choices for analgesics.

(6) When in doubt about a sports injury, ask for help. Have a low threshold for ordering x-ray studies, especially if there is marked swelling, marked tenderness, hemarthrosis, or deformity. Order AP and lateral views and, in the case of long bones, views of the joint above and below the injured area. *Always* review the films with a radiologist if the injury is severe or if the patient has marked symptoms but the x-ray study looks negative.

C. BIBLIOGRAPHY

School Health

AAP Committee on School Health: Do not resuscitate orders in schools, *Pediatrics* 105:878, 2000.

AAP Committee on School Health: Guidelines for urgent care in school, *Pediatrics* 86:999, 1990.

AAP Committee on School Health: School health assessments, *Pediatrics* 105:875, 2000.

Children with health impairments in schools, *Pediatrics* 86:636, 1990.

Dworkin P: School failure, *Pediatr in Rev* 10:301, 1986.

Robinson J: Infectious diseases in schools and child-care facilities, *Pediatr in Rev* 22:39, 2001.

Giftedness

Jaffe A: The gifted child, *Pediatr in Rev* 21:240, 2000.

Robinson N, Olszewski-Kubilius P: Gifted and talented children—issues for pediatricians, *Pediatr in Rev* 17:427, 1996.

Learning Disorders

Bashin A et al: Language disorders in childhood and adolescence, *Pediatr Ann* 16:145, 1987.

Capin D: Developmental learning disorders—clues to their diagnosis and management, *Pediatr in Rev* 17:284, 1996.

Garnett K, Fleischner J: Mathematical disabilities, *Pediatr Ann* 16:159, 1987.

Gottesman R, Kelly M: Helping children with learning disabilities toward a brighter adulthood, *Contemp Pediatr* 17:42, 2000.

Nass R: Developmental dyslexia, *Pediatr in Rev* 13:231, 1992.

School Readiness, Placement, Failure

Bonny A, Britto M, Klostermann B et al: School disconnectedness—identifying adolescents at risk, *Pediatrics* 106:1017, 2000.

Casey P, Evans L: School readiness: an overview for pediatricians, *Pediatr in Rev* 14:4, 1993.

Attention Deficit Disorder/Attention Deficit Hyperactivity Disorder

AAP Subcommittee on Attention-Deficit/Hyperactivity Disorder; Committee on Quality Improvement: Clinical Practice Guideline: Treatment of the school-aged child with attention-deficit/hyperactivity disorder, *Pediatrics* 108:1033, 2001.

Culbert T et al: Children who have attentional disorders: interventions, *Pediatr in Rev* 15:5, 1994.

Hunt R, Paguin A, Payton K: An update on assessment and treatment of complex attention-deficit hyperactivity disorder, *Pediatr Ann* 30:162, 2001.

Miller K, Castellanos FX: Attention deficit/hyperactivity disorders, *Pediatr in Rev* 19:373, 1998.

Reiff M et al: Children who have attentional disorders: diagnosis and evaluation, *Pediatr in Rev* 14:455, 1993.

Schmitt B: The child with a short attention span (ADD), *Contemp Pediatr* 9:57, 1993.

Wender E: Managing stimulant medication for attention-deficit hyperactivity disorder, *Pediatr in Rev* 22:183, 2001.

Sports

AAP Committee on Sports Medicine and Fitness: Medical conditions affecting sports participation, *Pediatrics* 107:1205, 2001.

AAP Committee on Sports Medicine and Fitness, Committee on School Health: Physical fitness and activity in schools, *Pediatrics* 105:1156, 2000.

Andrews J: Making the most of the sports physical, *Contemp Pediatr* 14:183, 1997.

Berul C: Cardiac evaluation of the young athlete, *Pediatr Ann* 29:162, 2000.

Hergenroeder A: Prevention of sports injuries, *Pediatrics* 101:1057, 1998.

Huurman W, Ginsburg G: Musculoskeletal injury in children, *Pediatr in Rev* 18:429, 1997.

Luke A, Mitchell L: Sports injuries—emergency assessment and field-side care, *Pediatr in Rev* 20:291, 1999.

Metzl J: Preparticipation examination of the adolescent athlete, part 1, *Pediatr in Rev* 22:199, 2001.

Metzl J: Preparticipation examination of the adolescent athlete, part 2, *Pediatr in Rev* 22:227, 2001.

Perriello V, Barth J: Sports concussions—coming to the right conclusions, *Contemp Pediatr* 17:132, 2000.

Rome E: Sports-related injuries among adolescents—when do they occur and how can we prevent them? *Pediatr in Rev* 16:184, 1995.

Szer I: Musculoskeletal pain syndromes that affect adolescents, *Arch Pediatr Adolesc Med* 150:740, 1996.

19

SCHOOL HEALTH ISSUES

SEXUALLY TRANSMITTED DISEASES

A. GENERAL

The clinical presentation may include urethritis; vulvovaginitis, cervicitis, or dysuria in women; ulcerations on the penis, vulva, or vagina; inguinal lymphadenopathy; PID; epididymitis; proctitis; pharyngitis; arthritis; rash; and conjunctivitis. However, many individuals are asymptomatic. At least 20 different causative microorganisms are now recognized (bacteria, viruses, fungi, protozoa, arthropods). Some of these microorganisms are listed in the sections that follow.

20

B. GONORRHEA

1. May be seen at any age; suspect sexual abuse if prepubertal.
2. May be asymptomatic (more than 50% of females, 25% of males).
3. Culture cervix, urethra, pharynx, rectum, and inflamed joint if the index of suspicion is high.
4. Diagnosis
   a. Gram's stain showing greater than 8 gram-negative intracellular diplococci (more reliable on urethral swab of male; less reliable on endocervical swab of female). Confirm with culture.
   b. Send specimen to laboratory for culture immediately.
5. Screen for syphilis (VDRL, STS) on all patients suspected of having gonococcal infection. Consider other sexually transmitted infections (e.g., HSV, *Chlamydia, Trichomonas*).
6. Treatment (current recommendations reflect the increase in penicillinase-producing strains)
   a. Asymptomatic and uncomplicated gonorrhea infections (vaginitis, cervicitis, urethritis, proctitis, pharyngitis); patient weight greater than 45 kg
      (1) Cefixime 400 mg PO once (only advantage is oral dosing c/w ceftriaxone) *or*
      (2) Ceftriaxone 125 mg IM once *or*
      (3) Ciprofloxacin 500 mg PO once *or*
      (4) Ofloxacin 400 mg PO once
          plus
          Azithromycin 1 g PO once *or*
      (5) Doxycycline 100 mg PO bid × 7 days
      (6) Other alternatives
          (a) Spectinomycin 2 g IM (covers rectal, urethral, and cervical gonococcal infections) *or*
          (b) Ceftizoxime 1 g IM once *or*
          (c) Cefotaxime 500 mg IM once *or*
          (d) Cefotetan 1 g IM once *or*
          (e) Cefoxitin 2 g IM once with probenicid 1g PO *or*

          (f) Enoxacin 400 mg PO; lomefloxacin 400 mg PO; *or* norfloxacin 800 mg PO

    (7) None of these regimens treat *Chlamydia*. Always treat for *Chlamydia* when treating for gonococcal infection.

    (8) Prepubertal children (less than 45 kg)

          (a) Ceftriaxone 125 mg IM once; ceftriaxone 50 mg/kg (maximum 1 g) IM or IV qd × 7 days for bacteremia or arthritis. Increase to maximum of 2 g/d × 10 to 14 days for meningitis *or*

          (b) Spectinomycin 40 mg/kg (maximum 2 g) IM once

Note: **Follow-up culture is *mandatory*. Obtain it approximately 1 week after treatment is completed. Do not forget to treat contacts and to cover for *Chlamydia*.**

  b. Disseminated gonococcal infection: Symptoms include dermatitis, arthralgias, arthritis, and tenosynovitis

    (1) Ceftriaxone 1 g IM or IV qd *or.*

    (2) Cefotaxime 1 g IV q8h *or.*

    (3) Ceftizoxime 1 g IV q8h *or.*

    (4) Ciprofloxacin 500 mg IV q12h or ofloxacin 400 mg IV q12h (if allergic to beta-lactams) *or.*

    (5) Spectinomycin 2 g IM q12h (if allergic to beta-lactams).

    (6) All regimens should be continued for 24 to 48 hours after improvement begins. Treatment is then changed to one of the following oral drugs to complete a full week of treatment. Always treat presumptively for *Chlamydia trachomatis*.

          (a) Cefixime 400 mg PO bid *or*

          (b) Ciprofloxacin 500 mg PO bid *or*

          (c) Ofloxacin 400 mg PO bid

  c. Gonococcal meningitis or endocarditis: Ceftriaxone 1 to 2 g IV q12h. Therapy for meningitis is continued for 14 days; therapy for endocarditis is continued for 4 weeks. Seek advise from the appropriate specialist.

C. PELVIC INFLAMMATORY DISEASE (SALPINGITIS)

1. Many women have mild or subtle symptoms that do not readily indicate PID. Fever occurs in only 33% of patients. Patients may have lower abdominal pain, vaginal discharge, irregular bleeding, and cervical motion/adnexal tenderness. Risk of subsequent sterility exists. Remove IUD if present.

2. Minimum criteria for the diagnosis of PID include.

  a. Lower abdominal tenderness

  b. Adnexal tenderness

  c. Cervical motion tenderness

3. Additional criteria that support the diagnosis of PID include:

  a. Oral temperature greater than 38.3° C

  b. Abnormal cervical or vaginal discharge

    c.   Elevated ESR

    d.   Elevated CRP

    e.   Laboratory documentation of infection with *N. gonorrhoeae* or *C. trachomatis*

4. Cause: Often polymicrobial. The most common pathogens are *Neisseria gonorrhoeae, C. trachomatis,* and anaerobic bacteria (most commonly *Peptostreptococcus, Peptococcus,* and *Bacteroides* organisms). Other organisms include *Mycoplasma hominis* and *Ureaplasma urealyticum.*

5. Hospitalize the patient in the following circumstances:

    a.   Surgical emergency (e.g., ectopic pregnancy, appendicitis) is to be ruled out.

    b.   Patient is pregnant.

    c.   Patient has not responded to oral therapy.

    d.   Patient cannot follow outpatient regimen (especially if significant nausea or vomiting is present), cannot tolerate PO medications, or cannot return for follow-up in 48 to 72 hours.

    e.   Severe illness (T greater than 38.3° C; WBCs greater than 20,000; nausea/vomiting).

    f.   There is high suspicion of a pelvic abscess or the presence of an adnexal mass.

    g.   Patient is immunodeficient (e.g., has HIV infection with low CD4 counts, is receiving immunosuppresant therapy).

    h.   Patient is an adolescent. This is controversial but is safe and ensures that the patient will begin treatment properly.

6. Treatment

    a.   Outpatient

        (1)   Ofloxacin 400mg PO bid × 14 days and metronidazole 500 mg bid × 14 days *or*

        (2)   Ceftriaxone 250 mg IM once *or*

        (3)   Cefoxitin 2 g IM once and probenecid 1 g PO once *or*

        (4)   Another parenteral third-generation cephalosporin (e.g., ceftizoxime or cefotaxime)

        (5)   *Ceftriaxone,* cefoxitin, and other third-generation cephalosporins should be followed by PO doxycycline 100 mg bid × 14 days which will also treat bacterial vaginosis

    b.   Inpatient (gynecologist should be consulted)

        (1)   Cefotetan 2 g IV q12h *or* Cefoxitin 2 g IV q6h, *plus* doxycycline 100 mg IV bid until improvement, followed by PO doxycycline 100 mg bid to complete 14-day course.

        (2)   Alternative is IV clindamycin 900 mg q8h *plus* gentamicin 2 mg/kg once, followed by gentamicin 1.5 mg/kg q8h until improvement, followed by PO doxycycline 100 mg PO bid or clindamycin 450 mg qid to complete 14-day course.

        (3)   Limited data support the use of other parenteral regimens.

20

SEXUALLY TRANSMITTED DISEASES

   c. Miscellaneous
      (1) Treat contacts.
      (2) Get follow-up culture.

D. FITZ-HUGH–CURTIS SYNDROME

With Fitz-Hugh–Curtis syndrome, infection extends from salpingitis to the capsule and outer surface of the liver. Consider the diagnosis if patient has RUQ pain, palpable liver, abnormal LFTs, or adnexal/cervical motion tenderness. Treatment is as listed in Section C, Point 6b.

E. CHLAMYDIA INFECTION

1. May be found in mixed infections
2. Presents with urethritis, cervicitis, salpingitis, Fitz-Hugh–Curtis syndrome in females, inguinal lymphadenopathy, epididymitis, proctitis in males; commonly asymptomatic
3. Diagnosis: Culture in specific media, MicroTrak (direct fluorescent staining), ELISA, endocervical Gram's stain greater than 30 WBCs per oil immersion field, in males greater than 10 WBCs/HPF in first 15 ml of void
4. Treatment
   a. Adults and adolescents (nonpregnant)
      (1) Azithromycin 1 g PO once *or*
      (2) Doxycycline 100 mg bid × 7 days (not in pregnancy) *or*
      (3) Erythromycin base 500 mg qid × 7 days *or*
      (4) Erythromycin ethylsuccinate 800 mg PO qid × 7 days *or*
      (5) Ofloxacin 300 mg PO bid × 7 days
   b. Pregnancy
      (1) Erythromycin base 500 mg PO qid × 7 days *or*
      (2) Amoxicillin 500 mg tid × 7 days *or*
      (3) Erythromycin base 250 mg PO qid × 14 days *or*
      (4) Erythromycin ethylsuccinate 800 mg PO qid × 7 days *or*
      (5) Erythromycin ethylsuccinate 400 mg PO qid × 14 days *or*
      (6) Azithromycin 1 g PO once
   c. Children weighing less than 45 kg: Erythromycin base 50 mg/kg/d ÷ qid (maximum 2 g/d) × 10 to 14 days
   d. Children weighing more than 45 kg, less than 8 years of age: Azithromycin 1 g PO once
   e. Children weighing more than 45 kg, more than 8 years of age: Azithromycin 1 g PO once or doxycycline 100 mg PO bid × 7 days
5. Treatment for conjunctivitis and pneumonia in infancy
   a. Erythromycin 50 mg/kg/d ÷ qid × 10 to 14 days
   b. Topical ophthalmic therapy not needed
6. Be sure to contact and treat all sexual partners of the patient (or parent in the case of neonatal chlamydia infection)

F. SYPHILIS

1. Forms
a. Congenital: Mucocutaneous lesions, "snuffles," rash, bone changes (painful pseudoparalysis, dactylitis), hepatosplenomegaly, lymphadenopathy, fever, anemia, FTT. Infants may not always manifest symptoms.
   (1) Infected infants may be seronegative if maternal infection was late in gestation.
   (2) Infants should be treated at birth if maternal treatment was inadequate, unknown, with drugs other than penicillin, or if adequate follow-up cannot be ensured.
   (3) Always examine CSF before treatment.
b. Acquired syphilis
   (1) Primary stage: Chancre detectable in adolescents and adults, less common in children
   (2) Secondary stage: Rash, condylomata lata

2. Evaluation
a. Obtain serologic tests for VDRL or RPR, followed by confirmation with FTA-ABS.
b. CSF: Protein, cell count, VDRL. Perform darkfield microscopy for spirochetes.
c. Scrape any mucosal and cutaneous lesion and perform darkfield microscopy.
d. Perform bone x-ray examination, LFTs, CXR, eye examination, and auditory brainstem response for congenital infection.

3. Treatment
a. Congenital syphilis
   (1) Crystalline penicillin G 50,000 U/kg/dose q12h × first 7 days of life, then q8h for another 3 to 7 days or penicillin G procaine 50,000 U/kg/d IM qd × 10 days.
   (2) If more than 1 day of therapy is missed, the entire course should be restarted.
   (3) If CSF is initially positive, reexamine CSF q6mo until normal. Repeat if CSF serologic test remains positive 6 months after first therapy, if the blood serologic test remains positive 1 year after treatment, or if there is a fourfold rise in VDRL. The child should be retreated if the CSF cell count is abnormal after 2 years *or* if VDRL-CSF is still reactive after 6 months.
   (4) An infant successfully treated for congenital syphilis is *not* immune and may later contact acquired syphilis.
b. Acquired syphilis
   (1) Primary, secondary, or early latent syphilis (less than 1 year duration): Penicillin G benzathine 50,000 U/kg (maximum 2.4 million U) IM once, in two injection sites.
      (a) Alternate therapy if penicillin absolutely cannot be used: Doxycycline 100 mg PO bid × 2 weeks *or* tetracycline

20

SEXUALLY TRANSMITTED DISEASES

500 mg PO qid × 2 weeks for children more than 8 years of age

(b) Need follow-up serologic test: Successful outcome is a negative serologic test by 12 months for primary syphilis, by 24 months for secondary syphilis, and by 48 months for latent syphilis

(2) For late latent syphilis or syphilis of unknown duration (adult): Penicillin G benzathine 7.2 million units total, administered as three doses of 2.4 million units IM each at 1-week intervals.

(3) For late latent syphilis or syphilis of unknown duration (child): Penicillin G benzathine 50,000 U/kg IM, up to the adult dose of 2.4 million units, administered as three doses at 1-week intervals (total 150,000 U/kg up to the adult total of 7.2 million units).

(4) If penicillin allergy: Doxycycline 100 mg bid *or* tetracycline 500 mg PO qid for those older than 8 years. Both drugs should be administered for 2 weeks if the duration of infection is less than 1 year, and for 4 weeks if the duration is more than 1 year or of unknown duration. Repeat therapy if there is not a fourfold decrease in titer by 1 year after treatment or if clinical signs and symptoms persist.

Note: **Remember: Contact, evaluate, and treat all sexual partners!**

(5) For neurosyphilis: Aqueous penicillin G 3 to 4 million U IV q4h × 10 to 14 days or penicillin G procaine 2.4 million U IM qd plus probenecid 500 mg qid × 10 to 14 days. Either regimen is followed by penicillin G benzathine 2.4 million U IM weekly × 3 weeks.

(6) Follow-up and retreatment

(a) All patients with early syphilis and congenital syphilis should have repeat VDRL at 3, 6, and 12 months after treatment.

(b) VDRL should be nonreactive or reactive with a low titer within 1 year following successful therapy.

(c) The possibility of reinfection should be considered when a patient with early syphilis needs to be retreated. Retreatment should be considered in the following:

(i) Clinical signs of syphilis persist or recur.

(ii) There is a fourfold increase in VDRL titer.

(iii) High-titer VDRL fails to show a fourfold decrease in 1 year. Retreat according to the schedules recommended for syphilis of more than 1 year's duration.

G. HERPES SIMPLEX VIRUS

1. Patient may be asymptomatic or have painful ulcerations on genitalia. Ulcers between vaginal folds and the posterior cervix can be easily missed.

a. Cytologic tests (e.g., Pap or Tzanck smear) reveal multinucleated giant cells in approximately 75% of culture-positive specimens.

b. Viral medium is needed for culture.

2. Treatment of primary genital herpes in adolescents.

a. Acyclovir 400 mg PO tid × 7 to 10 days *or*

b. Acyclovir 200 mg PO 5 times/day × 7 to 10 days (adult dosage) *or*

c. Famcyclovir 250 mg PO tid × 7 to 10 days *or*

d. Valacyclovir 1 g PO bid × 7 to 10 days

e. The use of topical acyclovir is discouraged

3. Treatment of episodic recurrent herpes infection.

a. Acyclovir 400 mg PO tid × 5 days *or*

b. Acyclovir 200 mg 5 times/day × 5 days *or*

c. Acyclovir 800 mg PO bid × 5 days *or*

d. Famcyclovir 125 mg PO bid × 5 days *or*

e. Valacyclovir 500 mg PO bid × 5 days

4. Suppression of recurrent genital herpes.

a. Acyclovir 400 mg PO bid *or*

b. Famcyclovir 250 mg bid *or*

c. Valacyclovir 250 mg bid *or*

d. Valacyclovir 500 mg qd *or*

e. Valacyclovir 1000 mg qd

H. HEPATITIS B AND HEPATITIS C

1. Clinical: Jaundice, anorexia, vomiting, liver enlargement/tenderness. (See also Chapter 8.)

2. Chemistries: Increased LFTs and increased bilirubin; plus serologic findings for hepatitis B and C; if severe liver disease, PT/PTT may be prolonged.

3. Abnormal urine (increased bilirubin), abnormal stool (acholic).

4. Universal immunization of infants (and adolescents) against hepatitis B is recommended.

I. HUMAN PAPILLOMAVIRUS INFECTION

1. HPV causes warts known as condyloma acuminata; the incubation period is 1 to 6 months. Certain types are associated with genital neoplasia. Most cases in infants are secondary to perinatal transmission.

2. The wart has a cauliflower-like appearance (white or strawberry pink-red) and can be located on the genitalia, around the anus, or in and around the mouth. At the time of detection, the lesions may range in size from several millimeters to several centimeters because of confluence of multiple lesions.

3. PE and laboratory tests are necessary to rule out other venereal diseases. Investigate the possibility of sexual abuse.

4. Treatments vary by extent and location of lesions.

a. Podofilox 0.5% solution (patient can apply bid × 3 days, followed by 4 days of no treatment; can have a total of 4 cycles of such therapy), surface treated should not exceed 10 cm^2; *or*

20

SEXUALLY TRANSMITTED DISEASES

b. Imiquimod 5% cream (patient can apply 3 times/wk hs × 16 weeks, and wash off 6 to 10 hours later) *or*

c. Podophyllum 10% to 25% in compound tincture of benzoin, applied weekly (up to 6 weeks) by a health professional; area treated less than 10 cm^2 per session; not for internal lesions *or*

d. Tricholoracetic acid 80% to 90%, applied weekly (up to 6 weeks) by a health professional, to be followed by talc or baking soda to remove unreacted acid

5. Recalcitrant warts and those in the urethra, vagina, or rectum may require cryotherapy, excision, laser ablation, or electrocautery.

J. HIV DISEASE

See Chapter 22, Section A.

K. BIBLIOGRAPHY

General

CDC: 1998 guidelines for treatment of sexually transmitted diseases. 47:RR-1, 1-116.

Drugs for sexually transmitted infections, *The Med Letter* 41 (issue 1062), September 24, 1999.

Judson F, Ehret J: Laboratory diagnosis of sexually transmitted infections, *Pediatr Ann* 23:361, 1994.

Nyirjesy P: Vaginitis in the adolescent patient, *PCNA* 46:733, 1999.

Quinn T: Recent advances in diagnosis of sexually transmitted diseases, *Sex Transm Dis* 21(2 suppl):S19, 1994.

Gonorrhea

AAP Committee on Child Abuse and Neglect: Gonorrhea in prepubertal children, *Pediatrics* 101:134, 1998.

Darville T: Gonorrhea, *Pediatr in Rev* 20:125, 1999.

Sung L, MacDonald N: Gonorrhea—a pediatric perspective, *Pediatr in Rev* 19:13, 1998.

Chlamydia

Danville T: Chlamydia, *Pediatr in Rev* 19:85, 1998.

Grayston JT: *Chlamydia pneumoniae* (TWAR) infections in children, *Pediatr Infect Dis J* 13:675, 1994.

Hammerschlag M: *Chlamydia trachomatis* in children, *Pediatr Ann* 23:349, 1994.

Syphilis

Coles FB, Hipp S: Syphilis among adolescents, *Contemp Pediatr* 13:47, 1996.

Darville T: Syphilis, *Pediatr in Rev* 20:160, 1999.

Glaser J: Detecting congenital syphilis, *Contemp Pediatr* 11:57, 1994.

Sung L, MacDonald N: Syphilis—a pediatric perspective, *Pediatr in Rev* 19:17, 1998.

Herpes Simplex Virus

Abadie J: Acyclovir, *Pediatr in Rev* 18:70, 1997.

Annunziato P, Gershon A: Herpes simplex virus infections, *Pediatr in Rev* 17:415, 1996.

Murph J, Grose C: Routine acyclovir therapy, *Contemp Pediatr* 16:79, 1999.

Nelson C, Demmier G: Superficial HSV infection—how serious is it? What should you do? *Contemp Pediatr* 13:96, 1996.

Hepatitis

AAP Committee on Infectious Diseases: Update on timing of hepatitis B vaccination for premature infants and for children with lapsed immunizations, *Pediatrics* 94:403, 1994.

AAP Committee on Infectious Diseases: Hepatitis C infections, *Pediatrics* 101:481, 1998.

Shapiro C: Epidemiology of hepatitis B, *Pediatr Infect Dis J* 12:433, 1993.

Zellos A, Schwartz K: What's the latest on hepatitis C? *Contemp Pediatr* 15:39, 1998.

MINOR TRAUMA

A. MAMMALIAN BITES

Mammalian bites are common occurrences. In the United States, up to 1% of all emergency department visits are bite related. Disfigurement, functional impairment, and infection are all important complications of mammalian bites. Bite wounds that have an increased risk of subsequent infection are those that involve deep punctures, crushed tissue, substantial delay in primary care (more than 12 hours), or high-risk anatomic location (hands, feet). Rates of infection by biting species are: dogs (5% to 15%), humans (5% to 30%), cats (20% to 50%). Most infections following mammalian bites are polymicrobial in nature. A mixture of aerobes and anaerobes can generally be recovered. Regardless of the nature of the biting mammal, certain management principles apply.

1. Determine the circumstances of the attack and the identity of the biter. If the biter is a nonhuman, attempt to determine its species and rabies immunization status.
2. Examine the skin carefully, noting the location of the wound(s), and the length (or caliber) and depth.
3. Provide proper analgesia and, if needed, appropriate sedation.
4. Wash the wound with copious amounts of clean water or saline. Initial rinsing with tap water is acceptable. Detergents are often harmful to tissues and are generally not required to achieve adequate cleansing.
5. Judiciously debride devitalized tissue and remove all foreign material from the wound.
6. Examine for vascular, muscle, tendon, and nerve damage.
7. Repair deep and surface structures as appropriate.
8. Apply protective dressings and, when appropriate, splint and/or elevate the injured area.
9. Administer tetanus and/or rabies immunizations as needed.
10. Determine the need for administration of antibiotics.
11. Arrange for follow-up evaluation by the primary care physician within 24 to 36 hours.

B. MAMMALIAN BITES BY HUMANS

1. Bites by humans are of intermediate risk for subsequent infection (5% to 30%). When signs and symptoms of infection are present, broad-spectrum antibiotics should be administered. Bacteria that cause infection include streptococci, staphylococci, anaerobes, and (rarely) aerobic gram-negative organisms. Oral amoxicillin plus clavulanic acid or IV penicillin plus oxacillin are effective treatments for most of these infections. Penicillin-sensitive individuals can be treated with clindamycin. Continued cleansing is important adjunctive therapy.
2. The use of prophylactic antibiotics for human bites remains controversial. Abrasions due to human bites rarely if ever become

infected, and therefore do not require antibiotics. The rate of subsequent infection following human bites (deep) puncture wounds, and lacerations is considerable (up to 30%). Placement of sutures or other skin closures increases that risk. As a result, it is suggested that prophylactic antibiotics be administered to all children who sustain human bite wounds that have deep puncture components or require closure.

3. Closed-fist injuries, as often occur during fistfights, may appear benign but can lead to serious morbidity. Joint infection is one of the main concerns. As is the case for all open mammalian bite wounds, these require meticulous cleansing. They also require administration of broad-spectrum antibiotics.

4. Adolescents involved in sports also risk high-impact human bite injuries. A crush/laceration to the forehead of an opposing football player is a good example. For these injuries and other human bite wounds with crush components, the same approach as for closed-fist injuries applies.

5. Human bites can be closed with sutures or tape closures. As stated above, closure of human bite wounds increases infection rates. Closure interferes with drainage from the wound. Extensive cleansing of the wound should always precede wound closure. Human bite wounds should *never* be closed with occlusive means such as tissue adhesives.

6. Administer tetanus prophylaxis when appropriate.

7. Assure appropriate follow-up.

C. MAMMALIAN BITES BY ANIMALS (NONHUMAN)

1. It is important to determine the identity of the biting animal. Bites by wild carnivores require different management than those by wild rodents. Similarly, management of bites by "captive" domestic carnivores differs from that for strays. Most of the management differences involve need for administration of antibiotics or rabies prophylaxis.

2. Infection rates following mammalian bites by nonhumans vary by species. Dog bites have a relatively low risk of subsequent infection (less than 15%). Cat bites often become infected (up to 50%). Much of the difference in infection rates is attributable to the types of wounds inflicted. Dog bite wounds tend to be larger, more open, and easier to clean. Cat bite wounds are typically small caliber, deep punctures that are difficult to clean.

3. Studies have shown that the signs and symptoms of infection take several hours to become clinically evident. Redness, swelling, and tenderness due to infection from *P. multocida* take at least 8 hours, and generally 12 hours to develop. Those due to staphylococcal and streptococcal species take 3 to 6 hours longer.

4. Most infected nonhuman mammalian bite wounds involve multiple organisms of different identities (e.g., gram-positive, gram-negative,

anaerobic, aerobic). *Pasteurella multocida* is an extremely virulent organism that is commonly (up to 80%) isolated from infected cat bite wounds. *Pasteurella canis* is often found in infected dog bite wounds. From most infected dog or cat bite wounds, 5 to 7 different organisms can be isolated. These infections require broad-spectrum antibiotics. As for human bites, amoxicillin plus clavulinic acid, oxacillin plus penicillin, or clindamycin are effective for most.

5. Prophylactic antibiotics might be useful in some instances. They are generally recommended for bite wounds with deep puncture components, bites by cats, bites with crush components, full thickness bites located on the hands and feet, and bites requiring closure.

6. After thorough cleansing and (if needed) debridement, most lacerations can be closed with either sutures or tape closures. Due to the higher risk of infection and lesser cosmetic importance, puncture wounds *should not* be closed. Closure of deep lacerations on the hand, is controversial. Deep wounds in this location have the highest risk of subsequent infection. If primary closure is attempted, antibiotics should be administered. These and other high-risk (for infection) wounds can alternatively be managed with cleansing, packing, antibiotic administration, and delayed primary closure (36 to 48 hours later). As for bites by humans, bites by nonhumans should *never* be closed with tissue adhesives.

7. Administer tetanus prophylaxis when appropriate.

8. Assure appropriate follow-up.

D. POST-EXPOSURE RABIES PROPHYLAXIS

1. Most human rabies comes from contact with carnivorous wild animals (skunks, raccoons, woodchucks, coyotes, foxes) and bats. Although unusual, rabies does occur in domestic cats, dogs, and ferrets. Rodents (rats, squirrels, hamsters, mice) and lagomorphs (rabbits) generally are not considered to transmit rabies.

2. Rabid animals concentrate the rabies virus in their saliva. Outside of caves and laboratories (where airborne transmission is a concern), rabies is transmitted only by introducing the virus from the rabid animal's saliva into open cuts or wounds in the skin or onto mucous membranes.

3. Rabies prophylaxis should be provided to all children who sustain open bite wounds by rabies-prone animals, including wild carnivores, bats, and noncaptive domestic dogs and cats. Rabies prophylaxis can be avoided when bites do not break the skin surface, or when they are inflicted by domestic dogs, cats, or ferrets whose rabies vaccination status is known to be current. Although recommendations vary, most municipalities require revaccination of domestic pets every 2 years. If a biting dog, cat, or ferret is captive and able to be quarantined or observed, rabies prophylaxis can be initially omitted.

21

MINOR TRAUMA

4. The recommendations provided in Table 21-1 are only a guide. When determining the need for rabies prophylaxis, consider the animal species involved, the circumstances of the bite or other exposure (e.g., scratches, abrasions, open wounds, or mucous membranes contaminated with saliva or other potentially infectious material from a rabid animal), the vaccination status of the animal, and the presence of rabies in the region.

5. Exposure to a bat is often considered a rabies-prone event. Bat teeth are small caliber. Bat bites are often imperceptible. This is especially true if the exposure involves someone who is unable to provide a reliable history (e.g., an infant or young child, an intoxicated child, a mentally impaired child, or a child who was sleeping during the possible exposure to a bat). Even in the absence of demonstrable bite(s), such exposures should be considered rabies-prone.

6. If rabies prophylaxis is indicated, both passive and active immunization should be given. Passive immunization is with rabies immune globulin (RIG). Human diploid cell vaccine (HDCV) or another brand of active vaccine should be given as soon as possible, regardless of the interval between exposure and treatment.

TABLE 21-1
RABIES POST-EXPOSURE PROPHYLAXIS GUIDE

Animal Type	Evaluation and Disposition of Animal	Post-exposure Prophylaxis Recommendations
Dogs, cats and ferrets	Healthy and available for 10 days of observation	Prophylaxis only if animal develops signs of rabies*
	Rabid or suspected of being rabid†	Immediate immunization‡ and RIG
	Unknown (escaped)	Consult public health officials for advice
Bats, skunks, foxes, raccoons, and most other carnivores; woodchucks	Regarded as rabid, unless area is known to be free of rabies, or until animal is proven negative by lab tests†	Immediate immunization‡ and RIG
Livestock, rodents, and lagomorphs (rabbits and hares)	Consider individually	Consult public health officials. Bites by rodents and lagomorphs almost never require treatment.

From 2000 Red Book: Report of the Committee on Infectious Diseases, ed 25, Elk Grove Village, IL, 2000. American Academy of Pediatrics.

*During the 10-day holding period, at the first sign of rabies in the biting dog, cat, or ferret, treatment with Rabies Immune Globulin (human) (RIG) and vaccine should be initiated. The suspect animal should be euthanized immediately and tested.

†The animal should be euthanized and tested as soon as possible. Holding for observation is not recommended. Immunization is discontinued if immunofluorescent test of the animal is negative.

‡See text.

7. The single dose of RIG is 20 IU/kg. If possible, infiltrate the entire dose around the wound. When impractical to do so, administer the remaining RIG in a large muscle remote from the location of administration of the active vaccine. RIG provides passive immunity while the body mounts an active immune response. If RIG was not given when the HDCV vaccination was begun, it can be given until the eighth day after the first dose of vaccine was given. Thereafter, RIG is unnecessary because presumably an active antibody response to the vaccine has occurred.

8. HDCV (or other active vaccine) is administered as five separate doses. Each dose is 1 ml, regardless of the age or size of the patient. HDCV is given as an IM injection in the deltoid (anterior part of the thigh can also be used). HDCV is *never* administered in the gluteal area. HDCV induces an active immune response that requires approximately 7 to 10 days to develop and persists for 1 year or longer. The first dose should be administered as soon as possible after exposure; give additional doses 3, 7, 14, and 28 days after the first dose. A postvaccination serum specimen for rabies antibody testing is no longer necessary unless the patient is suspected of being immunocompromised (i.e., receiving steroids or immunosuppressive therapy essential for the treatment of another condition).

9. Many municipalities require that bites be reported to the animal warden or police. Whenever possible, those officials will have the owners or the animal pound watch the animal for signs of rabies for 10 days.

E. BURNS

1. Burns are classified according to the extent (depth and percent body surface area) of injury. First-degree burns involve only the epidermis. Second-degree burns extend into the dermis; third-degree burns extend into the subcutaneous tissues; and fourth-degree burns extend into muscle, tendons, or bone.

2. Most burns treated in emergency departments are partial-thickness, or second-degree burns. These involve destruction of the epidermis, and less than 50% of the dermis. Such burns often exhibit blisters, edema, and significant pain. The injured skin appears pink and moist and usually heals with minimal scarring.

3. Deep partial-thickness burns involve destruction of the epidermis and more than 50% of the dermis. The injured skin has a paler, drier appearance than more superficial injuries and is sometimes difficult to distinguish from full-thickness injuries. Thrombosed vessels often give deep partial-thickness burns a specked appearance. Some burns that initially appear to be partial-thickness can later be identified as full-thickness, especially if secondary damage from infection, trauma, or hypoperfusion occurs. Deep partial-thickness burns can take many weeks to heal. Significant scarring is common.

21

MINOR TRAUMA

4. Full-thickness burns involve complete destruction of the epidermis and dermis. Injured skin usually has a pale, charred, or leathery appearance. Destruction of cutaneous nerves in the dermis makes these injuries nonpainful. Full-thickness burns cannot reepithelialize, and must heal from the periphery.

5. All burns eventually become colonized by potentially pathogenic bacteria. Cleansing and debridement reduces substrate for bacterial proliferation. Aggressive topical antibacterial therapy, with or without systemic antibiotics, can reduce the number of bacteria but cannot sterilize the burn.

6. Children with first-degree burns (erythema only) may be treated with analgesics, cool compresses, anti-inflammatory creams and, if itching is a problem, oral antihistamines.

7. Children with second-degree burns (pain, blisters, with or without areas of blanching within the burn area) may need to be hospitalized if the burns involve the face, perineum, hands, or feet or if the total body surface area burned is greater than 5% in infants, greater than 10% in children, and greater than 15% in adolescents/adults.

a. The initial management of second-degree burns includes cleansing the area with saline, trimming broken blisters or ragged skin edges (leaving intact blisters alone), applying 1% silver sulfadiazine (Silvadene) or other similar agent, or a petroleum-impregnated covering (e.g., Xeroform) to a more superficial burn, and securing the burn with clean gauze (and elastic netting if necessary for the particular body part).

b. The patient should be seen daily until healing is well underway. Further debridement, if necessary, can be performed at these visits.

c. Burn cleansing and dressing may be done at home by capable caregivers. Using plain forceps, nonviable tissue should be completely removed before each redressing.

d. Systemic antibiotics should be instituted at the first sign of burn site infection. Remember that a thin rim of erythema at the periphery of the burn is to be expected during healing.

e. Analgesics (acetaminophen, codeine) should be administered for pain relief. For hospitalized patients, parenterally administered narcotics may be more effective than oral agents.

f. Once the burn has healed (7 to 14 days), an emollient should be applied to protect the new, fragile epidermis. Protection against strong sunlight should also be instituted.

g. Tetanus prophylaxis should be provided according to recommended standards.

8. For the management of children with extensive second-degree or deeper burns, refer to *The Harriet Lane Handbook*.

F. DENTAL TRAUMA

1. The various types of dental trauma are as follows:
a. Concussion: Injury to periodontal ligaments without displacement or mobility of the tooth. There is percussion sensitivity.
b. Subluxation: The tooth is mobile horizontally and is tender to percussion.
c. Displacement: The tooth is intruded into the socket, extruded lingually, or avulsed.
d. Fracture: In an enamel fracture, only an edge is missing. In crown fractures, there are cracks in the enamel but no tooth discoloration. In dentin fractures, there is a yellow discoloration (if the pulp is exposed, a pinkish color is obvious).
e. Mandibular fracture
   (1) Unilateral: Mandible deviates toward the affected side.
   (2) Bilateral: Mouth is gaping and malocclusion is present.
f. Maxillary fracture: Involvement of bony processes into which the teeth are embedded. Teeth may be displaced and mobile.
2. The PE of a child with suspected dental injury includes components that are not part of most routine examinations. After examining the face and lips for obvious traumatic lesions and asymmetries, it is important to do the following:
a. Palpate the mandible and maxilla for tenderness.
b. Instruct the patient to open and close the mouth so that asymmetric and unstable areas may be appreciated.
c. Examine the mouth for bleeding, swelling, and broken teeth.
d. With the patient biting down, ask if the bite feels normal.
e. Check each tooth individually for pain and mobility.
3. Some injuries require more urgent intervention than others.
a. Concussions and crown and enamel fractures require a timely dental referral.
b. Subluxations, displacements, and fractures with pulp exposure require an immediate dental referral.
c. Fractures of the upper or lower jaw require treatment by an oral surgeon.
d. Avulsed permanent tooth should be reimplanted. If on-site reimplantation is not possible, the tooth should be transported in a balanced salt solution (e.g., 3M Save-a-tooth solution). If that is not available, less ideal solutions such as milk or saline can be used. It is important to prevent the root surface from air drying in order to try to preserve the vitality of the periodontal ligament. The best prognosis exists if reimplantation is instituted within 1 hour of the injury. The tooth should be held by the crown (not the root), and gently rinsed under running water or saline. Do not scrub any part of the tooth. Do not reimplant primary teeth. Reimplanted teeth should be splinted by a dentist.

21

MINOR TRAUMA

G. FROSTNIP AND FROSTBITE

1. In *frostbite*, freezing of tissues occurs. Numbness is the most consistent early symptom of cold injury. If the area involved is rewarmed soon after the onset of numbness, a tingling sensation that resolves with further rewarming develops, and no permanent tissue damage results, the clinical situation is referred to as *frostnip*, and no further treatment is required. If the initial symptom of numbness is not acted on reasonably early, frostbite quickly ensues.

2. Frostbite most commonly involves the toes, fingers, ears, and nose. The initial appearance of the affected areas might be benign. Coloration varies from yellow-white to mottled blue. Skin consistency varies from doughy to stiff and frozen.

3. In most cases, rewarming results in initial hyperemia and return of at least some sensation. Edema develops after several hours and can last several weeks. Vesicles or bullae form in 6 to 24 hours. In superficial injuries, thin blebs form that are filled with clear or yellow fluid. In deeper injuries, thick-walled blebs filled with hemorrhagic fluid develop.

4. In more severe injuries, a hard, dark eschar forms in areas of devitalized tissue. This typically occurs 10 to 14 days after the injury. In severe cases, mummification of dead tissue can occur 3 to 4 weeks after injury.

5. With rewarming, superficially frostbitten areas become red, swollen, and painful. No cyanosis is present, and sensation is normal.

6. With rewarming, more deeply injured areas develop often severe, dull aching pain that, after several days, is replaced by throbbing pain. Residual tingling from local neuritis is common. Many patients describe an electric-current-like sensation that can persist for weeks. These symptoms are often exacerbated in warm environments. Some sensory symptoms persist for years after the injury.

7. Favorable prognostic signs include early return of sensation, return of relatively normal color and warmth, and large clear blebs that form early (and extend to the tips of the fingers when they are involved).

8. Unfavorable prognostic signs include residual nonblanching cyanosis after rewarming, lack of edema, and the late development of small hemorrhagic blebs (that do not extend to the tips of the digits, when involved).

9. Initial treatment involves rapidly warming in an environment where reexposure to freezing conditions will not occur. Immerse affected areas in tepid water (40° C to 43° C) for 20 to 40 minutes. Massage, application of ice water, and extreme heat are contraindicated, because all can increase tissue injury. If present, vesicles or bullae should be left intact and covered with gauze. Carefully cleanse the injured area with soap or antiseptic and apply sterile dressings. Analgesics are often required during rewarming. Plastic surgery consultation and hospitalization are necessary whenever there is deep frostbite.

H. INSECT REACTIONS

1. The reaction to insect bites or stings may be local (redness, pain, swelling at the site), systemic (urticaria, hypotension, wheezing, laryngeal edema, shock), or both. These reactions generally occur within 2 hours of the sting. Delayed reactions can occur as long as 1 week following the sting and include fever, arthralgias, urticaria and, rarely, neuritis or vasculitis.

2. When obtaining the history, always try to identify the stinging insect. Determine if there have been previous systemic (or local) reactions to stings and if there is a history of allergy.

3. Treatment for local reactions includes stinger removal, cleansing, and, when necessary, application of ice or cool compresses to the area. Antihistamines also can be administered to help provide relief of pruritus and swelling.

4. It is often difficult to distinguish local reactions from skin infections. This especially is true of insect bites in the region of the eye, where swelling and redness are common and evident components of any inflammatory response. For older wounds (e.g., more than 24 hours old) that are red and tender, and others that appear infected (tumor, rubor, dolor, calor), systemic antibiotics (e.g., cephalexin 25 to 50 mg/kg/d ÷ qid) should be given.

5. For mild systemic reactions that occur immediately (e.g., generalized urticaria), antihistamines, such as diphenhydramine (5 mg/kg/d ÷ qid) or hydroxyzine (2 mg/kg/d ÷ qid) may be given.

6. For anaphylactic reactions, epinephrine 0.01 mg/kg is given either SQ (0.01 ml/kg of 1:1000 solution) or IV (0.1 ml/kg of 1:10,000 solution). According to the extent of symptoms, the patient might also require IV fluids, nebulized albuterol, methylprednisolone 1 to 2 mg/kg IV, and diphenhydramine 1 mg/kg IV (see Chapter 22).

I. TICKS

1. Ticks are capable of transmitting a variety of infectious agents, including rickettsiae, bacteria, protozoa, viruses, and spirochetes. Among the most well-known tickborne diseases are RMSF, Lyme disease (see Chapter 16), ehrlichiosis, bebesiosis, tularemia, relapsing fever, Colorado tick fever, and tick paralysis.

2. Ticks produce saliva that can induce tissue destruction. Once attached to the skin, ticks should be promptly removed by applying steady, slow traction with forceps (or tweezers if at home). The tick should be grasped as close to the skin as possible and pulled directly upwards, avoiding twisting or jerking that might cause the mouth parts to break off. Care should be taken to not squeeze or crush the tick, since that can increase the transmission of infectious agents. An ulcer or granuloma may develop if the tick's mouth parts remain after removal. Such lesions often require intralesional steroids or excision.

21 MINOR TRAUMA

3. Children with evidence of RMSF (relapsing fever, rash, headache) require antibiotic therapy and proper supportive care. While tetracyclines should not be given routinely to children younger than 8 years of age, most experts consider doxycycline to be the drug of choice for treatment of RMSF in children of any age. IV chloramphenicol (50 to 100 mg/kg/d, maximum 4 g/d) is an alternative to doxycycline, but might be less effective. If used, serum drug levels should be checked to decrease the likelihood of toxic reactions to chloramphenicol. Therapy for RMSF is continued until the patient is afebrile for at least 2 or 3 days. Usually, for RMSF, antibiotic therapy is required for 7 to 10 days.

4. Tick paralysis is associated with the bite of the wood tick, deer tick, or dog tick. The engorged tick transmits a neurotoxin that can produce cerebellar dysfunction or ascending weakness. Following a 4- to 7-day latent period, restlessness, irritability and ascending flaccid paralysis develop. Symptoms can progress to respiratory paralysis and death, if the tick is not removed. Laboratory data are usually normal. The mechanism of action of the toxin is unknown. Management consists of removal of the tick and supportive care.

J. SPIDERS

1. There are more than 100,000 species of spiders. All are carnivorous and utilize venom to immobilize and kill their prey. Because most spider fangs are too short or fragile to penetrate human skin, and because their venom is generally mild, the risk of serious injury from spider bites is small. In the United States, two species of spiders (black widow and brown recluse) are capable of causing more severe reactions.

2. Black Widow Spiders

a. The black widow spider (*Latrodectus* species) is a shiny black animal, about the size of a quarter (1 to 1½ inches long). The mature female is four times the size of the male and has a red hourglass marking on its abdomen (some males do as well). The female is a threat to bite when she is guarding her egg sac or is provoked. Five *Latrodectus* species are found in the United Sates, with at least one species in every state except Alaska. The two most common species are *L mactans* and *L variolus.*

b. The black widow spider venom contains a neurotoxin that causes severe muscular cramps and pain 1 to 8 hours after the bite. No local symptoms are associated with the bite itself. Afflicted patients complain of pain in the abdomen, flanks, thighs, and chest. Children often develop nausea and vomiting. Respiratory distress, chills, urinary retention, and priapism can also occur. Cardiovascular collapse can lead to death. The overall mortality rate is 4% to 5%. In young children, mortality rates can be as high as 50%.

c. A clinical grading scale for *Latrodectus* envenomation has been developed by Clark. Grade 1 refers to generally asymptomatic patients who have normal vital signs and only local pain at the bite site. Grade 2 refers to patients with localized symptoms of muscular pain and diaphoresis, but normal vital signs. Grade 3 refers to patients with generalized muscular pain, abnormal vital signs, nausea, vomiting, headaches, and diaphoresis.

d. For children who weigh less than 40 kg, treatment with *Lactrodectus* antivenin (2.5 ml, one vial) should be initiated as soon as a bite is confirmed. Specific directions on the package insert, including skin testing for hypersensitivity to horse serum, should be followed. For those who weigh more than 40 kg, administration of antivenin is not as urgent. However, antivenin should be considered for those younger than 16 years and for those with respiratory distress or significant hypertension.

e. Calcium gluconate (0.1 ml/kg per dose, 10% solution) can be given to help control leg and abdominal cramps, but has limited efficacy. Methocarbamol is less effective than calcium gluconate. Muscle relaxants (e.g., benzodiazepines) have short-lived, variable effects.

3. Brown Recluse Spiders

a. Brown recluse spiders live primarily in the southern and midwestern states. They are small (1 to 1.5 cm in length), and have a brown violin-shaped marking on the dorsum of the cephalothorax. They attack only when provoked, and produce a cytotoxic venom that contains a substance similar to hyaluronidase.

b. The bite is initially innocuous, and usually goes unnoticed. Subsequent reactions range from mild to severe. Within 2 to 8 hours, the site of the bite becomes painful and erythematous, and a central blister or pustule appears. Subcutaneous discoloration develops within 24 hours, and spreads in size (up to 10 to 15 cm) over the next 3 to 4 days, at which point the pustule drains, unroofing an ulcer.

c. The amount of venom injected determines the degree of local reaction. If there is no evidence of necrosis within 72 hours of the bite, scar formation is minimal.

d. Small children are at greatest risk of developing systemic reactions to brown recluse venom. If systemic symptoms develop, they will manifest 24 to 48 hours after the bite. Fever, chills, malaise, nausea, vomiting, weakness, intravascular hemolysis, hematuria, and renal failure have been reported. No specific laboratory tests accurately identify brown recluse envenomation.

e. Spider bites are typically single lesions. When multiple lesions are found, one should consider other causes of injury.

f. Treatment varies according to the clinical stage of the bite. Single lesions with central hemorrhage, bullae, or necrosis should be measured. Lesions with areas of necrosis less than 2 cm can be observed and treated with local care.

g. Children with lesions that have areas of necrosis greater than 2 cm should receive antibiotics. Additional local treatment of these larger

MINOR TRAUMA

21

wounds varies according to the age of the bite. Necrotic areas should be conservatively debrided if lesions are 3 to 5 days old at the time of first presentation. For lesions less than 48 hours old, necrotic tissue should be excised. If the necrotic area (in lesions less than 48 hours old on initial presentation) continues to enlarge, but remains less than 2.5 cm when complete, it should be allowed to granulate. Skin grafting should be considered for larger lesions.

h. Studies have shown no significant alteration of necrosis by steroids or heparin. Although animal studies likewise do not support the use of dapsone or hyperbaric oxygen, dapsone continues to be used in adults. Dapsone should not be used in children due to the risk of methemoglobinemia.

i. Antivenom for brown recluse spider bites is not yet commercially available. The mainstay of treatment for systemic reactions is vigorous supportive care.

K. SNAKEBITES

Each year in the United States, there are approximately 45,000 snakebites. Of those, approximately 8000 are by poisonous snakes. Fortunately, most who are bitten by poisonous snakes recover. However, a small number of fatalities (9 to 15) are reported each year. The majority of deaths occur among children and the elderly; and among those for whom antivenin has not been given, has been administered late, or has been administered in insufficient quantities.

1. Only 20 of the 120 (or more) species of snakes indigenous to the United States are venomous. Most belong to the Crotalidae family (pit vipers), and include rattlesnakes, copperheads, and cottonmouths (water moccasins). The coral snake (Elapidae family) is the only other native poisonous snake.

2. Pit vipers are identified by a foramen or pit located between each eye and nostril. The pit is a heat-sensitive organ that enables the snake to locate warm-blooded prey. Pit vipers have triangular heads, elliptical pupils, and two curved canalized fangs. Nonvenomous snakes have rounded heads, round pupils, and no fangs.

3. Coral snakes are shy, nocturnal, and rarely bite humans. They have a pattern of red, yellow (or cream), and black rings. Red against yellow ("kill a fellow") are the markings of the coral snake. Red against black ("venom lack") are the markings of nonvenomous look-alikes. Coral snakes have black snouts and round pupils and lack facial pits.

4. Recently decapitated or dying snakes are still capable of inflicting bites. This is due to the still intact bite reflex.

5. Superficial lacerations produced by fangs usually do not result in envenomation because the discharge orifice of the fang lies slightly proximal to the tip.

6. The primary local signs and symptoms of most pit viper envenomations are fang punctures, pain, edema, and erythema or ecchymoses of the

bite site and adjacent tissues. The latter usually occur within 30 minutes of the bite and extend as the venom spreads. If erythema and edema have not manifested within 8 hours after a snakebite, it is safe to assume that envenomation has not occurred.

7. Other frequently reported signs and symptoms include tender regional lymphadenopathy, perioral paresthesias that extend to the face and scalp, and tingling of the fingertips and toes. Victims complain of a "minty," "rubbery," or "metallic" taste in the mouth and tingling of the lips.

8. Venom is a complex substance that affects every body tissue and organ, primarily or secondarily. The major pharmacologic effects of venom in humans are hypovolemic shock, hemorrhage, renal failure, pulmonary edema, and local tissue necrosis. Venom does not penetrate the blood-brain barrier.

9. Most authorities have adopted a simple and practical approach to grading *pit viper* envenomations: minimal, moderate, or severe. An envenomation might seem minimal when the patient is initially evaluated but can rapidly progress to severe in the absence of treatment with antivenin.

a. Minimal (pit viper) envemomations are confined to the site of the bite and are unassociated with any systemic symptoms, signs, or abnormal laboratory findings.

b. Moderate (pit viper) envenomations are those in which manifestations extend beyond the site of the bite, but without life-threatening symptoms or signs (e.g., nausea and vomiting, perioral paresthesias, fasciculations, or unusual tastes).

c. Severe (pit viper) envenomations usually result in swelling, ecchymoses, and bullous formation involving an entire extremity or part. They produce severe systemic signs and symptoms, such as dyspnea, tachypnea, respiratory failure, alteration in consciousness, and profound hypotension. Severe hemorrhage and markedly abnormal coagulation studies result.

10. Envenomations by Elapidae (coral snakes and cobras) differ markedly from those by pit vipers. There may be little or no swelling immediately after the bite. Occasionally, a delay of from 1 to 5 hours occurs before the onset of systemic signs and symptoms. Elapid venoms cause changes in nerve conduction and neuromuscular transmission that affect cranial nerves, resulting in ptosis, dysphagia, dysarthria, and intense salivation. Later findings include loss of deep tendon reflexes and respiratory depression.

11. The ultimate severity of any venomous snakebite depends on the quantity of the venom injected and the comparative toxicity of the venom. Influential factors include the size and species of snake; the number of fang punctures; and the age, size, and underlying medical condition of the victim. It is important to note that the potency of the

venom of an individual snake within a species can be up to five times greater than that of another of the same species.

12. Field treatment of a suspected snakebite begins with placing the patient at rest and keeping him or her warm and reassured. The area of the bite should be immobilized below the level of the heart. All rings or constricting items should be removed. Caffeine and alcohol enhance absorption of venom and should be avoided. The use of ice, tourniquets, incision and suction, and electric shock therapy *should be avoided.* The victim should be transported to the nearest medical facility as soon as possible.

13. Management in the ED.

a. The following historical information should be obtained: the time of the bite, the description of the snake, the type of field therapy (if any), and the patient's past medical history (including prior exposure to horse serum and prior snakebites and therapy).

b. The preliminary PE should include measurement of vital signs, inspection of the bite site for fang marks, evaluation of neurologic status, and an attempt to classify degree of envenomation. Circumferential measurements of the bitten extremity should be done every 15 minutes.

c. A skin test for hypersensitivity to horse serum should be done only if it is known that antivenin will be administered. In such cases, an intravenous line (or two) should also be placed.

d. A baseline urinalysis and CBC, platelet count, and coagulation studies and chemistries should be obtained. CBC, platelet count, and coagulation studies should be reassessed every 4 hours or after each course of antivenin, whichever is less. An ECG is recommended for adults older than 40 years of age.

e. Antivenin is the mainstay of treatment of significant venomous snakebites. Approximately 60% of venomous bites cause symptoms that require antivenin treatment. The purpose of the antivenin is to neutralize the venom at the site of the bite before the venom is absorbed. For many years, a polyvalent (horse-derived) antiserum has been used to treat Crotalidae envenomations. A newer Crotalidae antivenom (affinity-purified, mixed monospecific crotalid antivenom ovine Fab), is currently undergoing trials.

f. Antivenin is given to patients who have shown evidence of envenomation and progression within 30 to 60 minutes after being bitten. Once envenomation has been established, administration of antivenin should not be delayed. The effectiveness of antivenin is both dose- and time-related. It is most effective when given within 4 hours of the bite and less effective after 12 hours.

g. The dose of Crotalidae antivenin should be based on the amount of venom inoculated and the potency of the individual snake's venom. Both are difficult to determine. A general set of dosing guidelines is as follows: 5 vials for mild envenomations, 10 vials for moderate envenomations, 15 vials for severe envenomations, and 20 vials for those with cardiovascular collapse. For children, many experts recommend increasing antivenin doses by 50%, because of higher ratio of venom to body mass.

h. After a proven coral snake bite, 3 vials of antivenin (Micrurus, by Wyeth) should be administered. If symptoms evolve, 3 to 5 additional vials should be given.

i. Bacteria on fangs and in venom vary, but gram-negative and gram-positive rods are commonly present. Most experts recommend administration of a broad-spectrum antibiotic, such as a quinolone derivative, to patients with moderate or severe envenomations.

j. If there is any doubt regarding the severity of the envenomation, the patient should be monitored in an intensive care unit for at least 24 hours.

L. LACERATIONS

Lacerations occur commonly in childhood. Reports indicate that up to 7% of visits to urban pediatric emergency departments are by children with lacerations or puncture wounds. For these injuries, management issues generally concern wound closure and prevention of infection. Wound management guidelines are fairly straightforward. Best outcomes result from careful attention to simple principles. Universal precautions should be utilized to maintain a clean field and to prevent direct exposure to blood.

1. Determine the circumstances of the injury, including what material caused the laceration (e.g., glass, metal, plastic, wood), the relative amount of force involved, the time elapsed since the laceration occurred, where the injury transpired (e.g., outdoors, home), and the body part(s) injured.

2. Obtain a focused, pertinent medical history, including the patient's tetanus immunization status, other medical problems, known allergies, and medications.

3. Test the function of muscle(s), tendon(s), and nerve(s), and assess the vascular status in the immediate area of the injury.

4. Administer an appropriate anesthetic. A variety of agents, both injected and topical, can be used safely and effectively in children.

a. Administer 1% lidocaine (Xylocaine), a conventional local anesthetic that is injected around the wound margin through a 25-gauge or 27-gauge needle. Always aspirate before injection to avoid injection into a vessel. The duration of action of plain 1% lidocaine is about 90 minutes.

b. Alternatively, 1% lidocaine with epinephrine may be injected to decrease bleeding from injured tissues. Because epinephrine causes vasoconstriction, it should never be applied to body parts with limited (end-arterial) vascular supply, such as the nose, fingers, toes, or penis. Epinephrine extends the duration of action for lidocaine.

21

MINOR TRAUMA

c. LET has largely replaced TAC as the topical anesthetic of choice for minor wound repair. Gauze or cotton is saturated with LET, and then applied directly to the open wound. Within 15 to 20 minutes, effective anesthesia is usually obtained. At that point, vasoconstriction around the wound margin is usually visibly evident. As is true for injected epinephrine, LET should not be used on end organs. The duration of action for LET is about 45 minutes.

5. Some children also require a sedative. Again, a variety of safe and effective agents can be used.

a. To sedate younger children (preteens), many prefer to use ketamine (0.5 to 1 mg/kg IV). It has the advantage of providing sedation, analgesia, and amnesia. Conventional protocols call for premedication with atropine and midazolam to prevent side effects of the drug. However, some debate the need for premedication with midazolam. The effects of ketamine are seen within minutes of its administration. The sedative effects of ketamine last only 10 to 20 minutes. Analgesic effects last approximately 40 minutes.

b. Benzodiazepines alone are also commonly used to sedate children for procedures. Midazolam can be administered intravenously (0.1 mg/kg), orally (0.5 mg/kg), or intranasally (0.4 mg/kg). Its onset of action is approximately 1 to 5 minutes (IV), and its duration of action approximately 90 to 120 minutes. A reversing agent (flumazenil) is available if needed, but its effects are short-lived (30 to 60 minutes).

6. After the anesthetic and/or sedative have taken effect, the wound should be thoroughly irrigated. Drainage pads should be placed under the wound to collect run-off. Liquids that are tissue-friendly (e.g., sterile water or saline) should be used. Irrigation with at least 100 ml normal saline per 1 cm laceration (length) is recommended. To prevent exposure to body fluids, a syringe splash-guard or other protective device should be utilized.

7. Explore the wound for deep injury. Remove foreign bodies and dirt. Particularly dirty wounds (e.g., those with "road burn") might need to be scrubbed with a surgical sponge or brush. However, most can be adequately cleaned with proper irrigation.

8. Debridement of devitalized tissue helps to reduce infection rates. Judiciously debride *all* devitalized tissue, taking care to preserve all viable tissue.

9. Obtain an x-ray examination of the wound if there is *any* suspicion of residual metal pieces or glass. Metal and glass appear on x-ray study; wood and plastic generally do not. Studies have indicated that even when the bottom of a wound can be visualized, glass fragments can be "invisible" to the physician, but identifiable on radiograph.

10. A variety of sizes and types of suture materials are available. As needle size increases, radius increases. As suture size increases, caliber decreases. Needle size and shape are exactly as pictured on the outside of each packet.

a. Type of suture material:
   (1) Both nonabsorbable (monofilament nylon) and absorbable (polyglactin) material is available. Nonabsorbable material is used for most surface sutures. Nylon is stronger than absorbable material, but requires removal after initial wound healing. Some manufacturers produce pliabilized nylon, which has less memory than regular nylon, and is easier to manipulate with instruments. Blue polypropylene suture can be used instead of nylon, in areas where identification of the suture material at the time of removal might be difficult (e.g., scalp, eyebrows).
   (2) Absorbable material is used for subcutaneous sutures. Rapidly absorbing sutures (polyglactin 910) also can be used on surface areas where suture removal is difficult. Polyglactin 910 retains its strength for about 7 to 10 days. Since regular absorbable suture material often takes several weeks to weaken and "absorb," only rapidly absorbing material should be adapted to surface use.
   (3) Silk is more reactive than synthetic material, thereby limiting its usefulness in most repairs. Monofilament materials are preferred over braided or multifilament materials, which are thought to increase the risk of wound infection.
b. Size of suture: Most lacerations can be repaired using 4-0 or 5-0 suture material. The 4-0 suture is heavier caliber, and therefore stronger than 5-0. The 6-0 suture, which is lighter weight than 5-0, is often used for more delicate repairs, such as those on the face or nail bed. The 5-0 is easier to manipulate, and is perfectly adequate for facial repairs as well. For repairs of most other parts of the body, 4-0 suture is generally effective. Repairs of areas that are subject to greater amounts of tension or movement (e.g., lacerations of the thigh or knee) might require 3-0 suture.

11. Helpful suturing tips:
a. Avoid damaging the needle. The suture needle is hollow at the (swage) end that holds the suture material, and solid at the tip. To avoid bending (or straightening the curved needle), hold the needle between half to two thirds of the distance from the tip.
b. The width of the scar is primarily determined by the amount of tension on the wound at the time of closure. For wounds under greater tension, subcutaneous sutures can be helpful. Generally, such wounds should also have more sutures placed, and they should be placed closer to the wound edge.
c. Skin heights of opposing sides of the wound should be matched exactly, and wound edges should always be everted at the time of closure.
d. Tight sutures increase the risk of tissue ischemia and subsequent wound infection. It is important to anticipate swelling and closely approximate tissue, rather than tightly close it.

21

MINOR TRAUMA

e.   Space sutures appropriately, such that tissues are effectively approximated, and removal is facilitated. Avoid "micro-suturing," that necessitates invasive removal techniques.

12. Alternatives to sutures:

a.   Staples: Staples are inexpensive, disposable, and easy to apply. They are useful for repair of lacerations in cosmetically unimportant areas, such as the scalp, or for long linear lacerations. They are not recommended for use in the face, hands, or feet. Staples are generally left in place for a period similar to sutures in the same area. They are easily removed with a staple remover.

b.   Tape: Wound tape can be used as the sole method of closure for linear lacerations under minimal tension. Wound tape can also be used to reinforce other repairs. Tape will not effectively adhere to areas that are naturally moist or hairy. Tape should be applied to clean, dry skin that has been prepared with an adhesive (e.g., tincture of benzoin). The latter is a wound irritant and should not be spilled into the open wound. Tape closures might not be the best choice for repair of wounds in young children, who are apt to peel them off. Wound tape will "naturally" peel after several days.

c.   Tissue adhesive: Tissue adhesive (2-octyl cyanoacrylate) can be used for smaller wounds that are under minimal tension. Adhesives dry rapidly and can be difficult to apply. Care should be taken to limit contact of the glue to only the opposing skin surfaces, since it will adhere to eyelashes, examiners' fingers, gloves, and other objects as well as it will to skin. Tissue adhesive acts as an occlusive dressing over the wound. Therefore, tissue adhesive should *never* be utilized for repair of potentially contaminated wounds.

13. Wound dressings:

a.   Beyond its aesthetic appeal, a proper dressing provides several other functions, including: protection, absorption, compression, and immobilization.

b.   Dress the injured area in its position of function.

c.   Apply an antibiotic ointment when appropriate.

d.   Apply a three-layer dressing; tape appropriately.
   (1)   Nonadherent layer (e.g., telfa pad, vasoline gauze) applied to skin
   (2)   Absorbent layer of 4 × 4 gauze
   (3)   Protective layer of gauze wrap (e.g., kling bandage), elastic netting, or both

e.   Occasionally, an elastic bandage is needed for immobilization or hemostasis. Care should be taken to avoid excessive compression of the wrapped area.

f.   Immobilization is sometimes required if the laceration is in a mobile area. Splints can be incorporated into the protective layer of the dressing, or applied on top of the dressing. Splinting might need to be continued for a period of time after the sutures are removed.

Maguire J, Geha R: Bee, wasp, and hornet stings, *Pediatr Rev* 8:5, 1986.
Resiman RE: Insect stings, *N Engl J Med* 331:523, 1994.

Ticks and Spiders
Blackman JR: Spider bites, *Am J Fam Pract* 8:288, 1995.
Goldberg G: Stings and bites: emergencies and annoyances, *Contemp Pediatr* 2:32, 1985.
Rees R et al: The diagnosis and management of brown recluse spider bites, *Ann Emerg Med* 16:945, 1991.
Reeves JA et al: Black widow spider bite in a child. *Am J Emerg Med* 14:469, 1996.
Woestman R et al: The black widow: is she deadly to children? *Pediatr Emerg Care* 12:360, 1996.
Wright SW et al: Clinical presentation and outcome of brown recluse spider bite, *Ann Emerg Med* 30:28, 1997.

Snakebites
Dart RC et al: Affinity-purified, mixed monospecific crotalid antivenom ovine Fab for the treatment of crotalid venom poisoning, *Ann Emerg Med* 30:33, 1997.
Gold HS, Wingert WA: Snake venom poisoning in the United States: a review of therapeutic practice, *South Med J* 87:579, 1994.
Rudolph R et al: Snakebite treatment at a southeastern regional referral center, *Am Surg* 61:767, 1995.

Lacerations
Baker MD et al: Lacerations in urban children, *Am J Dis Child* 144:87, 1990.
Bruns WA et al: Laceration repair using tissue adhesive in a children's emergency department, *Pediatrics* 98:673, 1996.
Callahan JM, Baker MD: General wound management. In Henretig FM, King C, editors: *Textbook of Pediatric Emergency Procedures,* Baltimore, 1997:1125, Williams & Wilkins.
Kennedy RM, Luhmann JD: The "ouchless emergency department": getting closer: advances in decreasing distress during painful procedures in the emergency department, *Pediatr Clin North Am* 46:1215, 1999.
Liebelt EL: Reducing pain during procedures, *Curr Opin Pediatr* 8:436, 1996.

21 MINOR TRAUMA

MISCELLANEOUS DISEASES AND DISORDERS

1. The human T lymphotrophic virus type III (more commonly known as HIV) is the cause of AIDS. HIV infects the helper CD4 T lymphocytes, causing lymphocyte dysfunction with resultant immunodeficiency.

2. Because the virus incorporates its own DNA into the human host DNA, it can remain latent for many years, especially in lymphoid tissue.

3. Most HIV infections in infants and children are secondary to perinatal transmission from infected mothers. Before universal screening of blood and blood products, some children, especially those born prematurely and those with hemophilia, acquired their disease through transfusions with contaminated blood. Shared contaminated IV drug needles and unprotected sexual intercourse are the most common means of HIV spread in adults and adolescents. Young children have also been infected with HIV after sexual abuse (intercourse) by infected individuals.

4. Infants infected with HIV may have FTT, profound weight loss, developmental delay, or persistent oral candidiasis. Hepatosplenomegaly, generalized lymphadenopathy, chronic diarrhea, fever, malaise, and recurrent infections should also raise suspicions about HIV. Persistent parotitis and lymphoid interstitial pneumonia are peculiar to childhood AIDS.

5. The most common presentation of AIDS in older children, adolescents, and adults is *Pneumocystis carinii* pneumonia. Weight loss (or failure to gain adequate weight), growth delay, generalized lymphadenopathy, and hepatosplenomegaly can also be presenting signs. However, many children and adolescents infected with HIV have no gross signs or symptoms.

6. Opportunistic infections (e.g., CMV, herpes virus) are common.

7. The PE must be complete. AIDS is a multisystem disease, and there are often multiple abnormal physical findings.

8. Laboratory tests to support a clinical diagnosis include an ELISA screen for HIV antibodies (with the Western blot test to confirm a positive ELISA). Infants born to HIV-positive mothers have passively transferred maternal antibodies and may test falsely positive well into the second year of life. An HIV culture, PCR, or both can be used to document true infection. If an individual is known to be HIV positive, a quantitative test ("viral load") helps to assess success of therapy in controlling the infection.

9. Other tests to assess immune function include a CBC with differential, CD4 count, CD4/CD8 (T cell) ratio, T-cell function tests, and serum immunoglobulins. Remember, CD4 counts normally vary by age and

are highest during infancy. LFTs and a CXR may be helpful, depending on the presentation.

10. Therapy

a. In general, all HIV-positive patients are treated. Formerly, it was thought that asymptomatic HIV-positive children would not need therapy until they became symptomatic or until they showed laboratory evidence of disease progression (decreasing CD4 counts, increasing viral load). Now, it is believed that early treatment will preserve immune function, decrease the likelihood of resistance, and prolong life.

b. That said, the choice of drugs must be carefully considered because of the significant side-effects associated with most of them. In addition, since HIV care in children is an evolving art with new medications every year, the long-term effects of some of these medications are completely unknown.

c. Antiretroviral drugs interfere with viral replication; they suppress rather than kill the virus. Indications for use are symptomatic disease or CD4 counts (cells/cc): less than 1750 if patient is less than 1 year of age, less than 1000 if patient is 1 to 6 years of age, and less than 500 if patient is older than 6 years of age.

d. There are several classes of approved antiretroviral drugs for children. Not all drugs available for adults have been approved for children, although pediatric specialists in HIV care have used most of these drugs when left with few options. A child or adolescent who is HIV positive should *always* be managed by a specialist with expertise in this field, and any recommendations of drug choice should be at his or her discretion.

e. Two classes of antiretroviral medications are the nucleoside reverse transcriptase inhibitors (NRTIs) and the nonnucleoside reverse transcriptase inhibitors (NNRTIs). They inhibit viral reverse transcriptase, which makes a cDNA copy of the viral genomic RNA. NRTIs lack a hydroxyl group and prevent the addition of another nucleotide to create a complete cDNA molecule. NNRTIs interfere with binding at the active site of reverse transcriptase.

(1) The NRTIs are zidovudine (AZT, Retrovir), stavudine (d4T, Zerit), didanosine (ddI, Videx), lamivudine (3TC, Epivir), and Abacavir (Ziagen). Not all are approved for children. Always check the most recent dosage recommendations.

(a) AZT is associated with myelosuppression and liver dysfunction; thus LFTs and CBCs must be regularly monitored. AZT comes in liquid and capsule form, and its dosage in HIV-positive children is 180 mg/m^2/dose q8h or 240 mg/m^2/dose q8h. AZT is also used during pregnancy to reduce the chance of viral transmission from mother to fetus. When used during pregnancy, it is important to continue AZT therapy in the neonate for 6 weeks after birth at a dosage of 2 mg/kg/dose PO q6h.

(b) ddI is an alternative to AZT. Its advantage is that it is not myelosuppressive. It is used when a child cannot tolerate AZT or clinically worsens while on AZT; it is also used in combination with AZT when lower doses of AZT are indicated because of associated side-effects. The pediatric dosage is 100 mg/m^2/dose q12h given on an empty stomach. The use of ddI has been associated with pancreatitis and (uncommonly) peripheral retinal depigmentation. Peripheral neuropathy (paresthesias) may also occur. Children receiving ddI should have frequent serum amylase and lipase determinations, an ophthalmology evaluation before and q6mo thereafter or as needed, and prompt evaluation if there is any tingling, numbness, or pain in the hands or feet.

(c) 3TC is often used in combination with AZT. It should not be used in any patient with pancreatitis or at risk to develop it. It comes in liquid and tablet form, and its pediatric dosage is 4 mg/kg (maximum 150 mg) bid. Its use in children has been associated with pancreatitis; monitoring serum amylase is essential.

(d) d4T comes in liquid and capsule form. Although it has been associated with peripheral neuropathy and pancreatitis in adults, the incidence of these side effects is not as high in children. The pediatric dose is 1 mg/kg/dose (maximum 30 mg) q12h.

(2) NNRTIs include nevirapine (NVP, Viramune), delavirdine (DLV, Rescriptor), and efavirenz (Sustiva). Not all are approved for children. Always check the most recent dosage recommendations.

    (a) NVP is associated with hepatitis and a significant rash that might progress to a Stevens-Johnson syndrome. Its dose is 120 mg/m^2 qd × the first 14 days and then 120 mg/m^2 bid thereafter (if tolerated).

    (b) DLV is associated with a rash. An optimal pediatric dose has not yet been determined.

    (c) Efavirenz comes in liquid and tablet form. It is associated with rash, nightmares, dizziness, and effects on the developing fetus.

(3) Protease inhibitors (PIs) cleave viral polyprotein into the subunits required to make a fully mature (i.e., infectious) virion. PIs include nelfinavir (NFV, Viracept), ritonavir (RTV, Norvir), indinavir (IND, Crixivan), saquinavir (SQV, Fortovase), and Amprenavir. Not all have been approved for children.

    (a) NFV comes in powder or tablet form. It has a graduated dose schedule based on weight. It is associated with GI symptoms and rash.

22

MISCELLANEOUS DISEASES AND DISORDERS

    (b) RTV comes in (foul-tasting) liquid and pill form. After a lower lead-in dose, its usual dose is 350 mg/m^2 bid. It is associated with increased LFTs and GI symptoms.

    (c) IND must be given on an empty stomach and has a propensity to crystallize in renal tubules leading to renal stones. Its use is limited in children.

    (d) SQV is usually given with RTV because the latter increases its serum levels. Its use in children is limited. SQV is associated with GI symptoms.

    (e) Amprenavir is a new drug, given bid; optimal dosage has not yet been determined. It is associated with GI symptoms.

  f. Most HIV-positive individuals begin with two NRTIs and one PI, but various combinations of drugs have been used. Monotherapy is *not* an option because of the very real likelihood of the development of resistance. Once resistance has developed, it is likely to be present for life.

  g. Other therapies include prophylaxis against *P. carinii* with TMP/SMZ, dapsone, or aerosolized pentamidine. Initiation of prophylaxis is based on CD4 counts. Prophylaxis should be initiated if CD4 counts (cells/cc) are less than 1500 if patient is younger than 1 year of age, less than 750 if patient is 1 to 2 years of age, less than 500 if patient is 2 to 6 years of age, and less than 200 if patient is older than 6 years of age. TMP/SMZ is the drug of choice, but its use is contraindicated when there is a history of sulfa allergy or G-6-PD deficiency. It is not used in infants younger than 6 weeks of age. Dose is 75 mg/m^2/dose bid.

  h. In HIV-positive persons, infections must be treated aggressively; IVIG (400 mg/kg/dose) might be needed q28d in patients with recurrent serious bacterial infections.

  i. If neutropenia is a problem due to needed antiretroviral therapy, G-CSF therapy should be considered.

  j. VZIG must be administered if there is exposure to varicella.

  k. Acyclovir is indicated for clinical varicella and severe herpes infections.

11. Avoid OPV in infected infants, children, and their contacts, and in indeterminant children with HIV-positive household members; primary immunization against polio is with IPV.

12. DTP, *Haemophilus influenzae* type B, hepatitis B, pneumococcus, influenza, and MMR vaccines should be given at the usual schedules and intervals. Varicella vaccine is not usually given.

13. TB screening should be carried out on schedule. An anergy skin-test panel is helpful in interpreting PPD test results, especially in patients with low CD4 counts.

14. Involve social services and religious support systems (if present) as early as possible to assist the family and patient. After all, these families must face the very difficult issues of terminally ill family members, their subsequent deaths, and surrogate care for other children. There is still a strong social stigma against those with HIV

infection that makes it difficult for family members to speak openly about their experiences and their fears. Provide as much support as possible.

15. Occupational exposure to HIV can occur (e.g., needle stick); exposure to HIV in children can occur through breast-feeding, human bites, sexual abuse, and sticking oneself with a needle or syringe, especially those found in the street. The likelihood of infection after an exposure is related to the type of exposure, the amount of blood entering the person's body, and the viral load in that specimen of blood. Seek assistance from a specialist in HIV care or infectious disease, or the local Health Department. Ordinarily, prophylaxis after exposure should start as soon as possible but within 48 hours; therapy should continue for 28 days. Most authorities recommend 2 NRTIs and a PI for post-exposure prophylaxis.

16. The best way to "cure" AIDS is to prevent it. Persons who are engaging in sexual intercourse and do not know their partner's HIV status should use condoms; abstinence is preferable and is the only certain way to prevent the sexual transmission of HIV. Other ways to prevent AIDS include the cessation of IV needle sharing and *universal* testing of blood and blood products for HIV. Because AZT has been shown to reduce transmission of the virus from mother to fetus, AZT therapy is indicated in pregnant women who are HIV positive.

B. CHEST PAIN

1. Chest pain is a relatively uncommon presenting complaint in young children but becomes more common as children age. It can be functional, herald serious disease, or have a significance somewhere in between.

2. Important historical information includes the following:

a. The onset, duration, recurrence, location, radiation, and quality (sharp vs. dull) of the pain

b. Relationship to rest, exercise, and eating

c. Precipitating factors

d. Actions or medications that worsen or improve the pain

e. History of similar pain or of being awakened from sleep by pain

f. Other concomitant symptoms: Diaphoresis, nausea, vomiting, dyspnea, coughing, wheezing, vertigo, syncope, palpitations, skin color changes

g. Presence of fever, respiratory symptoms, and myalgias (especially if pain is acute)

h. Symptoms of indigestion

i. The possibility of foreign-body aspiration

j. A history of trauma

k. A history of a heart murmur, cardiac disease or surgery, sickle cell disease, chronic respiratory disease

l. Psychosomatic symptoms: Is the child under stress?

m. Medication or illicit drug use

22

MISCELLANEOUS DISEASES AND DISORDERS

n. Family history of angina, cardiac disease, death (especially if recent) from cardiac causes

3. The PE should be complete, with special emphasis on the following:

a. Vital signs

b. General appearance: Frightened, in pain, indifferent

c. Skin: Cyanosis, pallor

d. Respiratory examination: Rate, depth, symmetry of respirations; splinting; rales; wheezes; area of decreased breath sounds

e. Cardiac examination: PMI, rate, regularity of rhythm, murmurs, rub, gallop, assessment of pulse equality and strength, palpation of chest and neck for thrills, auscultation of neck for bruits (remember to auscultate with the patient both in the supine and sitting positions)

f. Chest wall: Areas of tenderness, asymmetry, inflammation; palpation of ribs, intercostal spaces, upper abdomen, and vertebral bodies to determine direct or referred areas of tenderness

4. Causes of chest pain

a. Cardiac: Suggested by pain associated with exercise, palpitations, color change, syncope, vertigo

    (1) Ischemia: Squeezing pain, tachypnea, tachycardia, gallop, rales, wheezing, CHF, shock

    (2) Left ventricular outflow obstruction: Especially pain precipitated by exercise when cardiac oxygen demand is not met by the supply; aortic valve or subvalvular stenosis (harsh systolic murmur varying little with maneuvers that alter ventricular filling); idiopathic hypertrophic subaortic stenosis (murmur softens during Valsalva's maneuver; pansystolic murmur with S4; ECG *may* show septal Q wave)

    (3) Coronary artery disease: Compression, fistula secondary to collagen-vascular disease or Kawasaki disease; systolic/continuous murmur, gallop; ECG may show infarction or ST-T wave changes

    (4) Mitral valve prolapse: Usually asymptomatic; midsystolic click or late systolic murmur (altered by position); ECG may show T wave changes, U wave, tachycardia

    (5) Dissecting aortic aneurysm: Acute, sharp, "tearing" pain

    (6) Arrhythmias: Palpitations, chest pain, dizziness; may be tachycardia, bradycardia, or varying rhythms

    (7) Pericardial infection, inflammation, or infiltration by tumor: Sharp pain exacerbated by inspiration, cough, movement; friction rub heard on auscultation; ECG may show ST elevation and low QRS voltage

b. Pulmonary

    (1) Pneumonia: Rales, decreased breath sounds, tachypnea, cough, respiratory distress

    (2) Asthma (exercise induced): May have pain in the absence of wheezing

       (3)   Pleurisy: Sharp pain aggravated by cough/inspiration

       (4)   Pneumothorax: Sharp pain, dyspnea, area(s) of decreased breath sounds

       (5)   Pulmonary infarction: Intense pain, respiratory distress; may be cyanosis and shock

c.   Gastrointestinal

       (1)   Esophageal reflux: Substernal pain that is worse after eating or when supine, aerophagia, belching

       (2)   Esophagitis: Similar pain as in reflux but may be more intense

       (3)   Hiatal hernia

       (4)   Mallory-Weiss syndrome: Acute onset, substernal pain; blood commonly in vomitus or stool

       (5)   Gastric spasm, inflammation, ulcer: Lower chest or epigastric pain elicited by direct palpation

       (6)   Duodenal ulcer

       (7)   Biliary/pancreatic disease

d.   Mediastinal diseases

       (1)   Pneumomediastinum

       (2)   Tumors

       (3)   Mediastinitis

e.   Chest wall disorders

       (1)   Costochondritis: Tender costochondral junctions

       (2)   Trauma: May be able to reproduce pain with palpation over affected area

       (3)   Breast development

       (4)   Slipping rib syndrome

f.   Emotional

       (1)   Pain is vague, fleeting, and localized over the heart or left arm.

       (2)   Pain is not precipitated by exercise; it may occur at rest.

       (3)   Other psychosomatic symptoms may be present.

g.   Precordial catch syndrome

       (1)   Sharp pain below left sternal border or left breast without radiation

       (2)   Relieved by change of position, chest massage, or deep inspiration

h.   Miscellaneous

       (1)   Chest wall zoster

       (2)   Malignancies

       (3)   Hemoglobinopathies

       (4)   Collagen-vascular diseases

       (5)   Spinal root irritations

       (6)   Drug abuse (especially inhaled cocaine)

5.   Laboratory tests should be dictated by the history and physical findings as follows:

a.   If a cardiac cause for pain is suspected (e.g., pain with exercise, palpitations, color change, syncope), an ECG, ECHO, and prompt referral to a cardiologist are in order.

22

MISCELLANEOUS DISEASES AND DISORDERS

b. If a pulmonary cause is likely, a CXR and preexertional and postexertional pulmonary function testing may be useful.

c. Even after a complete evaluation, a specific cause is not found in 30% to 50% of cases.

6. Treatment is directed toward the underlying cause of the chest pain.

C. FAILURE TO THRIVE

1. FTT is defined as weight less than the third percentile *or* less than 80% of ideal weight *or* weight that decreases by at least two percentile lines on a growth chart. The height and head circumference usually are not affected as much as the weight.

a. There is an equal race and sex incidence.

b. Most patients are younger than 24 to 36 months of age.

c. FTT may be the reason for presentation or may be an "incidental" finding when the child has an acute illness.

2. Important historical information includes the following:

a. Prenatal, birth, neonatal histories, especially maternal exposure to drugs, cigarettes, infectious agents, and risk factors for HIV

b. Sleep, bowel, and bladder habits

c. Developmental history: Is delay present? If so, is it global or local?

d. Feeding history: "Average" day diet recall, type of formula used and how it is prepared, amount of formula/milk ingested each day, amount and types of other fluids ingested each day, amount and types of solids ingested each day

e. Presence of "meal battles," feeding difficulties, tongue thrusting, choking, diaphoresis, color changes, regurgitation

f. How child is fed: Can the child feed himself or herself? Can the child drink from a cup?

g. Presence of infectious disease symptoms (which ones?), chronic medical conditions, long-term medication use

h. Medical history

i. Review of systems

j. Family history, especially heights/weights of parents, siblings, grandparents; chronic illness in parents (could be undiagnosed HIV infection)

k. Social history: Child's affect and behavior, parental history of abuse or FTT, family's financial and living conditions, parents' social supports, parents' bond with child, other caretakers of child; was this child planned?

3. A complete, meticulous PE is *mandatory!*

a. Particular attention should be given to growth parameters; weight, height, and head circumference should be measured and plotted against the child's age.

    (1) Weight, height, and head circumference less than the third percentile: Usually in utero insult; however, may represent severe, prolonged caloric deprivation

  (2) Weight and height less than the third percentile, head circumference normal: Endocrinopathies, structural dystrophies, constitutional short stature

  (3) Weight less than the third percentile, height and head circumference normal: Caloric deprivation (poor intake vs. poor utilization), nonorganic FTT

b. Child's appearance: Clean vs. dirty, small vs. scrawny, fearful vs. too trusting, clinging, avoiding mother, avoiding eye contact

c. Skin: Dirty, rashes, chronic conditions such as eczema, signs of abuse

d. Muscle mass: Decreased, with little fat

e. Head: Asymmetries; overriding/separated sutures; size, shape, texture of fontanelle; flattened or balding occiput; signs of trauma; transilluminate infant's head

f. Mouth: Tongue thrust, enlarged tongue, teeth (number, condition)

g. Cardiopulmonary: Any abnormality

h. Abdomen: Organomegaly, protuberance

i. Extremities: Length relative to length of trunk

j. Neurologic/developmental assessment

4. Causes

a. Organic (30% to 40% of cases)

  (1) GI (40% of all organic FTT): Most commonly clefts, chalasia, gastroesophageal reflux, celiac disease, Crohn's disease, Hirschsprung's disease, cystic fibrosis, liver disease

  (2) Renal: Remember renal tubular acidosis in addition to more obvious diseases

  (3) CNS: Some 20% of all organic FTT

  (4) Cardiac disease: Usually obvious

  (5) Endocrine: Diabetes mellitus, diabetes insipidus, thyroid disease (hyperthyroidism or hypothyroidism), adrenal disorders, hypopituitarism (congenital or acquired)

  (6) Chronic infections (e.g., HIV) and toxin exposure (e.g., lead poisoning)

b. Nonorganic (perhaps 75% to 90% of all FTT cases in some series; may be as low as 10% to 15% depending on population)

  (1) May be "hyperalert" with minimal vocalization vs. a heightened response to strangers

  (2) Pale, loss of muscle mass

  (3) May have tonic immobility (flexed)

  (4) History of feeding problems; difficult temperament; being unplanned/unwanted, the youngest; parental history of abuse, FTT, depression; lack of involved father; distant/overwrought mother; lack of social supports; poor preventive health care (delinquent immunizations); history of multiple medical providers

  (5) If such patients are hospitalized, two thirds improve away from home; however, they may require *3 to 4 weeks!*

22

MISCELLANEOUS DISEASES AND DISORDERS

      (6)   Usually decreased growth hormone and serum iron parameters, delayed bone age

5. Evaluation

a. Immediate hospitalization is advisable if abuse or neglect is suspected, if the child is ill, or if treatable organic disease is present. Probably should hospitalize any child with FTT within 1 to 2 months of growth deceleration.

b. Investigate organic and nonorganic causes simultaneously (preferably with a supportive, multidisciplinary approach).

c. Perform a complete history/PE/developmental assessment.

d. Initial laboratory tests: CBC with differential, serum electrolytes, BUN, creatinine, and glucose; U/A and culture; stool examination for reducing substances and fat; PPD, with or without CXR.

e. Other tests as dictated by history/PE: Radiographic assessment of GI tract, GU tract; ECG; bone age (unreliable if very young); sweat test; and HIV testing. The less evident an organic cause is at presentation, the less likely laboratory tests are to find one. One study examined 185 children with FTT who received 2607 laboratory tests; only 10 (0.4%) established a diagnosis and only 26 (1.0%) supported a diagnosis.

f. Calorie count, observed feeding trial.

6. Treatment is directed toward the underlying cause. Children with nonorganic FTT and their parents merit family counseling or psychotherapy. Unfortunately, only 33% of children are normal at follow-up 5 to 10 years later, and 50% are delayed or experience learning problems, personal problems, or both.

D. HYPERTENSION

1. BP measurement is a necessary part of the PE.

a. In neonates, infants, and toddlers, BP may be more easily measured by an oscillometric method than by auscultation.

b. The manual method is preferred in older children and adolescents.

    (1)   The child is seated with the right arm at heart level.

    (2)   The blood pressure cuff is wrapped around the upper part of the arm; the bladder should encircle the arm and cover it at a minimum two thirds of its length. The cuff is inflated to approximately 2 mm Hg above the point at which the radial pulse disappears.

    (3)   The cuff is deflated slowly and deliberately while observing the manometer (aneroid or mercury).

    (4)   Auscultation over the brachial artery reveals the onset of an audible tapping sound (systolic pressure, Korotkoff I sound); further deflation and auscultation reveal a muffled sound (Korotkoff IV) and, finally, its disappearance (Korotkoff V).

    (5)   Because there is debate as to which sound (IV or V) truly represents diastole, both are recorded (e.g., 110/70/64).

    (6)   Because some children have heart sounds audible throughout the cuff's deflation, the Korotkoff IV sound has been used in age- and sex-appropriate BP standards.

2. Inaccurate BP measurements occur when the cuff size is incorrect (especially too small); when the patient is moving, crying, or upset; or when the equipment is not calibrated correctly. Observer bias also occurs.

3. A healthy child is said to have high normal BP when he or she has either a systolic or diastolic pressure between the 90th and 95th percentiles for age and sex. If a child's systolic or diastolic pressures equal or exceed the 95th percentile on three separate occasions, he or she has persistently elevated blood pressure (hypertension). Thus multiple measurements are needed to confirm the diagnosis of hypertension.

4. Causes

a. Renal: Acute glomerulonephritis, hemolytic-uremic syndrome, nephrosis, lupus, trauma, obstructive uropathy, congenital disorders (polycystic renal disease, dysplasia, hypoplasia), tumors, lead nephropathy, mercury poisoning, radiation nephritis, S/P GU surgery/renal transplant/renal rejection, end-stage renal disease.

b. Vascular: Renal arterial disease, renal vein thrombosis, renal artery stenosis, aortitis, aortic coarctation either in the thoracic or abdominal areas.

c. Endocrine: Primary hyperparathyroidism, primary hyperthyroidism, pheochromocytoma, neuroblastoma, Cushing's syndrome, adrenogenital syndrome (11-hydroxylase and 17-hydroxylase deficiencies), primary aldosteronism.

d. Chemical agents: Therapy with sympathomimetics, steroids, or oral contraceptives; amphetamine or cocaine abuse.

e. Miscellaneous: Collagen-vascular disease, poliomyelitis, Guillain-Barré syndrome, dysautonomia, porphyria, hypercalcemia, Stevens-Johnson syndrome, burns, malignancies, SBE, increased intracranial pressure, neurofibromatosis.

f. Primary hypertension occurs in the absence of conditions known to elevate blood pressure. Both genetics and environment (e.g., high salt intake) may play a role in its genesis. Many children are asymptomatic; symptoms when present include frontal headaches, epistaxis, and nervousness. Obesity may be present in as many as 50% of the children.

5. When a child has a persistently elevated BP, important historical information includes the following:

a. The child's birth history

b. Presence of chronic conditions or chronic or recurrent symptoms (headache, epistaxis)

c. Long-term use of medications

22

MISCELLANEOUS DISEASES AND DISORDERS

    d. Growth pattern

    e. Urinary tract infections or disorders

    f. Diet history

    g. Family history of hypertension or its complications (renal disease, myocardial infarction, stroke)

    h. Lifestyle and stressors

    i. Hospitalizations and surgeries

6. The PE must be complete because many causes of secondary hypertension have characteristic physical findings. Check for the presence of an abdominal bruit or café-au-lait spots. Special emphasis is placed on the BP measured in both arms and one leg (to R/O coarctation) and in the right arm with the patient in the supine, sitting, and standing positions. A fundoscopic examination (an abnormal examination indicates that hypertension has been present more than 1 year) and a complete cardiac examination are mandatory.

7. Laboratory tests are dictated by the history and physical findings. A routine U/A and serum creatinine, BUN, electrolytes, uric acid, and CBC determinations are useful screens. If the patient is obese, a fasting cholesterol (and its fractions) and high- and low-density lipoprotein levels are also useful. In any child for whom drug therapy is considered, a baseline ECHO is needed to assess chronicity of the hypertension. A CXR, renal ultrasound, renal imaging, head CT scan, and peripheral plasma renin activity assessment should also be considered.

8. Management (children and adolescents)

a. Secondary hypertension: Treat the underlying condition, if possible. Drug therapy might be necessary to control the hypertension.

b. Primary hypertension

    (1) Weight loss to achieve ideal weight.

    (2) Proper exercise.

    (3) Limited salt intake.

    (4) Avoidance of sympathomimetics, alcohol, and tobacco.

    (5) Try to maintain a positive attitude with regard to stressors and patience with therapy.

Note: **Hypertension in children and adolescents was previously initially treated with diuretics and, if diuretic therapy was unsuccessful, beta-adrenergic blockers. Angiotension-converting enzyme inhibitors (ACE drugs) and calcium channel blockers are now available and are considered first-line drugs.**

    (6) ACE drugs (e.g., enalapril) interfere with the enzymatic conversion of angiotensin I to angiotension II, a major vasoconstrictor. Thus they cause vasodilation and decreased vascular resistance, with more pronounced effects in preterm infants.

        (a) The dosage of enalapril is 0.08 mg/kg/d (maximum 0.6 mg/kg/d) for children. These dosages can be divided q12h or qd. An initial dosage for adolescents is 2.5 mg qd, which may be increased gradually to 20 mg.

(b) Serum BUN, creatinine, potassium, and CBC should be monitored during therapy for any patient with renal disease who is treated with an ACE inhibitor.

(7) Calcium channel blockers (e.g., amlodipine, nifedipine) inhibit the inward flux of Ca across the cell membrane of smooth muscle cells of resistance arterioles, thereby diminishing vascular smooth muscle tone. Thus they are potent vasodilators.

(a) The dosage of amlodipine is 0.1 to 0.3 mg/kg/dose (maximum 0.6 mg/kg/d ÷ bid or qd).

(b) Common side effects are headaches, palpitations, and flushing.

(8) Diuretics can be useful in hypertensive patients with renal disease. They produce an increase in urine volume and Na excretion, which results in decreased extracellular and plasma volume, body weight, and cardiac output.

(9) Beta-adrenergic–blocking drugs (such as propranolol) were at one time used as first-line therapy for hypertension. However, side effects associated with their use (bradycardia, exacerbation of asthma symptoms, CNS effects, sleep disturbances, altered glucose and lipid metabolism) and the efficacy of ACE drugs and calcium channel blockers has rendered beta-blockers less desirable as long-term therapy for hypertension.

(10) A hypertensive crisis (abrupt, marked elevation in BP) can occur in renal disease, hemolytic-uremic syndrome, renal vascular disease, pheochromocytoma, renin-secreting tumors, and severe CNS disease. Symptoms include headaches, epistaxis, diplopia, seizures, CHF, facial palsy, edema, and hypertensive retinopathy. The primary goal of drug therapy is to reduce BP at a rate that minimizes complications while ensuring adequate blood supply to vital organs. The following is a list of useful drugs:

(a) Labetalol 0.5 to 2.0 mg/kg/h by a continuous infusion gives a more constant response. The onset of action is within 5 minutes. The duration of action is during its infusion.

(b) Sodium nitroprusside (0.5 to 8 mcg/kg/min IV; usual dose, 3 mcg/kg/min) can be used to emergently treat severe hypertension in children with normal to only moderately decreased renal function. The onset of action is 30 to 60 seconds, but BP begins to rise again within seconds of discontinuing the drug.

(c) Nicardipine (1 to 4 mcg/kg/min) may also be used; initial onset of action is within 1 minute, with a duration of action of approximately 3 hours.

22

MISCELLANEOUS DISEASES AND DISORDERS

E. KAWASAKI DISEASE

1. KD is an acute vasculitis of unknown etiology. Patients are usually less than 5 years of age (peak incidence 18 to 24 months) with a male-female ratio of 1.5:1. There is a 0.15% mortality rate in the subacute or early convalescent stage, usually from cardiovascular complications.

2. The diagnosis is based on a constellation of characteristic clinical signs and symptoms and laboratory abnormalities. There is a triphasic clinical course.

a. Acute febrile stage (days 1 through 15): Fever plus at least four of the five starred features should be present to establish the diagnosis. The fever is high and spiking (greater than 40° C) and only temporarily responsive to antipyretics. Fever should be present for at least 5 days before a diagnosis of KD is confirmed, but the disease should be considered earlier if other characteristic features are present.

   *(1) Conjunctival injection usually occurs within 2 to 3 days of fever onset; it is bilateral, painless, nonpurulent, and especially marked in the bulbar conjunctivae.

   *(2) Oral mucosal findings occur within 1 to 3 days of fever onset and involve reddened fissured lips, a reddened oropharynx, and a "strawberry" tongue.

   *(3) Rash occurs with the onset of fever and takes several forms (erythematous, irregular plaques that are partially confluent; morbilliform eruption; scarlatiniform; urticarial). The rash occurs principally on the face and trunk but may be accentuated in the perineum; it is *never* vesicular, bullous, petechial, purpuric, or crusting.

   *(4) Extremity changes occur within several days of the onset of fever. The palms and soles develop diffuse erythema, often accompanied by indurative edema and tenderness; the skin of the dorsum of the hands and feet can appear shiny and stretched.

Note: **Not all patients have edema; it is more common in infants.**

   *(5) Lymphadenopathy is the least common major feature; it is usually not generalized but is often a solitary cervical node (greater than 1.5 cm in diameter) that is often tender but rarely fluctuant.

   (6) Behavior changes: Irritability, lethargy, mood lability.

   (7) Abdominal pain, diarrhea, vomiting, liver inflammation, anorexia, mild jaundice, hydrops of the gallbladder.

   (8) GU signs and symptoms (sterile pyuria, urethritis, hematuria).

   (9) Cough, rhinorrhea.

   (10) Joint involvement (late in first stage).

   (11) Cardiovascular involvement (perivasculitis and microvasculitis of coronary arteries, pancarditis), tachycardia.

   (12) Significant laboratory findings: Elevated ESR and CRP, pyuria, elevated WBC count with shift to the left, CSF mononuclear pleocytosis, thrombocytosis (end of this stage), negative cultures.

Note: **Patients with fever and fewer than four of the starred features can be considered for therapy with IV immune globulin, as can those with fewer than 5 days of fever if other signs are characteristic.**

b. Subacute stage (days 14 to 21): Fever, rash, and lymphadenopathy subside. Conjunctivae may still be red; oral mucosal changes are still present. Peripheral extremities begin to desquamate, starting periungually and moving proximally between days 10 and 20. Anorexia and mood changes are still present.

   (1) Joint involvement: Arthralgias/arthritis in large joints (knees, hips, elbows). Effusion(s) may be present.

   (2) Cardiac disease: Improving pancarditis; coronary arteries demonstrate persistent panvasculitis and may demonstrate areas of thrombosis. Coronary artery aneurysms develop in 20% of untreated patients. Clinically, there may be tachycardia, a gallop, muffled heart sounds, minor ECG changes (prolonged PR interval, ST-T wave changes). More severely ill children may have cardiomyopathy with CHF, pericardial effusion, and mitral valve insufficiency. Sudden death may result from aneurysm rupture or coronary artery occlusion.

   (3) Significant laboratory findings: Test results abnormal in the first stage are usually still abnormal; thrombocytosis (usually 600,000 to 1,000,000); mild anemia; elevated AST, CPK, and LDH (if myocarditis).

c. Convalescent stage (up to 3 months after onset): Eyes, oral mucosa, extremities, mood, joint symptoms, and appetite are improving or normal. Early in this stage, coronary artery inflammation is still present; sudden death is still a threat. Most abnormal laboratory values have normalized by the end of this stage.

3. Differential diagnosis in early stage

a. KD may be confused with measles, group A streptococcal infection (scarlet fever), Epstein-Barr virus, leptospirosis, drug eruption, erythema multiforme, Stevens-Johnson syndrome, toxic shock syndrome (staphylococcus), acrodynia, JRA, SLE, RF, and serum sickness.

b. Discrete intraoral lesions, purulent conjunctivitis, exudative pharyngitis, splenomegaly, and generalized adenopathy are distinctly uncommon in patients with KD and, when present, suggest an alternate diagnosis.

4. Risk factors have been identified to detect children most likely to develop coronary aneurysms or thrombosis. Children with 5 factors or less generally do well; those with greater than 9 are at high risk.

a. Male gender

b. Age less than 1 year

c. Duration of initial fever longer than 15 days

d. Recrudescent rash

e. WBCs greater than 30,000

22

MISCELLANEOUS DISEASES AND DISORDERS

  f. Westergren sedimentation rate greater than 100
  g. Presence of cardiomegaly
  h. Presence of arrhythmias
  i. Recrudescent fever
  j. Evidence of myocardial infarction
  k. Prolonged QR interval
  l. Hemoglobin less than 10
  m. Elevated ESR longer than 5 weeks
 5. Management
  a. Acute stage
   (1) Appropriate workup to rule out sepsis, meningitis (if indicated), treatable infections.
   (2) Baseline CBC, ESR, CRP, U/A; consider liver/cardiac enzymes, CXR, ECG.
   (3) Immune globulin at a dose of 2 g/kg should be given as a single IV infusion over 10 to 12 hours as soon as possible after the diagnosis has been established. Retreatment with IV immune globulin (same dose) may be needed for those with persistent fever or symptoms. The prevalence of coronary abnormalities is only 2% among patients treated with aspirin and IV immune globulin.
   (4) Give aspirin 100 mg/kg/d ÷ qid until the patient is afebrile for 24 hours (some recommend this dose until the fourteenth day of illness) followed by 3 to 10 mg/kg once daily until platelet count and ESR return to normal (usually 3 months after the onset of illness).
   (5) The child may need to be hospitalized for IV immune globulin; if not hospitalized, the child needs to be seen 2 to 4 times/week.
   (6) If an outpatient develops cardiac symptoms or abnormalities, he or she should be hospitalized immediately.
   (7) Do not use steroids! They increase platelet counts and are associated with a higher incidence of coronary aneurysms.
   (8) A two-dimensional ECHO may be indicated during the acute phase in some patients but is usually obtained 4 to 8 weeks after the onset of symptoms. ECHO detects proximal coronary artery dilation and aneurysms with high sensitivity and specificity.
  b. Subacute stage
   (1) After day 14, the aspirin dosage should be reduced to 3 to 10 mg/kg/d given as a single daily dose.
   (2) Clinical status, CBC, platelet count, and ECG should be serially monitored.
   (3) Repeat ECHO (compare with initial one); if baseline and 3 to 6 week ECHO show no evidence of coronary abnormality, further imaging is unnecessary.
   (4) Provide supportive therapy.
   (5) If patient has CHF, provide appropriate therapy.

(6) Perform a coronary angiogram if the child has an infarction or coronary vessel damage.

c. Convalescent stage

(1) Aspirin therapy is stopped if no abnormalities are found on ECHO at 3 months; follow-up is individualized.

(2) Children with evidence of aneurysms should have serial ECHOs to assess aneurysm change. Patients who develop giant coronary aneurysms (internal diameter 8 mm or greater) are at the greatest risk for coronary thrombosis, stenosis, and myocardial infarction.

(3) Long-term therapy for high-risk children with cardiac abnormalities includes low-dose aspirin, either alone or with dipyridamole.

(4) Children with increasing cardiac symptoms or vessel involvement may require coronary artery bypass grafting.

F. LEAD POISONING

1. Sources of lead

a. Lead-based paint (the most common high-dose source of lead exposure for children): Window wells and sills are areas with high concentrations of lead dust (increased concern during home renovation and remodeling)

b. Soil and dust

c. Drinking water

d. Parental occupations and hobbies (furniture refinishing, making stained glass, working in a smelter or battery factory)

e. Air (much lower now that lead has been removed from gasoline)

f. Food (lead in soil or in lead soldered cans)

g. Imported ceramic objects, especially if used to hold foods or fluids for consumption

h. Cosmetic eye decorations containing kohl; medications from foreign countries

2. High-risk children

a. Children less than 72 months of age (and especially 12 to 36 months of age) who experience the following situations:

(1) Live in or are frequent visitors to deteriorated housing built before 1960

(2) Live in old houses with recent, ongoing, or planned renovation

(3) Live near lead smelters, battery recycling plants, or other industries likely to result in atmospheric lead release

(4) Have parents or other household members who participate in a lead-related occupation or hobby

b. Siblings, housemates, and playmates of children with lead poisoning

3. Symptoms of lead poisoning

a. Most children with elevated lead levels are asymptomatic and can only be identified by blood lead levels

22

MISCELLANEOUS DISEASES AND DISORDERS

b. Mild to moderate lead poisoning may be associated with learning/behavior problems, fatigue, malaise, anorexia, irritability, headache, abdominal pain, sporadic vomiting, and constipation.

c. Severe poisoning is associated with clumsiness, ataxia, paresis, sensorium changes, vomiting, coma, convulsions, and signs of increased intracranial pressure. The possibility of lead encephalopathy should be considered in the differential diagnosis of children presenting with coma and convulsions of unknown etiology.

d. Consider the possibility of lead poisoning in the child with developmental delay (especially language delay), FTT, ingestions, and parasitic infestation.

4. Screening

a. Screening should vary according to the prevalence of lead poisoning in an area. Universal screening by blood lead levels (BLL) is recommended in high risk areas defined as (1) greater than 12% of 1- and 2-year-old children have BLL greater than 10 mcg/dL, or (2) the prevalence of BLL is unknown, but more than 27% of housing was built before 1950. Local health departments have developed (are developing) data by zip codes and census tracts. Children should have blood lead testing at 9 to 12 months of age and again at 2 years of age. More frequent testing needs to take place if the BLL is greater than 9 mcg/dL. In addition, any child 36 to 72 months of age who has not previously been tested should be tested.

b. For children who do not meet the above high-risk criteria, targeted screening can take place. The decision to perform a lead test on a child should be based in part on the responses to a community-specific risk assessment questionnaire, which should include these questions:

(1) Does your child live in or regularly visit a house or child-care facility built before 1950?

(2) Does your child live in or regularly visit a house or child-care facility built before 1978 that is being or has recently (within the last 6 months) been renovated or remodeled?

(3) Does your child have a sibling or playmate who has or did have lead poisoning?

Children whose parents answer "yes" or "not sure" to any of these three risk-assessment questions should be considered for screening.

c. Follow-up screening is based on risk assessment and initial blood lead results. Children with developmental delay and frequent hand-to-mouth activity may be at increased risk.

d. Assessment of a blood lead level is the primary screening method. Unless contamination of capillary blood samples can be prevented, lead levels should be determined on venous samples whenever practical. All capillary specimen results should be considered presumptive and must be confirmed on a venous sample.

e. In patients with elevated blood-lead levels, an x-ray study of the abdomen can provide information about ingested lead paint chips, and x-ray studies of the long bones can provide information about the chronicity of the poisoning.

f. All children with blood-lead levels 20 mcg/dL or greater should be tested for iron deficiency, preferably with serum iron, iron-binding capacity, and serum ferritin.

5. Interpretation of blood-lead test results and follow-up recommendations: Classification is based on blood-lead concentration (Table 22-1).

6. Treatment

Note: Several drugs are used in the treatment of lead poisoning. They bind or chelate lead and deplete the soft and hard (skeletal) tissues of lead. All have potentially serious side effects and must be used with caution. The effect of chelation on neurodevelopmental toxicity in asymptomatic children is controversial. Chelation therapy may be dangerous if the child is not removed from the source of lead exposure.

a. Blood lead 25 to 44 mcg/dL (asymptomatic): Chelation has been controversial at this blood-lead level. A placebo-controlled trial of DMSA

TABLE 22-1

INTERPRETATION OF BLOOD-LEAD CONCENTRATIONS IN CHILDREN

Class	Blood-Lead Concentration (mcg/dL)	Comment
I	≤9	A child in Class I is not considered to be lead-poisoned.
IIA	10-14	Many children (or a large proportion of children) with blood-lead levels in this range should trigger community-wide childhood lead poisoning-prevention activities. Children in this range may need to be rescreened more often.
IIB	15-19	A child in Class IIB should receive nutritional and educational interventions and more frequent screening. If the blood-lead level persists in this range, environmental investigation and intervention should be done.
III	20-44	A child in Class III should receive environmental evaluation and remediation and a medical evaluation. Such a child may need pharmacologic treatment for lead poisoning.
IV	45-69	A child in Class IV needs both medical and environmental interventions, including chelation therapy.
V	≥70	A child with Class V lead poisoning is a medical emergency. Medical and environmental management must begin immediately.

22

MISCELLANEOUS DISEASES AND DISORDERS

in infants and toddlers with blood lead levels in this range showed no improvement in cognition, behavior, or neuropsychologic function over a period of 36 months.

b. Blood lead 45 to 69 mcg/dL (asymptomatic): Chelation therapy may be carried out with DMSA (succimer) at 1050 mg/m^2/d divided q8h × 5 days, and then 700 mg/m^2/d divided q12h × 14 days *or* calcium EDTA for 5 days at a daily dosage of 1000 mg/m^2 IV by continuous infusion or in two divided doses per day through a heparin lock over 30 to 60 minutes; it can also be given IM if mixed with procaine. However, EDTA efficacy is improved with a continuous IV delivery. Monitor renal and hepatic function and serum electrolytes. A second course of treatment may be needed if the BLL rebounds to 45 mcg/dL within 7 to 14 days after treatment. It is important to remove the child from the lead environment.

Note: Because of dose-related renal toxicity, calcium EDTA should never be given to patients with renal impairment or in the absence of adequate urine flow. When using calcium EDTA, monitor U/A, serum BUN, and creatinine.

c. Blood lead 70 mcg/dL or greater (asymptomatic): Chelation therapy should be carried out using both calcium EDTA and DMSA (see dosages earlier) *or* calcium EDTA and dimercaprol (BAL) at 300 mg/m^2/d parenterally × 5 days. The first dose of BAL should always precede the first dose of calcium EDTA by at least 4 hours. Renal and hepatic function and serum electrolytes need to be monitored. A second course of therapy with calcium EDTA alone may be required if the BLL rebounds to 45 to 69 mcg/dL within 5 to 7 days after treatment. If the rebound is to 70 mcg/dL or greater, BAL plus calcium EDTA should be used.

Note: BAL (prepared in peanut oil solution) should not be used in children who are allergic to peanuts or peanut products. Medicinal iron should not be administered during BAL therapy. Except in life-threatening situations, BAL should not be used in children with G-6-PD deficiency (may induce hemolysis).

d. Symptomatic lead poisoning
   (1) Refer the patient to a pediatric center that has expertise in the treatment of lead poisoning.
   (2) The patient needs chelation with calcium EDTA plus BAL and careful monitoring.

e. A few additional comments on succimer (2,3 dimercaptosuccinic acid; DMSA; Chemet), an oral agent.
   (1) Succimer should be administered only in a lead-free environment because it may increase GI absorption of lead.
   (2) A treatment course lasts 19 days. Start with a dosage of 350 mg/m^2 q8h × 5 days and then reduce dosage to 350 mg/m^2 q12h for an additional 2 weeks. There is approximately a 60% reduction in blood-lead concentration during treatment.

(a) A child with a history of constipation should have an enema before starting treatment.

(b) Young children who cannot swallow capsules can be given succimer by separating the capsule and sprinkling the beads on soft food or by putting them in a spoon and following with a fruit drink. Succimer can be used in children with G-6-PD deficiency and can be given concomitantly with iron. It is contraindicated in children with an allergy to sulfa or mercaptan.

(c) Maintain adequate hydration; use with caution in patients with compromised renal function.

(3) Adverse events

(a) Such events are uncommon but include malaise, nausea, vomiting, diarrhea, anorexia, rash, reversible neutropenia, and transient increases in serum transaminases and alkaline phosphatase.

(b) Serum transaminases should be monitored before initiating treatment and at least weekly during treatment. Also monitor U/A, CBC, serum BUN, and creatinine.

(4) Follow-up

(a) BLL should be monitored weekly until stable. Rebound elevations of 60% to 70% are common secondary to redistribution of lead from bone stores; levels plateau 2 to 3 weeks after discontinuing treatment. Repeated courses of succimer, usually at 4-week intervals, may be necessary. The end point of therapy is a post-rebound BLL of less than 15 mcg/dL.

(b) The safety of uninterrupted dosing for longer than 3 weeks has not been established and is not recommended.

7. Interventions to reduce lead exposure

a. Whenever possible, remove child from lead source; consider different residence, day-care, relative's home, etc.

b. Prevent access to peeling paint or chewable surfaces. Move cribs and playpens away from surfaces containing lead paint. Stabilize or cover lead paint. Put furniture in front of leaded areas to block accessibility.

c. Wet-mop floors and wet-clean window sills and wells and horizontal surfaces weekly with detergent. Use two buckets, one with detergent and one with rinse water, changing the rinse water frequently and disposing of the water in a toilet or laundry sink.

d. Avoid dry dusting, sweeping, and vacuuming hard surfaces; consider use of a HEPA vacuum.

e. Wash child's hands and face before meals.

f. Wash toys and pacifiers often.

g. Encourage regular meals and shakes low in fat and high in iron, calcium, and vitamin C.

22

MISCELLANEOUS DISEASES AND DISORDERS

h. Use cold water for cooking; run water for 2 to 3 minutes in the morning before using.

i. When a dwelling is being abated for lead or renovations are taking place, the child should be temporarily relocated to avoid exposure to lead dust.

G. LYMPHADENOPATHY

1. General guidelines

In the evaluation of a child with lymphadenopathy, the following points can be helpful in the differential diagnosis:

a. Size: Nodes less than 3 mm in diameter are normal. Up to 12 years of age, cervical and inguinal nodes up to 1 cm and epitrochlear nodes up to 0.5 cm may be normal. Nodes greater than 2 cm may indicate a granulomatous disease or tumor.

b. Node location
   (1) Hodgkin's disease: Supraclavicular and lower neck
   (2) Cat-scratch disease: Preauricular, axillary, inguinal, epitrochlear
   (3) Reactive hyperplasia: Inguinal, submental, posterior cervical
   (4) Atypical mycobacterium: Upper cervical, submandibular, preauricular

Note: **Generalized adenopathy usually results from generalized disease.**

c. Duration: Not too helpful in suggesting a diagnosis. Biopsy is indicated if the node increases after a 2-week follow-up *or* has not decreased after 4 to 6 weeks.

d. Consistency
   (1) Matted or fixed nodes: Neoplasm or granulomatous disease
   (2) Tender nodes with overlying erythema: Bacterial adenitis; the more tender the node, the less ominous the prognosis

e. Age
   (1) Patient less than 4 years of age: Reactive hyperplasia, atypical mycobacterium, acute pyogenic cervical lymphadenitis
   (2) Patient more than 8 years of age: Reactive hyperplasia, cat-scratch disease, Hodgkin's disease (especially in teenagers)

f. Associated signs and symptoms: Liver/spleen enlargement, prolonged fever, and weight loss suggest a serious systemic illness (malignancy).

2. History

a. Exposure to TB, cats? Medication history (e.g., phenytoin [Dilantin])? Periodontal disease?

b. The most common cause of cervical adenopathy in children is bacterial or viral infection in the ENT area.

c. Generalized adenopathy (two or more noncontiguous lymph node groups) usually results from reactive hyperplasia and is by far the most common diagnosis in children who undergo biopsy.

d. If the patient is febrile longer than 1 week, rule out mononucleosis, CMV, toxoplasmosis, and KD.

e. Ask about the possibility of HIV infection.

3. Workup

a. History, PE, CBC, ESR, PPD, monospot test, TC, viral titers, chest x-ray; if multiple enlarged nodes, HIV PCR (infant) or antibody (older than 18 months of age).

b. The role of needle aspiration is controversial; the most significant treatable conditions are best diagnosed by open biopsy.

4. Timing of lymph node biopsy. In general, indications for biopsy include the following:

a. Unexplained fever and weight loss

b. Fixation of node to overlying skin or underlying tissue

c. Supraclavicular location

d. Abnormal chest x-ray (strongest predictor of serious disease)

e. Increase in size of node after several weeks of observation

5. The following scoring system may be useful in adolescents:

Abnormal CXR	5 points
Lymph node >2 cm	3 points
ENT symptoms	−3 points
Constant	−2 points

a. If score is greater than 0, biopsy probably will lead to treatment.

b. If score is less than 0, watch; biopsy probably will not alter treatment.

c. The greater the score, the more likely it is to be correct.

6. Even after biopsy, a specific cause may be established in only 40% of children. The most common histologic diagnoses are reactive hyperplasia, neoplastic disease, and granulomatous disease.

Note: Approximately 20% of children who initially have a nondiagnostic biopsy eventually develop a specific pathologic process. Patients need close follow-up.

7. Specific causes of lymphadenopathy

a. Atypical mycobacterium

    (1) Usually mycobacterium avium complex; acquired from environmental sources. Human contact does not play a role in transmission.

    (2) It commonly occurs between 1 and 6 years of age.

    (3) Nodes are unilateral, firm, mobile, and without tenderness but may be fluctuant.

        (a) The overlying skin may become violaceous and thin. If untreated, the lymphadenitis may resolve, but often progresses to spontaneous drainage with sinus tract formation and scarring.

        (b) The usual location is preauricular, upper anterior cervical, or submandibular.

    (4) Systemic and pulmonary manifestations are uncommon.

    (5) The CXR is negative. The PPD is negative or weakly positive, but NTM-specific antigens, particularly PPD-B, can be diagnostically helpful.

      (6)   Diagnosis: Confirmed by positive AFB culture from node but is present in only 50% of cases. A positive AFB smear and characteristic histopathology are helpful but not diagnostic.

      (7)   Treatment: Total excision; anti-TB drugs are ineffective. Avoid I&D or needle aspiration (may lead to chronic draining sinus tract).

b.   Lymphoma

      (1)   Patients more than 8 years of age; usually teenagers

      (2)   Rubbery, matted or fixed, nontender nodes

      (3)   Supraclavicular and lower cervical location

      (4)   Liver/spleen enlargement, fever, weight loss, anemia, abnormal CXR (mediastinal or hilar adenopathy)

      (5)   Diagnosis: Biopsy

c.   Cat-scratch disease

      (1)   Unilateral, subacute regional lymphadenitis; parotid, preauricular, axillary, epitrochlear, inguinal; suppurative in 15% of cases; may be accompanied by malaise, fatigue, low-grade fever.

      (2)   History of cat (often kitten) exposure; crusted papule or vesiculopustule at inoculation site distal to node. Negative laboratory results for other causes of lymphadenopathy.

      (3)   May be positive cat-scratch skin test, but antigen is not standardized or licensed.

      (4)   Biopsy of node shows multiple nonnecrotizing granulomas and microabscesses; positive Warthin-Starry silver stain.

      (5)   Etiologic agent: *Rochalimaea henselae.*

      (6)   Diagnosis: Suggested by clinical features; can be confirmed by demonstrating elevated antibody titer to *R. henselae* or the presence of *R. henselae* DNA (by PCR) in purulent material aspirated from suppurative node.

      (7)   Treatment: Most cases resolve spontaneously within several months. Rifampin, ciprofloxacin, TMP/SMZ, and gentamicin may be effective but are indicated only in patients with severe disease. Avoid I&D of nodes because it may lead to chronic draining sinus tract.

Note: Other presentations of cat-scratch disease include Parinaud's oculoglandular syndrome, erythema nodosum, encephalopathy, osteolytic lesions, and multiple hepatic abscesses. Patients with hepatic abscesses have prolonged fever, abdominal pain, hepatomegaly, with or without splenomegaly, with or without regional lymphadenopathy, and scattered hyperechoic hepatic lesions on CT scan or ultrasound.

d.   Viral

      (1)   Any age

      (2)   Discrete, mobile, soft consistency; no redness or warmth; may be tender

      (3)   Upper anterior cervical, posterior cervical, generalized

   (4) Associated fever, malaise, URI symptoms; liver/spleen enlargement

   (5) Diagnosis: Serologic studies

Note: CMV and toxoplasmosis may be indistinguishable from Epstein-Barr virus infection.

 e. Bacterial

   (1) Any age, but usually the patient is less than 5 years of age

   (2) Discrete, red, warm, tender; may be fluctulant

   (3) Upper anterior cervical, posterior cervical, inguinal, occasionally axillary

   (4) May have associated systemic symptoms

   (5) Diagnosis: Cultures of throat, skin, or other obvious site; needle biopsy of node

   (6) Treatment: Broad-spectrum antibiotic that includes penicillinase-producing *S. aureus* coverage

H. STINGING INSECT REACTIONS (BEES, YELLOW JACKETS, WASPS, HORNETS, FIRE ANTS)

1. Small local reaction

 a. Small scattered hives with erythema, pain, and pruritus; lasts several hours.

 b. Treatment: Cold compress. Carefully remove stinger (honeybee) by scraping the sting site with the edge of a credit card.

2. Large local reaction

 a. Swelling at sting site greater than 5 cm; may involve entire extremity. Reaction peaks at 48 to 72 hours and may last as long as 1 week.

 b. Treatment: Ice, oral antihistamine, analgesic, oral prednisone burst if severe swelling (see Chapter 21, Section H).

3. Mild systemic reaction

 a. Generalized urticaria, erythema, pruritus, and angioedema (in children, 70% of systemic reactions to stings are cutaneous).

 b. Treatment: SQ epinephrine 1:1000, 0.01 ml/kg up to 0.3 ml, may repeat in 15 minutes; PO antihistamine.

 c. Skin testing and immunotherapy are not indicated.

 d. Patients with a history of prior reaction should have an epinephrine kit available for self-injection (Epipen, AnaKit), especially when away from access to medical care. However, among children with a generalized cutaneous reaction, the reaction with another sting is almost never more severe than the previous reaction.

 e. Careful instructions regarding insect avoidance.

4. Life-threatening systemic reaction

 a. Laryngeal edema, bronchospasm, hypotension; often accompanied by cutaneous manifestations.

 b. Treatment: SQ epinephrine 1:1000, 0.01 ml/kg up to 0.3 ml, oxygen, volume expanders, pressor agents, airway support, inhaled beta-2-agonist.

22

MISCELLANEOUS DISEASES AND DISORDERS

c. Steroids are not generally effective (delayed onset of action) but are usually given by IV route.

d. Patient should be referred to an allergist for skin testing and possible venom immunotherapy.

e. Patient should always carry an epinephrine self-injector (Epipen, AnaKit). Patient, family, and caregivers such as school personnel should be carefully instructed in the use of the injector device.

5. Unusual reactions following insect stings include serum sickness, vasculitis, encephalitis, nephritis, and Guillain-Barré syndrome.

Note: In general, stinging insect reactions are rarely fatal in children, and severe reactions tend to diminish over time.

I. BIBLIOGRAPHY

AIDS

AAP Committee on Pediatric AIDS: Evaluation and medical treatment of the HIV-exposed infant, *Pediatrics* 99:909, 1997.

AAP Committee on Pediatric AIDS: Issues related to HIV transmission in schools, child care, medical settings, and community, *Pediatrics* 104:318, 1999.

AAP Committee on Pediatric AIDS: Surveillance of pediatric HIV infection, *Pediatrics* 101:305, 1998.

AAP Committee on Sports Medicine: HIV and other blood-borne viral pathogens in the athletic setting, *Pediatrics* 104:1400, 1999.

Butz A, Joyner M, Friedman D et al: Primary care for children with HIV infection, *J Pediatr Hlth Care* 12:10, 1998.

Grubman S, Gross E, Lerner-Weiss N et al: Older children and adolescents living with perinatally acquired HIV infection, *Pediatrics* 95:657, 1995.

Kline M: Oral manifestations of pediatric HIV infection: a review of the literature, *Pediatrics:* 97:380, 1996.

Kline M, VanDyke R, Lindsey J et al: A randomized comparative trial of stavudine (d4T) vs zidovudine (AZT) in children with HIV infection, *Pediatrics* 101:214, 1998.

Melvin A, Tamura G, House K et al: Lack of detection of HIV-1 in the saliva of infected children and adolescents, *Arch Pediatr Adolesc Med* 151:228, 1997.

Mueller B et al: Clinical and pharmacokinetic evaluation of long-term therapy with didanosine in children with HIV infection, *Pediatrics* 94:724, 1994.

Chest Pain

Brown R: Recurrent chest pain in adolescents, *Pediatr Ann* 20:194, 1991.

Selbst S: Chest pain in children, *Pediatr in Rev* 18:169, 1997.

Failure to Thrive

Careaga MG, Kerner JA: A gastroenterologist's approach to failure to thrive, *Pediatr Ann* 29:558, 2000.

Frank D et al: Failure to thrive: mystery, myth, and method, *Contemp Pediatr* 8:114, 1993.

Schwartz ID: Failure to thrive—an old nemesis in the new millennium, *Pediatr in Rev* 21:257, 2000.

Zenel J: Failure to thrive—a general pediatrician's perspective, *Pediatr in Rev* 18:371, 1997.

Hypertension

Adelman RD, Coppo R, Dillon MJ: The emergency management of severe hypertension, *Pediatr Nephrol* 14:422, 2000.

Bartosh S, Aronson A: Childhood hypertension, *PCNA* 46:235, 1999.

Daniels S: The diagnosis of hypertension in children—an update, *Pediatr in Rev* 18:131, 1997.

Flynn J, Pasko D: Calcium channel blockers—pharmacology and place in therapy of pediatric hypertension., *Pediatr Nephr* 15:302, 2000.

Groshong T: Hypertensive crisis in children, *Pediatr Ann* 25:368, 1996.

Hohn A: Diagnosis and management of hypertension in childhood, *Pediatr Ann* 26:105, 1997.

Rosner B: Blood pressure nomograms for children and adolescents by height, sex, and age in the U.S., *J Pediatr* 123:871, 1993.

Sardegna K, Loggie J: Hypertension in teens, *Contemp Pediatr* 13:96, 1996.
Sinaiko A: Treatment of hypertension in children, *Pediatr Nephrol* 8:603, 1994.
Temple M, Nahata M: Treatment of pediatric hypertension, *Pharmacotherapy* 20:140, 2000.
Varon J, Marik P: The diagnosis and management of hypertensive crises, *Chest* 118:214, 2000.

Kawasaki Disease
Curtis N, Levin M: Kawasaki disease thirty years on, *Curr Op in Pediatr* 10:24, 1998.
Feit L: Keeping up with Kawasaki syndrome, *Contemp Pediatr* 12:37, 1995.
Pahl E: Kawasaki disease—cardiac sequelae and management, *Pediatr Ann* 26:112, 1997.
Rowley A, Shulman S: Kawasaki syndrome, *PCNA* 46:313, 1999.
Shulman ST et al: Kawasaki disease, *PCNA* 42:1205, 1995.

Lead Poisoning
American Academy of Pediatrics—Committee on Drugs: Treatment guidelines for lead exposure in children, *Pediatrics* 96:155, 1995.
American Academy of Pediatrics—Committee on Environmental Health: Screening for elevated blood lead levels, *Pediatrics* 101:1072, 1998.
Markowitz M: Lead poisoning, *Pediatr in Rev* 21:327, 2000.
Markowitz M: Lead poisoning—a disease for the next millennium, *Curr Prob in Pediatr* 30:62, 2000.
Rogan WJ et al: The effect of chelation therapy with succimer on neuropsychological development in children exposed to lead, *N Engl J Med* 344:1421, 2001.

Lymphadenopathy
Kelly CS, Kelly R: Lymphadenopathy in children, *PCNA* 45:875, 1998.
Peters T, Edwards K: Cervical lymphadenopathy and adenitis, *Pediatr in Rev* 21:399, 2000.

Stinging Insect Reactions
Müller U et al: Emergency treatment of allergic reactions to hymenoptera stings, *Clin Exp Allergy* 21:281, 1991.
Reisman RE: Natural history of insect sting allergy: relationship of severity of symptoms of initial sting anaphylaxis to re-sting reactions, *J Allergy Clin Immunol* 90:335, 1992.

22

MISCELLANEOUS DISEASES AND DISORDERS

CHRONIC, CATASTROPHIC, AND TERMINAL CONDITIONS

A. GENERAL ISSUES

1. Family issues
a. The occurrence of a chronic condition, catastrophic injury, sequelae of an illness, or a terminal illness is devastating for patient and family alike. One of the most helpful things that such families report is the presence of a caring physician who has known the patient and family over a long period of time. Such a person knows both the strengths of the patient and family and also the challenges they face.
b. Many parents report that the most important things that a physician can give them are respect, sensitivity, support, time to hear their concerns and answer their questions, information about their child's condition, and information about support groups in their community. Parents report dissatisfaction with care when the provider makes insensitive remarks or has a negative attitude toward the condition in question, fails to give sufficient information to parents or excludes them from decision making, makes inadequate referrals (too few, too late), or provides poor medical care.
c. The patient's regular physician might have to serve not only as medical caregiver but also as the patient's (and family's) advocate as they traverse the complicated health care system to obtain optimum care. This includes handling issues with insurance companies as to what is needed and what should and should not be covered, orchestrating specialist care, and obtaining medical equipment for home use, for instance.
d. The patient's regular physician must keep in close contact with any specialists who are involved in his or her patient's care. Thus, the regular physician cannot simply leave decisions about medications and therapies solely to the "experts," for the primary care physician *is* the expert for a given family.
e. It is important to remember that in cases of chronic, catastrophic, and terminal conditions the entire family is affected, regardless of the age of the ill or injured patient. Furthermore, the reactions of each person in the family will differ by age, gender, relationship to the patient, psychologic strengths and coping strategies, and the type of condition that is present. See Section E.
f. Not all families which have a member with a chronic, catastrophic, or terminal condition will be permanently adversely affected. Family functioning is affected by family size, family values, marital stability, innate coping skills, presence of antecedent family problems, connectedness to others outside the family, resources available (e.g., financial, community, emotional, religious), amount of information

about the condition in question, and ability of family members to share each other's concerns and feelings, especially the ill child's comfort in such sharing.

2. Physician issues
a. Primary care physicians can also be affected by the presence of certain conditions in their patients. Particularly stressful or painful reactions can be expected when the condition is fatal, preventable, the result of error or oversight, or when a given patient or family is close to the physician. Also potentially difficult are situations in which the affected patient is close in age to a physician's own children.

B. CHRONIC ILLNESS

1. General comments
a. From the adult point of view, the impact of a chronic illness depends on its persistence, severity, and ability to shorten the life of the affected child or adolescent. This is not necessarily true for children or adolescents, who consider many conditions that are minor but obvious (e.g., acne, eczema) as severe and worse than much more serious conditions that are "invisible" (e.g., diabetes).
b. Likewise, any therapeutic modality that makes the child or adolescent feel different (e.g., special diet, limitation of activity, daily medications by any route) is usually perceived as indicating a more serious condition than less obvious therapies.
c. After the diagnosis of a chronic condition, many children and adolescents need time to adjust to the new reality about themselves. Adjustment times cannot be predicted and depend on the condition in question (and its severity, persistence, or tendency toward exacerbations/worsening), age at diagnosis, impact on the patient's daily activities, support systems in place, and psychologic coping skills possessed by the patient and close family members.

2. Physical issues
a. Many chronic conditions have enormous impact on the physical development of a child or adolescent. Growth in weight and height may be delayed or stunted. Developmental milestones, attained at an earlier age, might be lost or never developed at all. The ability to care for oneself might be limited. Puberty might be delayed.
b. Some chronic conditions leave obvious scars on the body either because of their intrinsic effects or because of their treatments (e.g., a gastrostomy [GT] tube). Other conditions leave the child or adolescent weakened during times of flare-ups, thus interfering with his or her usual activities.
c. Other medical problems occur because of the side effects of needed medications (e.g., anemia, loss of appetite, gastric upset) or the impact of a special diet.

3. Psychosocial issues (by age)
a. Infancy and toddlerhood

(1) Infants and toddlers might have to endure prolonged separation from their parents or other primary caregivers, thus interfering with the normal bonding that occurs in healthy relationships; this causes emotional distress. Instances in which the parent is present but unavailable (e.g., a parent who cannot hold his or her restrained infant, a parent who cannot rescue the toddler who is having a procedure in the parent's presence) can also cause emotional distress.

(2) Infants and toddlers might have to undergo many painful procedures or operations. Because they cannot adequately express the degree of their pain and cannot understand why they must undergo repeated noxious stimuli, they experience psychologic suffering.

(3) The diets and activities of infants and toddlers may be severely limited, also causing them to suffer.

(4) The loss of familiar persons (e.g., siblings) and environments (e.g., one's room) contribute to a young child's loss of equilibrium.

b. Preschool and school-age children

(1) Children might have to endure prolonged separation from their parents or other primary caregivers, but unlike their younger siblings, they can understand a bit about why this is so. However, just because children ask questions does not imply that they *really* comprehend what they are being told. In addition, children may not ask questions but "pick up" information, which they may misinterpret. Sometimes, what they "hear" or imagine is far worse than reality. Efforts should be made to elicit their understanding of their condition, treatments, and prognosis, especially as they mature.

(2) The loss of normal activities will affect children, and this is especially true when they cannot be with their friends in the neighborhood or at school. When children must miss school, *every* attempt should be made to help them keep up with their assignments and to keep in contact with schoolmates. Friends should be invited to visit, call, e-mail, or write. The ill child should be encouraged to initiate some of these contacts.

(3) A child's diet might need to be radically altered. It is expected that most children will exhibit some defiance in this area, attempting to ingest foods that are forbidden or to refuse foods that are needed. Firmness, tempered with reasonable allowances for special treats, is usually the most successful approach. Depending on the condition in question (especially if certain medications are taken), some foods might have an unpleasant effect on a child's digestive system. Not all of these can be predicted, but those that can be predicted should be discussed with both child and parent.

23

CHRONIC, CATASTROPHIC, AND TERMINAL CONDITIONS

(4) The child needs to maintain as much normalcy in his or her life as possible. This includes favorite activities in or outside the home. If multiple activities must be curtailed without other activities to take their place, children may react to limitations with anger or continuous attempts to thwart them. For that reason, limitations on activities, diet, and so forth must be explained fully to the child, at an age-appropriate level, giving him or her the opportunity to ask questions, suggest alternatives, and voice displeasure.

(5) Many children with chronic illnesses take their medications without any problem. Others require coaxing, while still others refuse them. However, all children forget to take their medications at some time or another, and this is to be expected. An occasional lapse in medication adherence should be approached sympathetically and gently. After all, it *is* difficult to adhere 100% of the time. More frequent lapses should be investigated promptly to determine the reason. For example, does the medication make the child feel badly? Has he or she heard (rightly or wrongly) that this medication might cause some sort of problem? Does it taste bad? Is it hard to take? Is the child denying his or her illness and thinks that the medication is unnecessary? Is the child subject to ridicule because he or she must take a medication?

(6) When a chronic condition is first diagnosed, many children and adolescents undergo a period of grieving over the loss of their once-healthy selves, the loss of a healthy future, or just fear. They might become sad and weepy or angry and acting out. Sometimes, they are just sullen. In extreme cases, professional psychologic help might be warranted. Most children, however, do not require a professional in order to help them adjust to a chronic condition, but they *do* need someone to whom they can speak openly about their anger, fears, questions, and concerns.

(7) While some investigators believe that the likelihood of behavior problems increases in the presence of chronic conditions, others note that such problems are not necessarily a certainty, but are related to the parent–child bond, the mother's mental health, the prognosis of the child's condition, and the home milieu.

c. Adolescents

(1) Adolescents feel different from their peers, and usually dislike this difference. Hence, they may try to downplay dietary or activity restrictions or "forget" to take medications when they are around friends. This is to be expected. They need to understand fully why the restrictions are placed on them and the consequences of ignoring those restrictions (or neglecting to take medications).

(2) Such adolescents need to engage in as many of their usual activities as possible, including school (or keeping up with schoolwork if they must miss classes), hobbies, social

connections, and sports (if applicable). If the primary physician is unsure as to whether a certain activity is permitted, consultation with the condition-specific specialist involved is in order.

(3) Keep dietary restrictions to those most needed so that the adolescent can enjoy going out with friends without undue embarrassment.

(4) Appreciate that the adolescent with a chronic condition may be grieving about his or her health. This might be manifested by anger about his or her limitations (with accompanying behavior problems), the prospect of a future marked with remissions and exacerbations of the condition, and, perhaps, the prospect of a shortened life. Adolescents who are angry might fail to adhere to needed regimens, or they might exhibit acting-out behaviors. Grief may also be manifested as sadness or depression. Adolescents who are saddened by their condition might fail to adhere, especially if they think that their plight is hopeless. Asking questions of the adolescent to permit him or her to voice concerns, questions, anger, sadness, and so on is the best way to elicit what is motivating him or her to act in the way he or she does. Professional help may be needed, especially if the adolescent is engaging in risky behaviors such as sexual promiscuity, alcohol ingestion, drug use, or illegal activities. However, even adolescents not exhibiting these behaviors need someone to whom they can talk openly without fear of recrimination.

(5) Adolescents should have reliable friends with whom they can communicate in person, by phone, by e-mail, or in writing.

(6) Always answer all questions honestly and as fully as the adolescent needs them answered.

(7) Concerns about sexuality and attractiveness to others often surface. Many adolescents with chronic conditions worry that they will be unable to marry or have children because of their disease. These concerns must be taken seriously and be approached with great gentleness and reassurance.

4. Spiritual issues

a. For many children and adolescents raised in Western religious traditions, there are a number of spiritual issues that arise with a new (or continuing) diagnosis of a chronic condition, especially in times of flare-ups. These vary by age.

(1) "Why me?" Most children and adolescents fear being different from peers. Chronic conditions make them different. Children who believe in God may question why God would let them be different or suffer. This question is more common in elementary school-age children and adolescents than in preschoolers.

(2) "Is God mad at me?" "Am I being punished?" Following from the first question, children might think that they have done something

terribly wrong to merit such a condition. If children think that they are being punished for something they have done, they may resist taking their medications or getting better in the fear that such "trying to get out of it" might anger God who was punishing them in the first place. This question is common in children (of all ages) and adolescents, especially those who have been raised with an image of God as punitive.

(3) "If I pray real hard, will God make me all better?" "Why does God make some people better, but not me?" These questions are common in elementary school-age children and adolescents, and stem from their great desire for fairness. After all, if God makes one person better, why not another? Does that mean that God likes one better than another? Furthermore, bargaining is common in those of all ages who are facing loss. One makes a bargain with God that if one does a particular thing, then God should honor that person's request.

(4) "Am I going to die?" "Will I be alone?" These issues are both practical and spiritual and depend, in large part, on the child's or adolescent's ideas about the afterlife and who might be present there. Frequently, these questions surface after a particularly severe exacerbation of a chronic condition. These questions are posed by elementary school-age children and adolescents—both those who believe in God and those who do not. After all, death is the great unknown that each person must encounter alone. It is natural, then, that children and adolescents (who are so interested in their social world) would be afraid of both the experience and having to do it alone.

b. The assistance of a person well equipped to explore such issues with children and adolescents should be sought, for these questions generally do arise in some form. This need not be the health professional. Under no circumstances should a health professional squelch such questions because of discomfort in answering them, as this makes the young patient feel more alone than ever or confirms the view that the condition is punishment.

5. Ethical issues

a. Certain ethical issues arise during the diagnosis and treatment of a chronic condition, or with regard to participation in research trials.

(1) The main ethical issue is whether a patient should know the nature of his or her chronic condition. On the one hand, the patient might be more motivated to take medications and follow regimens if their purpose is better understood. On the other hand, knowledge of the nature of a condition, especially if it is progressive or fatal, might lead to despair. This must be approached on a case-by-case basis, but, in general, patients old enough to ask meaningful questions or obtain information on their own should be given as much information as they can

understand and tolerate. This will include elementary school-age children and adolescents. Under *no* circumstance should a health care professional participate in a lie to the patient.

(2) After disclosure of the condition, children and adolescents frequently want to know if they will get better, get worse, or die. Information should be honestly given at an age-appropriate level, answering their specific question(s). It is not necessary to provide information for which the patient has not asked or to overwhelm the child or adolescent with facts that he or she cannot fully understand.

(3) Children and adolescents generally want to know whether they will have to take medicine(s) or whether they will have to have certain tests. Specific questions should be answered honestly, but sympathetically. For example, if medications must be taken, say so and state why they are necessary. If blood testing must be done at each visit, say so and explain how those tests help to keep the patient as healthy as possible. The reason for the medication should not be falsified, and its importance should be neither minimized nor exaggerated.

(4) When regimens fail or need to be changed, the patient needs to understand the reasons for such alterations in therapy in an age-appropriate manner. If nonadherence is part of the problem, this, too, must be broached sympathetically but openly. "Scare tactics" do not usually work, because change in behavior comes from within, not from without.

(5) When a chronic condition has entered its terminal phase, different issues must be faced (see Section D).

(6) When patient and parent disagree on a course of therapy, each side must be approached with kindness and honesty, regardless of whose side the health professional favors. When children are very young, they have little role in determining their course of therapy. As they mature, their opinions and wishes increasingly must be taken into account. Sometimes, the use of a trusted neutral third party might help both sides see the value of each other's position.

(7) Involvement in research projects is a common ethical issue. Ideally, parents should give consent *and* pediatric patients should give assent to involvement in studies; this will be dependent on the age and ability of the patient to understand what is required. In the best case, some direct benefit would be likely for the child or adolescent who participates in a research study; in many cases, no direct benefit is likely (e.g., child is a control in a study looking at different therapeutic regimens), or there is a possibility that harm may occur *without direct benefit* to the patient (e.g., child is a control who will receive radiation to compare his or her anatomy to that of other children with a certain condition). In

23

CHRONIC, CATASTROPHIC, AND TERMINAL CONDITIONS

these latter cases, it is most prudent for the health care provider to advocate for the child or adolescent and honor his or her request *not* to be involved even if the parent wishes involvement. This is especially true if the child or adolescent feels this way after several attempts to elicit their assent.

b. Whenever there is a serious disagreement between patient and parent about a course of therapy, the services of an ethics committee or consultant should be sought.

6. Chronic medications, procedures, and visits to health professionals

a. Most children and adolescents with chronic conditions resist taking their medications, at least occasionally. This is also true of special diets, procedures, and other regimens. Such behavior is to be expected and approached sympathetically. It *is* hard to be young and unable to keep up with one's peers, have to eat special foods (or avoid others), have to undergo certain procedures regularly (e.g., nebulizations), or have to take medications. All of these remind the child or adolescent with a chronic condition that he or she is different. The reasons for the special diet, procedures, or medications must be clearly explained to the patient in an age-appropriate manner. Better yet is to show how adherence to these regimens is keeping the child or adolescent healthier.

b. Visits to health professionals might be welcomed by the young patient or feared because of what might be found or the very real potential of pain (e.g., a venipuncture). A sympathetic approach is best, acknowledging that some patients really do not like coming to see the doctor and being open to the possibility that this might be the case with a given child or adolescent. Keeping the lines of communication open with these young patients and eliciting their opinions of how visits could be better for them might go a long way in increasing their degree of comfort.

7. Hospitalizations

a. Being hospitalized is a major blow for many children and adolescents, who fear that their condition is worsening or that they may be dying. This is especially true if the disease exacerbation has been frightening or severe. Health professionals (and parents) may contribute to this mind-set by whispering around such patients, wearing worried looks, refusing to answer questions, looking away from patients, or avoiding them.

b. Hospitalization is a time when honesty (tempered with kindness and reassurance) is of paramount importance. Health professionals should engage their patient in conversations about their condition so that unrealistic fears can be minimized by accurate information. Fears should always be addressed and never trivialized.

c. The hospitalized child or adolescent is part of the team and should know the treatment strategy—why this hospitalization occurred, what is being done to make him or her better, the measures to prevent another hospitalization for this same reason, and his or her role in all this.

d. Some children and adolescents *like* to be hospitalized because of deplorable living conditions at home, or because they feel more secure with the level of care (and love) given in a hospital compared to that given at home. They might exaggerate symptoms simply to get admitted. Such children benefit from the services of mental health professionals and social work assessment of their home and caregivers.

C. CATASTROPHIC INJURIES

1. General comments
a. Catastrophic injuries are those that cause devastating and permanent sequelae to at least one major organ system.
b. Common catastrophic injuries are those to brain and spinal cord, vital internal organs, or limbs requiring amputation. Such injuries leave the affected person with deficits in cognition, self-care, ambulation, or even vital functioning such as breathing on one's own.
c. Common etiologies include motor vehicle accidents, drowning, diving accidents, sports injuries, gunshot injuries, burns, electrocution (via a faulty electrical appliance, downed wires, or, much more rarely, lightning), and child abuse.
d. Such injuries may leave the person completely technology dependent (ventilator, feeding by pump), whether or not he or she is in a vegetative state. Even with less life-threatening injuries, months (or years) of rehabilitation or numerous surgeries, each with its own sequelae and recovery time, may be needed.
e. Injuries and their sequelae not only impact the affected person but also the entire family, placing enormous strain on family reserves (emotional and material).

2. Physical issues
a. Depending on the age of the injured child and the type of injury sustained, physical development may be arrested or may regress. For example, an infant seriously injured by abuse might eventually reach physical milestones, but at a much slower rate (and much later) than usual. An older child with the same injury might demonstrate loss of motor abilities that are never fully recovered. Although prognosis is highly dependent on the type and severity of the injury sustained, in general, younger children seem to make better recoveries physically than do older children and adolescents.
b. Injuries to the brain may have far-reaching effects, such as loss of abilities to breathe independently; swallow or eat without choking; clear airway secretions; see, hear, speak, or move independently; or reach puberty.
c. Injuries to the spinal cord also have far-reaching effects, but these effects are dependent on the area of cord injured. Upper cord injuries

CHRONIC, CATASTROPHIC, AND TERMINAL CONDITIONS

23

may cause complete paralysis and sensory deficits below the shoulders (including the diaphragm, necessitating reliance on a ventilator), while lower cord injuries may cause paralysis and sensory deficits in the legs and, with certain injuries, inability to control urination or defecation.

d.   Regardless of injury and sequelae, the child or adolescent with physical impairment after an injury will benefit from the services of a physical therapist, occupational therapist, or both. These professionals should be enlisted early in the recuperation process. They can assess baseline abilities, gauge which regimens are most likely to make an impact, and monitor progress.

e.   Those with catastrophic injuries often experience much physical pain because of their injuries, needed therapies, or multiple surgeries. For severe pain, simple analgesics will not suffice and should not be relied upon out of fear of creating addiction to more potent analgesics. Pain management should be approached with the assistance of a pediatric professional well versed in this area. Failure to appreciate a child's or adolescent's degree of pain *and to do something about relieving it* might mean the difference between cooperation with therapeutic regimens leading to optimal recovery and failure to cooperate leading to a poorer outcome.

3.   Emotional/psychologic development

a.   The older an injured person is, the more cognizant he or she is of previous abilities and current deficits and limitations. Hence, older children and adolescents have the capacity to suffer more (and despair) than do infants and younger children. One moment, they were completely well; the next moment, they were seriously injured.

b.   Because infants are at an early stage of development, they do not realize what they have lost or what others their age can do. The same is true of toddlers and younger preschoolers. In some ways, this makes their recovery easier.

c.   Infants and toddlers need the security of trusted adults around them, especially during painful procedures.

d.   Preschoolers also need trusted adults with them. They need their questions and concerns addressed and their fears taken seriously. Because preschoolers can communicate verbally, parents, other caregivers, and health professionals should attempt to ease their suffering through comforting words and gentle explanations. This is especially true when procedures are painful or medications are distasteful.

e.   Elementary school-age children are fully aware of what they used to be able to do and what they can no longer do. In addition to needing the presence of trusted adults, they need their fears addressed sympathetically, without any ridicule or minimization of these fears. They will have many questions, and failure to address these questions might lead them to imagine scenarios even worse than reality. These children are very afraid that no one will ever like them again or want to play with them because they are different. They might wonder if they will ever go to school again. Children with greater insight will wonder if they will ever grow up, go to college, get a job, or marry because of their current limitations.

(1) Even if the prognosis is guarded, not all information needs to be presented at once when such questions are raised. Such children need to be encouraged, but they do not need to hear lies from the people they most trust.

(2) Other elementary school-age children completely deny their new limitations or injuries, and may, if they are able, push themselves too hard (e.g., in physical therapy sessions) or might have completely unrealistic expectations of recovery time. Elementary school-age children can have a range of emotional responses to their condition ranging from open tearfulness to anger and defiance to sullen silence.

f. Adolescents face all the issues previously described and have their own set of concerns. If their ability to think has been preserved, adolescents suffer greatly as they ponder either an uncertain future or one that will be full of pain and limitations. They are the age group most likely to feel guilt about their injuries, especially if they played a role in the injury in question (e.g., a teen who drove while inebriated and is now a paraplegic, the teen who had been warned repeatedly not to dive into the water and who is now paralyzed and ventilator-dependent), or the killing or injury of someone else as a result of the injury. It is not unusual for such teens to feel hopelessness and to think about suicide.

(1) Adolescents face the very real prospect of having their plans for life altered drastically. At a time when they are trying to achieve independence, they may now need parents for even the most simple of self-care tasks such as toileting, washing, feeding. They might despair, "Who will take care of me if my parents die?" "Who would ever want to marry me?" "How will I ever support myself?" "Will I be homeless?"

(2) If the adolescent is capable, he or she might express denial or depression by acting-out behaviors or unrealistically pushing physical limits. If capable, such adolescents might become involved in substance abuse as a way to escape.

g. Because nearly all children and adolescents with catastrophic injuries will experience great emotional suffering, they should receive intensive mental health services early in their treatment.

4. Spiritual issues

a. Children raised in a religious tradition and old enough to pose questions will frequently ask, "Why did God let this happen to me? Doesn't God like me? Is God mad at me?"

b. Children and adolescents who played a role in their injuries (e.g., the paralyzed child struck by a car who was warned repeatedly to stay in his yard, the adolescent who drove while inebriated) might wonder,

23

CHRONIC, CATASTROPHIC, AND TERMINAL CONDITIONS

"Am I being punished? Is God doing this because I broke the rules?" These questions also occur during painful therapies. Such questions are more common among children whose image of God is one of a judge or dispenser of punishment compared to those whose internal image of God is more loving and kindly.

c. Faced with their injuries and their painful recoveries, many children attempt to bargain with God: "If you let me walk tomorrow morning, I promise I'll never disobey my folks (or drink or act stupid, etc.) again." When such bargains are not met, children and adolescents can become depressed or angry with God. They may refuse to pray or even talk about God. This bargaining is not unique to children and adolescents; adults do it, also. In addition, it is not unique even towards God, as children and adolescents may attempt to bargain with their health professionals, ("If you let me go home tomorrow morning, I promise I'll take my medicine."). They become angry when their "deal" is not accepted, or when they have kept their part of the deal, but they still do not receive what they most want (e.g., the child takes her medicine, but still cannot go home because of fever).

d. Children and adolescents may fear that they will die and that they will die alone, without anyone to support them. Depending on their views of the afterlife, they might welcome it as a relief from their suffering or fear it because they expect to be punished. This is true even of children and adolescents who have been raised in atheistic environments.

e. Because of the spiritual issues evoked by catastrophic injury, a professional with experience in this area, *especially with children and adolescents,* should be involved as soon as feasible for all such children and adolescents. This professional is *not* necessarily the health professional. It is not this professional's role to proselytize, convert, or berate; neither is it the role of anyone visiting the child or adolescent to do so.

5. Ethical issues

a. Although involvement in a research study might be an ethical issue in catastrophic injury, the more likely ethical issue is a difference of opinion as to which therapy to pursue or whether to pursue any therapy. These are emotionally laden issues that can tear families apart.

b. Such issues are even more emotionally charged when what the injured child or adolescent wants to do (or to have done) differs from what the parent wants. If children or adolescents are old enough to express wishes, they should always be allowed to do so, and *they should be heard with respect both by parents and by health professionals.* After all, they are the ones who are experiencing the suffering firsthand. That does not mean that their views should necessarily prevail in all cases, because they may not have sufficient information or understanding to make an informed decision about their care (or about their involvement in a research study). Hence, they *must* be given sufficient information and assisted in their understanding of their situation. This may be best done by a parent, health care professional, or another trusted adult.

c. If there is disagreement over involvement in a research study that is not necessarily beneficial to the child or adolescent in question, and he or she has strong feelings against participation, his or her wishes should be honored. If there is disagreement over involvement in a study that is likely to benefit the patient, or if there is disagreement over the course of therapy, especially whether to "go on," the services of a hospital ethicist or ethics committee should be sought. However, the role of the patient's primary health care provider should not be minimized in such cases, because that person often knows the family best.

6. Chronic procedures, medications, visits to health professionals, and hospitalizations

a. Because recuperation from a catastrophic injury might require multiple surgeries (each with its own sequelae), frequent (painful) procedures, and daily medications, the affected child or adolescent might express anger, fear, or avoidance with regard to them. This is to be expected. The wise health professional will openly and sympathetically discuss these feelings.

b. Children and adolescents might also resist or react very negatively to visiting certain health professionals because they fear that the visits will result in further painful procedures or finding something else that is "wrong." They might make up excuses to avoid the visit.

c. A sympathetic approach is best to elicit the greatest degree of cooperation from such patients, but this road might be long and hard. After all, these patients remember a time when they were healthy, and they desperately want to return to those days. Each new procedure, hospitalization, and surgery reminds them how unlikely that outcome is.

d. Child life specialists can offer great assistance in this area; with more severely impacted patients, the services of a mental health professional are essential. These professionals can also assist with patients who *want* to be hospitalized or undergo procedures. Such patients generally demonstrate great anxiety and seek to control it, paradoxically, by seeking that which gives them the most anxiety.

D. TERMINAL ILLNESS

1. General comments

a. When children and adolescents are faced with a terminal condition, some common concerns arise regardless of the illness, as well as some concerns that are unique to specific illnesses. The common concerns are discussed later. Examples of specific concerns are inability to breathe in cystic fibrosis or other chronic lung diseases, progressive loss of movement in degenerative diseases, and intractable pain in metastatic cancer.

23

CHRONIC, CATASTROPHIC, AND TERMINAL CONDITIONS

b.   Terminal illnesses not only affect those who have them but also their families and friends (see Section E).

2.   Physical issues

a.   Depending on the age of the patient, the disease in question, and its stage, physical development might be arrested or delayed. Hence, normal developmental milestones might not be reached, or milestones once attained might be lost. In children old enough to understand how healthy they were previously and certainly in adolescents, this limitation in abilities or diminution in stamina might be very hard to accept. If the terminal illness is associated with pain, this, too, is depressing and exhausting.

b.   One's physical condition is affected by one's state of health, diet, activity, and effects of medications. A child or adolescent who is very ill might not want to eat and might not have the energy to be active. Needed medications might have profound side effects that further weaken the patient or make him or her feel more ill.

c.   Very ill children and adolescents look different than their healthier peers; they might be thinner and their color might be less robust. This will affect their self-esteem.

d.   Very ill preteens and teens might not reach puberty and might be embarrassed about their lack of development, certain that no one finds them attractive.

3.   Psychosocial and emotional issues

a.   Kubler-Ross described stages of dying, and these stages can be seen in older children and adolescents as well as in adults. Not every dying person traverses the stages in the order given, and not every dying person experiences each stage. Nevertheless, knowledge of these stages is valuable in better understanding the dynamics of dying or encountering any significant loss.

(1)   Denial: Refusal to believe the news, including responses such as "The diagnosis is incorrect," or "This is all a joke" (or a dream).

(2)   Anger: Directed at others, It's someone else's fault (e.g., the doctor missed the diagnosis earlier; the parents, not the ill child or adolescent, made a mistake).

(3)   Bargaining: Deals made with various people. For example, "If I get better, I promise to always eat properly, take my medicine, do my homework without complaining."

(4)   Sadness or depression directed at self: For example, "No matter what I do, I'm not getting better but worse. It's hopeless."

(5)   Acceptance: Openness to the dying process; willingness to seek closure of this life; looking forward to the next life (if there is a belief in an afterlife).

b.   Infants and toddlers react with anxiety to separation from parents and to the constant flow of strangers in their lives. Thus, they experience not only physical pain but emotional pain as well. The physical pain results from the disease process itself and also the iatrogenic pain of needed procedures to treat the illness. Physical pain must be adequately managed at all times.

c. Preschoolers fear separation from loved ones and the intrusion of strangers (usually those who want to cause them pain) in their lives. They become angry about repeated procedures and may display tantrums. Regression to an earlier (healthier, happier) stage of life is common, which is frequently associated with more infantile behaviors. Depending on the patient's degree of illness and pain, temperament, his or her frustration level and tolerance for pain, and coping strategies, the preschooler might respond with tears, anger, or silence. Preschoolers may try to bargain their way to health. They also have many questions that they will not ask if they think the questions are unacceptable. Fears are common—both realistic and unrealistic ones. A major concern is continued pain that no one is able to relieve. Pain must always be managed properly.

d. Many of the dynamics present for younger children also exist for elementary school-age children. They fear separation, strangers, and pain. They, too, need optimal pain management. They fear the loss of their energy, appetite, former abilities, usual activities, and social circles, and they especially miss school and other activities in which they routinely engaged. These children understand that they look different than they used to. They worry that they are ugly, with the result that no one will like them or play with them any longer. Because of this fear and because of their diminished energy, they have ambivalence about visitors—they want people to visit and show that they care, but they do not want people to see them as they are. Thus, they may be short-tempered or sullen, depending on their pre-illness temperament. They need friends to visit (if possible), call, send e-mails, or write to them. Seriously ill children might talk about dying and usually know that they are dying before adults have said so. Like younger children, they, too, are inhibited from asking questions if they believe that the questions are not welcomed. They, too, have both rational and irrational fears. Children of this age speak often about the unfairness of their situation and try to bargain themselves into health again.

e. Adolescents are similar to adults in their experience with the dying process. They may deny the seriousness of their illnesses, sometimes engaging in risk-taking behaviors to demonstrate how healthy they really are. Such young people may become angry at others for letting them get sick or for failing to meet their needs. They bargain in an attempt to buy more time. When they realize that their efforts are futile, they become saddened and depressed; in their hopelessness, they might even talk of suicide. Adolescents understand that they will be cheated out of a full life—they will not become adults, live independently, go to college, get a job, get married, or have children of their own. In fact, instead of independence, they might have to depend on their parents to meet their most basic needs. When they think of their healthy peers, it is no wonder that terminally ill adolescents are angry, sullen, or weepy. Although they need the company of these peers, especially in this most vulnerable time in their lives, they sometimes push them away because they fear rejection based on their appearance or limited abilities. When friends do not come to visit, they are likely to become more lonely than ever. They resent having to depend on their parents for company. These adolescents need friends who will visit (if possible), write, call, or send e-mails.

4. Spiritual issues

a. As in other conditions in this chapter, the question "Why me?" haunts dying older children and adolescents. Those who have been raised in a religious tradition might ask the question invoking God: "Why does God want me to die? Why won't God make me better?"

b. If a dying child or adolescent has prayed to or bargained with God to get better, and this has not occurred, he or she might understandably become confused or demoralized. "Why doesn't God hear my prayers? Doesn't God love me?"

c. If a dying child or adolescent has been raised with an image of God as a judge or dispenser of punishment, he or she might believe that the terminal illness is a punishment for real (or imagined) wrongs done, even years earlier.

d. Even children and adolescents raised without religion fear death because of its finality, although they might welcome it if they see it bringing an end to their suffering. If they have no belief in an afterlife, they may fear that they will become "nothing"; if they do believe in an afterlife, they might fear what the afterlife will be and whether they will be alone there.

e. Children and adolescents who have been raised in a particular religious tradition might be inclined to pray for family members, especially if they believe that their family will not be able to go on without them. Family members are usually unaware of these prayers.

f. Dying children and adolescents benefit from the presence of a trusted person who is skilled in discussing spiritual issues with children and adolescents; this is not necessarily a parent, his or her own pastor, or health professional.

5. Ethical issues

a. In the case of terminal illness, ethical issues usually revolve around whether or not to try another treatment (established or experimental) and whether or not to give a "do not resuscitate" status to a child or adolescent.

b. Adolescents and children who are old enough to understand their illness, treatment options, and prognosis should be permitted to give their own opinions about these matters. These opinions should be respectfully heard and considered, even if adults do not agree with them. Health professionals have an ethical responsibility to make sure that children and adolescents understand the salient issues to the best of their abilities.

c. When there is serious disagreement between parent and child or adolescent on the future course of therapy, a concerned but neutral third party should be sought. This might be a relative, the primary health care provider, or an ethicist. Whatever the identity of the person, he or she should be committed to bringing the two sides together without forcing one side to take the other's position. In all cases, concern for the dying child's or adolescent's degree of suffering, pain, and fatigue should be taken into account along with the chances for success of any potential treatment.

d. Although younger children might not be able to make an informed decision because their decisions are based on the present, older children and adolescents should be invited to assist adults in decision making on their behalf. For example, if a certain procedure is likely to provide a favorable benefit-to-burden ratio, parents and medical providers must act in the child's or adolescent's behalf *and explain their decisions to the one who is most affected by them.* Whenever possible, even young patients (not to mention the older ones), should be given choices about *something* in terms of their care, and their choices should be honored. For example, children could be asked with which liquid they want to take their medications, or whether they would like to go to the playroom before or after their procedure. Such choices give a child a sense of active involvement in their care.

6. Hospice care

a. Sometimes the care of a dying child or adolescent becomes too great, and parents will need, at the very least, respite care. Such care permits the family to have a break from the enormous physical, psychologic, and spiritual work of care while, at the same time, ensuring quality care for the dying family member.

b. Many families appreciate the services of a home hospice team that visits the dying child or adolescent daily, answers questions, adjusts pain medications, and offers support. Many parents report that providing terminal care at home (with adequate support) decreased their sense of isolation and hopelessness.

c. Some families cannot care for a dying child or adolescent in their home and opt for hospice care in an outside facility. Usually there is a great deal of guilt, at least initially, associated with this decision because parents feel like failures in terms of their inability to meet their child's needs. Such parents (and siblings) need much emotional support because, for some families, this *is* the correct decision. Such support can be given by the child's or adolescent's usual health care provider, the specialist caring for the patient, or a member of the hospice team.

d. If at all possible, try to be with the family and the terminally ill child or adolescent at the time of his or her death. If that is impossible, make contact with the family soon after the death to show your concern and to determine what assistance family members might need. If at all possible, try to attend the funeral. Parents have noted how much it meant to them that their child's physician took the time to be with them at such an important moment of their lives. Keep in contact with the family after the funeral is over. Be cognizant that parents and other siblings may need help in handling their grief. Be prepared to offer suggestions or make referrals.

E. PARENTAL AND SIBLING REACTIONS

1. Breaking bad news to those involved
   a. Parents
      (1) Parents differ in their responses to receiving bad news about their children. Some parents cry openly, while others remain silent. Still others become angry. Although women are usually stereotyped as weepy and men as strong and silent, in truth each parent's response is unique.
      (2) Always try to deliver such news in person, in a private space, and to both parents simultaneously; it makes miscommunication between the parents less likely.
      (3) After delivering the news, allow some silent time for parents to process what they have heard. Do not keep speaking and do not bombard them with questions.
      (4) If unsure that the message has been heard properly, repeat it.
      (5) Do not become defensive if a parent displays anger or is insulting. This may be his or her maladaptive way of coping with bad news. Remain calm. If it seems that there is a risk of physical danger, try to move toward the door. Get help.
      (6) Allow questions, and answer them gently and honestly. If parents have no questions, request that they write down any questions that may arise after they leave and call later with these questions.
      (7) Reassure parents that they will not be abandoned in their time of need. Provide the names of groups or individuals who might be resources for them with regard to the newly diagnosed condition.
      (8) If a parent is single, make sure that he or she has a support person with whom to share the news. Ideally, this person should be present when the news is being delivered.
      (9) When informing parents that a child or adolescent has died, be very aware that, in their grief and shock, they might react irrationally and say inappropriate things. They might also deny what they are hearing. Always use simple language and repeat the message until you are sure that it has been heard.
   b. Siblings
      (1) Permit parents to decide who should be the one to inform siblings about their ill brother or sister.
      (2) Depending on the news delivered, the way it was delivered, and the age of the sibling, the reaction may be nonchalance, laughter,

anger, fear, or weepiness. Individuals sometimes mask their true reactions. Siblings need space to optimally deal with the news.

(3) Siblings should be given as much information (in an age-appropriate manner) as they truly need and *no more*. Questions should be answered but not "over-answered." Remember, "I don't know" is an acceptable answer. Frequently, questions will seem self-centered, especially if the healthy sibling asks whether he or she is now going to get sick or die, or whether either will happen to a parent. Occasionally, questions will seem macabre, as when a sibling asks if he or she can have the bedroom of a dying (or newly deceased) child or adolescent. These questions are not necessarily hard-hearted, but are usually the result of being immature and not really knowing what to say.

(4) Siblings should be reassured that they will not be abandoned and that if they have questions, they can always ask them. Expect that questions and concerns will arise.

(5) Be aware that the illness, injury, or death of a child or adolescent will turn a sibling's world upside down. Be prepared for tantrums, change in school performance, change in functioning with friends, and mood swings. Many siblings experience sleep disturbances, separation problems, anxiety, fear, guilt (especially if they battled with the ill child or wished he or she was dead or would leave), or refuse to speak about a deceased sibling. Such problems are more likely when there have been antecedent behavior problems, a turbulent relation with the ill or deceased sibling, lack of support from parents or other family members, or lack of supportive social outlets outside the family. In the case of a death, there is a greater likelihood of behavior problems if the death was unexpected (e.g., suicide, motor vehicle accident).

(6) In the case of a death, be aware that children may have a strongly negative reaction to comments made by adults in an effort to be helpful or consoling. For example, "Your little brother died because God needed another angel in heaven." This comment can be construed to mean that the living child was not good enough to be an angel or that God kills people when another angel is needed. Both can evoke fear. As another example: "Grandma has gone to sleep for a long time." This comment can elicit a fear of going to bed in a child who was very close to the deceased. It is far better to use the word *died* than euphemisms.

c. The ill, injured, or dying child or adolescent

(1) Permit parents to decide who should relay information to the ill child or adolescent.

(2) In two-parent families, both should be present when disclosure is occurring.

23

CHRONIC, CATASTROPHIC, AND TERMINAL CONDITIONS

    (3)   In single-parent families, the parent should be present no matter who is doing the disclosure.

    (4)   Depending on the news delivered, the way it was delivered, and the age of the child or adolescent, the reaction may be nonchalance, laughter, anger, fear, or weepiness.

    (5)   The child or adolescent should be given as much information as he or she needs and no more. Questions should not be "over-answered." It is OK to say, "I don't know" if that is the most honest answer.

    (6)   Children and adolescents should be reassured that they will not be abandoned and that they can always speak freely about their fears and concerns. They should be invited to ask questions whenever they have them. They are likely to ask questions—over and over again.

    (7)   Children and adolescents receiving "bad news" experience a massive shift in their moorings. As such, they may demonstrate mood swings, tantrums, change in school performance, functioning with friends, and any of the other behaviors described in Sections B and C.

2. The need for support

a.   Regardless of the circumstances, all families need support in times of most chronic illnesses (especially exacerbations), catastrophic illnesses or injuries, and terminal illnesses. The types of support most needed vary by the condition and its severity, innate family resources, and family dynamics.

b.   Assess whether a given family has support among its members—both in the home and outside of the home.

c.   Determine whether the family has an active social network and how that network can support family members. Do not forget a family's parish or religious congregation as a potential source of support.

d.   Become acquainted with specific support groups in the community and provide families with points of contact. Try to identify support groups for children and adolescents as well as for adults.

e.   Offer yourself or your office as medical support for a family struggling with a chronic, catastrophic, or terminal condition.

3. Common reactions—adults

a.   A number of the reactions to bad news are identical to the stages of dying described by Kubler-Ross.

    (1)   Denial: Parents and other caregivers might believe that test results were erroneous or that the health professional making the diagnosis was incompetent. Although seeking a second opinion is a reasonable reaction to the diagnosis of a chronic, catastrophic, or terminal condition, frenzied "doctor shopping" is not. The wise health professional assists parents in procuring a competent second opinion.

(2) Anger: Parents and other caregivers might blame the doctor, hospital, school, local industries, or community for the chronic, catastrophic, or terminal condition. Litigation might be threatened. The wise health professional sympathizes with parental anger and does not become defensive (even when the anger is directed at him or her).

(3) Bargaining: Parents and other caregivers might believe that their actions somehow caused their child's or adolescent's condition. They might try to bargain with the doctor or God in an attempt to improve the situation. ("If she makes it, I promise that I'll never smoke around her again.") The wise health professional supports a parent in his or her desire for improved health, but makes no guarantees.

(4) Sadness or depression: Parents and other caregivers might reach the point where all seems hopeless, nothing will ever improve, and they might as well give up. Self-blame might also be present. The wise health professional understands these feelings. However, he or she is also aware that a depressed parent is usually not emotionally available to a child or adolescent who needs him or her the most (not to mention other children in the family) and will suggest professional mental help for parents so incapacitated.

(5) Acceptance: Many parents reach the point at which they accept their child's condition, all the while working valiantly to maximize his or her health or, in the case of a dying child, to make the final days as comfortable as possible. The wise health professional applauds these efforts and offers himself or herself as a support or resource to such parents.

b. Other common reactions

(1) Guilt: Many parents blame themselves for their child's or adolescent's condition, even if they could not have possibly played a role in its occurrence. Health professionals need to work with such parents to reinforce the idea that the condition was not caused by them in any way.

(2) Blame: Some parents blame each other for their child's or adolescent's condition, suggesting that if the other were a better parent, the child or adolescent would not be ill. Such blaming tears marriages apart. Health professionals must be alert to such behavior, counsel parents when it is present, and refer parents to mental health professionals when the difficulties are marked.

(3) Spoiling: Many parents spoil their ill child because he or she is "so sick." This behavior can also extend to surviving siblings, who do not receive the discipline they need. Such parents are not doing their children any favors, because the harshness of reality always emerges. Health professionals can be alert to such

behavior on the part of parents and can counsel against it, suggesting reasonable limits on activities or desires.

(4) Overprotecting: Many parents overprotect their ill child. Surviving siblings may also be overprotected, and they may become "vulnerable." Although this is understandable, it is not healthy to squelch a young person's sense of identity or independence. He or she needs these to have a healthy sense of self-esteem, especially in the midst of one's own (or a sibling's) illness. Health professionals must be alert to such parental behaviors and suggest ways that parents can encourage age-appropriate independence and identity, even in the midst of a chronic or life-threatening illness.

(5) Indifference or ignoring: Some parents respond to bad news by laughing it off, minimizing it, or simply ignoring it. They might act as if everyone is making a big fuss over nothing. Although they do not deny that a condition is present, they might deny its seriousness, or busy themselves in their work. Health professionals need to watch for this type of behavior, which is nonsupportive of the ill child or adolescent (and, often, the other spouse as well). Mental health counseling might be needed.

(6) Isolation: Some parents involute during times of crisis and prefer to handle everything alone. They may expect this of their children also. Such families usually have a history of "staying to themselves" even in the best of times. Isolation is a defense mechanism that is rarely helpful in times of serious stress—especially involving children and adolescents. Mental health intervention is indicated.

(7) Marital discord: The presence of a severe chronic or terminal condition in a child may change the way many parents communicate with each other (and with the other children). Each will grieve in his or her own way. They may blame each other for the condition. Professional counseling may be in order.

(8) Miscellaneous: Anorexia, sleep disturbances, restlessness, forgetfulness, anxiety, depression.

4. Common reactions—children and adolescents

a. Kubler-Ross's stages are also experienced by children and adolescents. Some of the stages are more likely to be experienced if ill children and adolescents see their parents manifesting the same reactions.

(1) Denial: The young person believes it's all a mistake—the doctors are dumb, or the tests are wrong. Health professionals need to work with parents to ensure that children and adolescents come to an understanding that they (or their sibling) really are ill. Ideally, parents come to that stage before the child or adolescent.

(2) Anger: The young person believes that the diagnosed condition is the fault of someone else (even a parent or sibling). Health professionals (with parents) can help children and adolescents

better understand that sometimes things happen that are nobody's fault.

(3) Bargaining: The young person believes that if he or she promises to do something (eat better, sleep more, do homework, obey parents) that the condition will get better or go away completely. Health professionals and parents need to help an ill young person see that such behaviors are good in themselves and *might* help him or her feel better (depending on the activity), but that there are no guarantees to perfect health.

(4) Sadness or depression: The young person understands that the condition is not going away and might only get worse. He or she might refuse to take medications or undergo procedures with a "What's the use?" attitude. Health professionals and parents can support these young people in the best way they can and secure mental health input when the problem is overwhelming or pervasive.

(5) Acceptance: The young person comes to accept his or her level of health, tries to follow medical recommendations as well as possible, and tries to make the most of each day. Health professionals and parents can fully support the efforts of these young people.

b. Other reactions are also common.

(1) Guilt: Many young people feel they are to blame for their own condition (or for their sibling's condition). Good, age-appropriate explanations of the cause of the condition presented with time for questions usually helps to minimize guilt, although such explanation might need to be repeated over and over again for maximum effect.

(2) Blame: Many young people blame others for their condition, creating guilt. Children may blame parents or siblings. Good, age-appropriate explanations of the cause of the condition presented with time for questions usually helps to minimize blame. Repeat explanations as necessary.

(3) Spoiled: Many young people with chronic or life-threatening conditions get their own way because of others' guilt or because they are believed to have "little time left." Some of these children and adolescents become tyrannical, expecting everyone to meet their every need. This places a strain on parents and siblings alike. Likewise, surviving siblings may receive less discipline because of parental fatigue, depression, or need. Health professionals can work with parents to set reasonable limits and can model such limit setting in the office or hospital. They can also explain why such behavior is unacceptable.

(4) Vulnerability: Some young people with chronic life-threatening conditions have been so overprotected by parents or other caregivers that they are literally afraid to move on their own,

23

CHRONIC, CATASTROPHIC, AND TERMINAL CONDITIONS

afraid that something even worse will happen to them than what they are already experiencing. Likewise, this can happen to surviving siblings. Health professionals can encourage such young people to do things for themselves, giving such encouragement in the presence of parents and other caregivers.

(5) Resentment: Children and adolescents with chronic or life-threatening conditions might resent their healthier siblings and peers. Siblings might resent the ill child or adolescent because they seem to get all the attention; sometimes they act out or engage in risk-taking behaviors just to get their parents' attention. Even after a death, surviving children may resent the dead child if the parents tend to idealize him or her. Health professionals can counsel parents to cherish their surviving children. Health care professionals can urge parents to talk with siblings who are not ill to help them see that resentment makes everyone unhappy and that healthy and ill siblings need to work with each other to ensure harmony. Healthy siblings *may* need some quality parental time, and the ill child *may* need to accept that. Healthy siblings need to know that there will be times when the parent's place *is* with the ill sibling, and the ill child or adolescent needs to know that, when a parent's presence is crucial, he or she *will* be there.

(6) Indifference or ignoring: Some healthy siblings act as if they are unaware of their ill sibling's condition, or they minimize it to their friends, even to the point of making jokes about it. Health professionals can help parents understand that this might be a defense mechanism, and that such healthy siblings are not callous or cruel. Health professionals can also speak with the healthy siblings to assess their understanding of their ill sibling's condition, offering explanations whenever possible.

(7) Isolation: Many ill children or adolescents will want to isolate themselves during an illness because of how they feel, look, or speak or because of any odors or equipment to which they are attached. Their healthy siblings may also isolate themselves from friends because they feel "different" having an ill sibling or one who has died. Health professionals can assist both groups in becoming more comfortable with the condition.

(8) Risk taking: Many ill young people engage in risky behaviors (e.g., drinking, smoking, drug use, illegal activities) to prove to themselves, their parents, or their friends that they are not as ill as everyone believes them to be. Surviving siblings may also act out. Such behavior is more likely if previous behavior problems, a turbulent relationship with the deceased, or a stormy relationship with the parents is involved. The primary medical provider should discuss the young person's behavior with him or her; in many cases, the services of a mental health professional are needed.

F. BIBLIOGRAPHY

Chronic Conditions

Garwick A, Kohrman C, Wolman C et al: Families' recommendations for improving services for children with chronic conditions, *Arch Pedaitr Adolesc Med* 152:440, 1998.

Garwick A, Patterson J, Bennett F et al: Parents' perception of helpful vs unhelpful types of support in managing the care of preschoolers with chronic conditions, *Pediatrics* 152:663, 1998.

Goldberg S: Chronic illness and early development—parent-child relationships, *Pediatr Ann* 119:35, 1990.

Jessop D, Stein R: Providing comprehensive health care to children with chronic illness, *Pediatrics* 93:602, 1994.

Leonard B: Siblings of chronically ill children—a question of vulnerability vs resilience, *Pediatr Ann* 20:501, 1991.

Noll R, Garstein M, Vannatta K et al: Social, emotional, and behavioral functioning of children with cancer, *Pediatrics* 103:71, 1999.

Perrin E, Lewkowicz C, Young M: Shared vision—concordance among fathers, mothers, and pediatricians about unmet needs of children with chronic health conditions, *Pediatrics* 105:277, 2001.

Perrin E, Sayer A, Willett J: Sticks and stones may break my bones . . . reasoning about illness causality and body functioning in children who have a chronic illness, *Pediatrics* 88:608, 1991.

Pless I, Power C, Peckham C: Long-term psychosocial sequelae of chronic physical disorders in childhood, *Pediatrics* 91:1131, 1993.

Silver E, Stein R, Bauman L: Sociodemographic and condition-related characteristics associated with conduct problems in school-aged children with chronic health conditions, *Arch Pediatr Adolesc Med* 153:815, 1999.

Thyen U, Kuhlthau K, Perrin J: Employment, child care, and mental health of mothers caring for children assisted by technology, *Pediatrics* 103:1235, 1999.

Terminal Conditions, Death, and Dying

AAP Committee on Psychosocial Aspects of Child and Family Health: The pediatrician and childhood bereavement, *Pediatrics* 89:516, 1992.

Fleischman A, Nolan K, Dubler N et al: Caring for gravely ill children, *Pediatrics* 94:433, 1994.

Hall J, Reyes H, Meller J et al: Traumatic death in urban children, revisited, *AJDC* 147:102, 1993.

Khanerja S, Milrod B: Educational needs among pediatricians regarding caring for terminally ill children, *Arch Pediatr Adolesc Med* 152:909, 1998.

Kubler-Ross E: *On children and death,* New York, 1983, Collier Books.

Partridge J, Wall S: Analgesia for dying infants whose life support is withdrawn or withheld, *Pediatrics* 99:76, 1997.

Vance JC, Najman JM, Thearle MJ et al: Psychologic changes in parents eight months after the loss of an infant from stillbirth, neonatal death, or SIDS—a longitudinal study, *Pediatrics* 96:933, 1995.

23

CHRONIC, CATASTROPHIC, AND TERMINAL CONDITIONS

INDEX

INDEX

INDEX